Management of Complex Cardiovascular Problems

THE EVIDENCE-BASED MEDICINE APPROACH

EDITED BY

Thach N. Nguyen, MD, FACC, FACP, FSCAI
Director of Cardiology
Community Health System
St Mary Medical Center
Hobart, IN, USA

Dayi Hu, MD
Dean of TongJi University School of Medicine
Shanghai, China

Moo-Hyun Kim, MD
Director of Cardiac Catheterization Laboratories
Vice Dean, Dong A University Medical School
Dong A University Medical Center
Busan, South Korea

Cindy L. Grines, MD
Editor-in-Chief, The Journal of Interventional Cardiology
Director of Cardiac Catheterization Laboratories
William Beaumont Hospital
Royal Oak, MI, USA

b Blackwell
Futura

To Pam Moyer

For the appreciation
of all your
lovely works

Spring 2008

© 2000, 2002 by Futura Publishing Company, Inc., New York
© 2007 by Blackwell Publishing
Blackwell Futura is an imprint of Blackwell Publishing

Blackwell Publishing, Inc., 350 Main Street, Malden, Massachusetts 02148-5020, USA
Blackwell Publishing Ltd, 9600 Garsington Road, Oxford OX4 2DQ, UK
Blackwell Science Asia Pty Ltd, 550 Swanston Street, Carlton, Victoria 3053, Australia

First published 2000
Second edition 2002
Third edition 2007

1   2007

ISBN: 978-1-4051-4031-7

Library of Congress Cataloging-in-Publication Data

Management of complex cardiovascular problems : the evidence-based medicine
approach / edited by Thach Nguyen ... [et al.]. -- 3rd ed.
     p. ; cm.
   Includes bibliographical references and index.
   ISBN-13: 978-1-4051-4031-7
   1.   Cardiovascular system--Diseases--Treatment. 2.   Heart--Diseases--Treatment. 3.
Evidence-based medicine. I. Nguyen, Thach.
   [DNLM: 1.   Cardiovascular Diseases--therapy. 2.   Evidence-Based Medicine.   WG 120
M266 2007]

RC671.M33 2007
616.1'2--dc22   2006034015

A catalogue record for this title is available from the British Library

Commissioning Editor: Gina Almond
Editorial Assistant: Victoria Pittman
Development Editor: Beckie Brand
Production Controller: Debbie Wyer

Set in 9.5/12pt Palatino by Charon Tec Ltd (A Macmillan Company), Chennai, India
www.charontec.com
Printed and bound in Singapore by Fabulous Printers Pte Ltd.

For further information on Blackwell Publishing, visit our website:
www.BlackwellCardiology.com

Contents

List of Contributors

Editors

Thach N. Nguyen, MD, FACC, FACP, FSCAI
Co-Editor, International Journal of Geriatric Cardiology; and Editorial Consultant, Journal of Interventional Cardiology; and Honorary Professor of Medicine, Capital University of Medical Sciences, Beijing, China; and Jiangsu Province Hospital, First Affiliated Hospital of Nanjing Medical University, Nanjing, China; and Beijing Friendship Hospital, Beijing, China; and The Institute of Geriatric Cardiology, Chinese PLA Hospital 301, Beijing, China; and Clinical Assistant Professor of Medicine, Indiana University; and Director of Cardiology, Community Healthcare System, St Mary Medical Center, Hobart, IN, USA

Dayi Hu, MD
Dean of Medical School of Shanghai, Tongji University; and Chief of Cardiology Department, People's Hospital of Peking, University of Beijing, China

Moo-Hyun Kim, MD
Director of Cardiac Catheterization Laboratories, Vice Dean, Dong A University Medical School, Dong A University Medical Center, Busan, Korea

Cindy L. Grines, MD
Editor-in-Chief, The Journal of Interventional Cardiology; and Director of Cardiac Catheterization Laboratories, Williams Beaumont Hospital, Royal Oak, MI, USA

Contributors

Bikash Agarwal, MD
Assistant Professor of Medicine, Indiana University School of Medicine; and Director, Hospitalist Program, St Anthony Memorial Hospital, Michigan City, IN, USA

Dao Duy An, MD, MSc Med
Vice Head of Cardiovascular and Geriatrics Ward, General Hospital of Kontum Province, Vietnam

Adolphus Anekwe, MD
Clinical Assistant Professor of Medicine, Indiana University Northwest Center for Medical Education; and Health Commissioner of the City of Gary, Consultant, Internal Medicine, IN, USA

Nikola Bakraceski, MD
Chief of Interventional Cardiology Department, Institute for Cardiovascular Diseases, Ohrid, Macedonia

Thomas Bump, MD
Electrophysiologist, Christ Hospital, Oak Lawn, IL, USA

Tan Huay Cheem, MD
Chief, Cardiac Department, National University Hospital; and Director, Cardiac Catheterisation Laboratory, National University Hospital, Singapore

Zhang Shuang Chuan, MD
Director & Professor of Pediatric Department, Peking University Shenzhen Hospital; and Guest Professor of Shenzhen Children's Hospital, Shenzhen, China

Nguyen Duc Cong, MD, PhD
Associate Professor, Vice Director, Department of Internal Medicine II, Hospital 103, Hadong City, Hatay Province, Vietnam

Heidi M. Connolly, MD, FACC
Professor of Medicine, Mayo Clinic College of Medicine, Rochester, MN, USA

Vijay Dave, MD
Director of Medical Education, Chairman,
Department of Medicine, Community
Healthcare System, St Mary Medical Center,
Hobart, IN, USA

Zee-Pin Ding, MBBS, MMed, FAMS
Consultant Cardiologist, Chief of
Echocardiography, National Heart Center,
Singapore

Vuong Duthinh, MD, PhD
Electrophysiology Consultant, Regional
Cardiology Associates, Grand Blanc, MI, USA

Kim Eagle, MD
Professor of Medicine, The University of Michigan
Cardiovascular Center, Ann Arbor, MI, USA

C. Michael Gibson, MS, MD
Director, TIMI Data Coordinating Center; *and*
Associate Professor Harvard Medical School; *and*
Chief of Clinical Research, Cardiovascular
Division, Beth Israel Deaconess Medical Center,
Boston, MA, USA

Felix Gozo, MD
Director of Cardiac Rehabilitation, St Mary
Medical Center, Hobart, IN, USA

Sim Kui Hian, MD
Chair, Medical Directorate; *and* Chair, Medical
Advisory Council; *and* Head, Department of
Cardiology; *and* Head, Clinical Research Centre
(CRC), Sarawak General Hospital, Malaysia; *and*
Adjunct Professor, Faculty of Medicine & Health
Sciences, University of Malaysia, Sarawak
(UNIMAS); *and* Vice President (2006–2008)
National Heart Association of Malaysia (NHAM)

Nguyen Lan Hieu, MD
Interventional Cardiology, Congenital Heart
Disease Program, Hanoi Medical University,
Vietnam Heart Institute, Hanoi, Vietnam

Pham Manh Hung, MD
Vice Director of the Interventional Laboratories,
Vietnam Heart Institute, Bach Mai Hospital,
Hanoi, Vietnam; *and* Secretary General of
the Vietnam National Heart Association,
Hanoi, Vietnam

Pham Nhu Hung, MD
Cardiology Consultant, Vietnam Heart Institute,
Hanoi, Vietnam

Jui-Sung Hung, MD, FACC, FAHA
Director, Central Taiwan Heart Institute; *and*
Professor of Medicine, China Medical University
and Chung Shan Medical University, Taichung,
Taiwan

David Jayakar, MD
Director of Cardiovascular Surgery, Community
Healthcare System, St Mary Medical Center,
Hobart, IN, USA

Pham Gia Khai, MD, PhD
Director, Vietnam Heart Institute, Bach
Mai Hospital; *and* Chief, Cardiology
Department, Hanoi Medical University, Hanoi,
Vietnam

Pham Quoc Khanh, MD
Director of Electrophysiology Laboratories,
Vietnam Heart Institute; *and* Vice President,
Vietnamese Interventional Cardiology Society,
Hanoi, Vietnam

Huynh Tuan Khanh, MD
Pediatric Cardiologist, Pediatric Hospital #2,
Hochiminh City, Vietnam

Gaurav Kumar, MD
Assistant in Medicine, Department of Medicine,
University of Illinois in Chicago, Chicago, IL,
USA

Rajiv Kumar
Third Year Medical Student, Indiana University
School of Medicine, Indianapolis, IN, USA

Chu-Pak Lau, MD
Division of Cardiology, Department of Medicine,
The University of Hong Kong, Queen Mary
Hospital, Hong Kong, China

**Kean-Wah Lau, MBBS, MMed, FRCP,
FACC**
Associate Professor of Medicine, National
University of Singapore; *and* Consultant
Cardiologist, Gleneagles Medical Center,
Singapore

Do Doan Loi, MD, PhD
Consultant in Cardiology, Vice Director of Bach
Mai General Hospital; *and* Deputy Dean of Hanoi
Medical University, Hanoi, Vietnam

Prakash Makam, MD
Director of Cardiovascular Research, Community
Healthcare System, Munster, IN, USA

Sundeep Mangla, MD
Director of Interventional Neuroradiology,
Director of Research, Department of Radiology,
Visiting Associate Professor of Radiology,
Neurosurgery, and Neurology, SUNY
Downstate Medical Center, Brooklyn, NY,
USA

Sanjeev V. Maniar, MD, ABPN
Neurology and Fellowship, Trained in EEG,
EMG and Intraoperative Epilepsy Monitoring,
Merrillville, IN, USA

Michael D. McGoon, MD
Professor of Medicine, Director, Pulmonary
Hypertension Clinic, Mayo Clinic College of
Medicine, Rochester, MN, USA

Huynh Van Minh, MD, PhD
Professor of Internal Medicine, Hue Medical
College; *and* Vice Director, Hue University
Hospital; *and* President, Vietnam Society of
Hypertension, Vietnam

James Nguyen, MD
Resident in Internal Medicine, Orlando Regional
Health Care, Orlando, FL, USA

Vo Thanh Nhan, MD, PhD
Associate Professor of Clinical Cardiology,
University of Medicine and Pharmacy;
and Director of Interventional Cardiology
and Cardiac Catheterization Laboratory,
Cho Ray Hospital, Ho Chi Minh City,
Vietnam

Olabode Oladeinde, MD, FACP
Internal Medicine Consultant, Department of
Medicine, Community Healthcare Systems,
St Mary Medical Center, Hobart, IN, USA

Brian Olshansky, MD
Professor of Medicine, Director, Cardiac
Electrophysiology, University of Iowa Hospitals,
Iowa City, IA, USA

Borce Petrovski, MD, PhD, FESC, FACC
Director of the Institute for Heart Diseases,
Clinical Center, University of St Ciril and
Metodius, Skopje, Macedonia

Hoang Pham, MD
Intern, Department of Medicine, Saint Vincent
Hospital, Worcester, MA, USA

Loan T. Pham, MD
Internal Medicine Consultant, Department of
Medicine, Kaiser Permanente Hospital, Fontana,
CA, USA

Ta Tien Phuoc, MD, PhD
Consultant in Cardiology, Chief of Clinical
Department, Bach Mai Hospital, Hanoi, Vietnam

Gianluca Rigatelli, MD, FACP, FACC, FESC, FSCAI
Director, Peripheral Vascular and Congenital
Heart Disease Interventions, Interventional
Cardiology Unit, Rovigo General Hospital,
Rovigo, Italy

Rupesh Shah, MD
Vice-Chair, Department of Medicine, Community
Healthcare System, St Mary Medical Center,
Hobart, IN, USA

Marc Simaga, MD
Neurology Consultant, North Indiana Neurology
Institute, Merrillville, IN, USA

Matthew J. Sorrentino, MD
Associate Professor of Medicine, Department of
Medicine, Section of Cardiology, University of
Chicago, Pritzker School of Medicine, Chicago,
IL, USA

Nguyen Hai Thuy, MD, PhD
Associate Professor of Medicine, Chief,
Department of Internal Medicine, Hue University
Hospital, Vietnam

Dat Nguyen Tran, MD
Resident-in-training, Denver, CO, USA

Huy Van Tran, MD, PhD, FACC, FESC
Department of Cardiology, Khanh Hoa Hospital;
and President, Khanh Hoa Heart Association; *and*
Vice President, Vietnamese Society of
Hypertension, Nha Trang, Vietnam

Hung-Fat Tse, MBBS, MD, FRCP, FACC
Professor of Medicine, Cardiology Division,
Department of Medicine, The University of
Hong Kong, Hong Kong, China

Norbert Lingling D. Uy, MD, FPCP, FPCC, FACC
Chief, Section of Cardiology, University of the
East Ramon Magsaysay Memorial Medical Center;
and Assistant Professor in Medicine, UERM
College of Medicine; *and* Consultant, Philippine
Heart Center and St. Luke's Heart Institute

Nguyen Lan Viet, MD, PhD
Professor of Medicine, Rector of Hanoi Medical University; *and* Vice Director, Vietnam National Heart Institute; *and* Vice President, Vietnam National Heart Association, Hanoi, Vietnam

Pham Nguyen Vinh, MD, PhD
Professor in Medicine, University Training Center; *and* Chief of Cardiology and Vice Director, Heart Institute of Ho Chi Minh City, Ho Chi Minh City, Vietnam

Shiwen Wang, MD, MCAE
Professor and Director, Institute of Geriatric Cardiology, General Hospital of Chinese PLA, Beijing, China

Abdul Wase, MD, FACP, FACC
Associate Clinical Professor of Medicine; *and* Director, Cardiology Fellowship Program, Wright State University School of Medicine; *and* Director, Electrophysiology, Good Samaritan Hospital, Dayton, OH, USA

Haiyun Wu, MD
Associate Professor, Institute of Geriatric Cardiology, General Hospital of Chinese PLA, Beijing, China

Foreword

The modern cardiologist is confronted with a bewildering amount of new information. At last count there were more than 100 cardiology journals. Many cardiology textbooks, covering every aspect of the field and dozens of symposia are published each year. The major cardiovascular centers all have their "in house" publications, which emphasize their local accomplishments. In addition, industry bombards cardiologists with many reviews, each placing the sponsor's project and trial in the best light.

What the practicing cardiologist really needs is a text that emphasizes unbiased, up to date information and that places this information into an appropriate context. The third edition of *Management of Complex Cardiovascular Problems: The Evidence-based Medicine Approach*, carefully edited by Dr Thach N. Nguyen and his co-Editors, does precisely this.

Particularly new, reader–friendly features are the boxes that distill the information that is presented in the text into several categories: *Critical Thinking* (new concepts); *Evidence-based Medicine* (the key results of important clinical trials); *Emerging Trends* (how new information may be applied to improve practice); *Clinical Pearls* (advice from master clinicians); *Real World Questions* (the most important questions facing practicing cardiologists – and their answers); and *Take Home Messages* (succinct summaries of each chapter).

This unique format provides busy cardiologists with an approach to deal with information overload and will thereby enhance the quality of care delivered to the cardiac patient. Thus, Dr Thach N. Nguyen and his talented authors have again provided us with important ammunition for the war against heart disease. This fine book describes clearly some of the most difficult problems that cardiovascular specialists face, and it provides enormously helpful directions in dealing with them. This eminently readable book should be equally valuable to practicing cardiologists in the front lines of the battle against the global scourge of cardiovascular disease and to trainees in the field.

Eugene Braunwald, MD
Distinguished Hersey Professor of Medicine
Harvard Medical School
Chairman, TIMI Study Group
Brigham and Women's Hospital

Acknowledgments

For the completion of this book, we owe much to our teachers, friends, colleagues, families, staff and patients. I (TNN) am indebted to Dr Eugene Braunwald, who wrote the Foreword, for his invaluable encouragement, very kind words and advice throughout my career. My deepest appreciation goes to my fellow Editors and Contributors and to my family, with the dedicated support (and my lost time always away with work) of SJ Morales, Chicago, IL; my parents Sau Nguyen and Hanh Tran, my family in Irvine, CA; and Milton Triana, Administrator of Community Healthcare System, St Mary Medical Center, Hobart, IN. It is a privilege having the special and kind support of Gina Almond and Beckie Brand from Blackwell, Oxford, UK. Special assistance was given by Cindy Macko at the Library of St Mary Medical Center, Hobart, IN and Yin Rong-Xiu at the Institute of Cardiovascular Disease, Capital University of Medical Sciences, Beijing, China. My appreciation for my staff, Carla, Brenda, Pat, Cindy, Christy, Jennie, Linda, Donna, Terrie, etc. – you all did a good job so I could finish my work early and spend more time reading, writing and editing.

Above all, we are indebted to our patients – the purpose of our care, the source of our quests, the inspiration of our daily work. To them we give our heartfelt thanks.

Preface

Cardiovascular disease is a major health, social and economic problem. On an individual basis, it limits the full development of a productive career, decreases the earning potential, dampens the prospect of a challenging lifestyle, and shortens life expectancy. In the macroeconomic aspect, cardiovascular disease contributes directly to work absenteeism, lower production output, and incurs a large and disproportionate share of healthcare expenses.

With recent advances in understanding the mechanism of disease and concurrent technology development, the management of cardiovascular disease has succeeded in decreasing mortality and improving morbidity. However, the problem of today's cardiologists is the fact that they are being bombarded by a never ending supply of new and heterogenous information. These publications range from the "must-read" weekly Journal of the American College of Cardiology, Circulation, New England Journal of Medicine, etc., to the free, throw-away printings from scientific or business sources. So keeping current in today's changing world of medicine and intelligently applying the new mainstream innovations, while staying emotionally stable, socially correct, financially successful, and navigating a mid-life crisis, is more than a major challenge for any practicing cardiology consultant.

Management of Complex Cardiovascular Problems: The Evidence-based Medicine Approach, Third Edition, brings together clinical consultants from different areas of expertise to address the day to day implications of conventional and frontline modalities of treatment for major cardiovascular problems. First, we identify the most clinically relevant questions that the consultants and their referring physicians would encounter at the bedside during their daily rounds. Then, in a frank and honest review and evaluation of related data of randomized trials or meta-analysis, we offer a wide range of solutions, incorporating evidence-based medical information, from conventional to investigational, into daily practice.

Each option is backed up by the abstract of a study or two from opposing views which have been well received or hotly debated by the cardiology community. However, not every modality of treatment or medication can or should be applied to every patient. Rather, it is an intelligent selection and application of the best modality of treatment. Because there are so many available options, we emphasize on ranking each drug or each modality of treatment by its utmost necessity. This method of assessing the management strategy helps the clinician to focus on the main treatment and its results while being able to add (or withdraw) a (few) secondary drug(s) or modality(ies) of treatment without deviating from the main problem that prompts the patient to come to the office or that the patient is being hospitalized for.

All the time, while scrutinizing the data from randomized trials or meta-analysis, we pay attention to the details, circumstances of occurrences, results in selected subsets of patients or subsets analysis. Besides reconfirming the data accepted by others, we may detect a trend which could lead to a different understanding or perspective of the problems, thus explaining the differences of the patients' outcomes. As we deduce a few lessons from these trials and apply them to patients, we give a personal touch to the management strategy and hopefully bring a happy ending to the cardiovascular problems of patients entrusted by society to our care.

This book (or any cardiology textbook) does not have all the answers, nor can we offer a perfect solution to every question, because clinical questions will always arise as long as the human body and physiology evolve. As many theories and hypotheses are being elegantly discussed, we present just a few principles and applications, which are the most likely treatments of the future. Following this principle, we channel our limited time, interest, and resources into a few promising treatments.

Even if we can suggest a best modality of treatment available for a specific problem, the correct political question continues to be which one is the best, for an affordable price, applying to the largest number of patients. None of us are living in Utopia, so the management offered in this book also tries to be cost-effective, keeping the expenditure of cardiac care within the national budget, as well as preventing it from bankrupting the health care system.

As editors and authors of this book, we hope we achieve our role as effective communicators to our readers, who are all friends and colleagues. We have tried to make the messages simple and easy to understand so they can be easily remembered and applied in the daily rounds of all of us. This is the one simple goal we have for ourselves and our readers.

CHAPTER 1

Acute Coronary Syndrome

Thach N. Nguyen, Tan Huay Cheem, Bikash Agarwal, Rupesh Shah, James Nguyen and Nguyen Lan Viet

Introduction

The definition of acute coronary syndrome (ACS) includes unstable angina (UA), non-ST segment elevation myocardial infarction (non-STEMI), and ST segment myocardial infarction (STEMI). However, in practice, ACS is used to indicate UA and non-STEMI. Their principal presentations are rest angina, new-onset angina, angina of increasing severity, postinfarction angina. Non-STEMI is defined as UA with positive cardiac biomarkers without ST segment elevation on the electrocardiogram (ECG). The factors which differentiate between low and high risk ACS by the thrombolysis in acute myocardial infarction (TIMI) risk scores are listed in Table 1.1. If there are less than two risk factors the

Table 1.1 TIMI risk score for acute coronary syndrome.

1. Age >65 years
2. Prior coronary stenosis >50%
3. Three or more risk factors for CAD (hypertension, hypercholesterolemia, family history of CAD, active smoking, diabetes)
4. Prior use of aspirin within last 7 days
5. ST segment depression
6. Elevated cardiac biomarkers
7. Two or more episodes of rest angina in the last 24 hours

CAD, coronary artery disease.

patient belongs to the low-risk group; from three to four risk factors the patient is of intermediate risk; and with more than four risk factors the patient belongs to the high risk group. Even without calculating the TIMI risk score, elevated troponin levels and ST-segment depression help to distinguish individuals at increased cardiovascular (CV) risk [1].

ACS is result of a mismatch between myocardial oxygen supply and demand. Occasionally, this is due to anemia, hyperthyroidism, infection, tachyarrhythmias, or valvular heart disease. However, the most common cause of change from stable CAD to ACS is disruption or fissuring of a vulnerable atherosclerotic plaque. This is followed by platelet-mediated thrombosis and vasoconstriction with or without elevation of cardiac markers. Not every elevation of CPK-MB or troponin is due to myocardial injury. Cardiac-specific troponin rises similarly to CK-MB but it is more specific for cardiac muscle and more sensitive (there is more of it in myocardial cells). Troponin also stays elevated long after CK-MB has returned to normal.

CRITICAL THINKING

Why does plaque rupture? A novel theory speculates that crystallization of cholesterol causes an increase in volume of the cholesterol content of a plaque and pierces the biological membrane into the arterial lumen. This is believed to be the mechanism of plaque rupture [2,3]. If it is true, there will be a whole new pharmacologic armamentarium (including red wine) to prevent crystallization of cholesterol and plaque rupture.

Because the pathophysiology of ACS is transient coronary occlusion with platelet-mediated thrombi, the present strategy for acute treatment of ACS is directed primarily at the platelet, the thrombus, and coronary artery vasoconstriction with aspirin, thienopyridines and heparin (Table 1.2).

Table 1.2 Management strategies for acute coronary syndrome.

1. Identify patients by risk profile for appropriate treatment
2. Administer evidence-based medicine treatment
3. Perform invasive studies and treatment if indicated
4. Initiate risk factor modification program (including exercise) in the hospital setting
5. Educate patients and family about risk modification program
6. Schedule follow-up for CAD and regular check-up for risk factor modification program

CAD, coronary artery disease.

Management

Aspirin

Three randomized trials have clearly demonstrated the benefit of aspirin in the management of ACS. The Veteran's Administration Cooperative Study [4] compared aspirin (324 mg daily for 12 weeks) to placebo in 1266 men. The incidence of death or myocardial infarction (MI) was 51% lower in the aspirin-treated patients. These results were confirmed in a Swedish trial [5] that compared a lower dose of aspirin (75 mg daily) to placebo in 796 men. A reduction in death or MI of 64% was observed at 3 months, and of 48% at 1 year. A similar result was achieved in a Canadian study [6] using a much higher dose of aspirin (1300 mg daily). These data are conclusive and justify the recommendation that all patients with ACS should receive regular aspirin as soon as possible, and that 80 mg should be continued daily for long-term management, unless a definite contraindication is present.

Thienopyridines

Clopidogrel, unlike aspirin, does not block cyclooxygenase, but interfere with ADP-mediated platelet activation. It exerts its therapeutic effect when more than 80% of platelets are inhibited. The clinical efficacy of clopidogrel was tested in the CURE trial.

Evidence-based Medicine: The CURE trial
Clopidogrel was studied in the Clopidogrel in Unstable Angina to Prevent Recurrent Events trial which randomized 12,562 patients with UA or non-STEMI to either clopidogrel and aspirin or placebo and aspirin. At 30 days, all patients, including the subgroup older than 65 years of age, had a significant relative risk reduction in the composite end point of death, non-fatal MI, and stroke. The impact of clopidogrel vs. placebo was as follows: low-risk group (TIMI score 0–2) 4.1% vs. 5.7% ($P < 0.04$), intermediate-risk group (TIMI score 3–4), 9.8% vs. 11.4% ($P < 0.03$), and high-risk group (TIMI score 5–7), 15.9% vs. 20.7% ($P < 0.004$) [7].

As a result, clopidogrel was indicated for patients with ACS. The patient should receive a 300–600 mg bolus dose in order to attain its therapeutic efficacy within 24 hours, and 75 mg/day for more than 9 months.

Unfractionated Heparin

Because plaque rupture and thrombosis are critical aspects of the pathophysi-ology of ACS, the efficacy of unfractionated heparin (UFH) has been tested by several randomized clinical trials. A meta-analysis of six randomized trials (1353 patients) by Oler *et al.* [8] demonstrated a 33% reduction in death or MI in patients treated with UFH and aspirin compared with patients treated with aspirin alone. Thus, intravenous UFH should be started as soon as possible, titrated to an aPTT of 1.5–2.5 times control. While rebound angina may occur after discontinuation of UFH, this phenomenon is reduced with concomitant aspirin use. However, the absorption of UFH is erratic, demanding frequent monitoring and titration, this is why its anticoagulant level is more likely to be outside the therapeutic and safety window.

Low Molecular Weight Heparins

The anticoagulant of low molecular weight heparins (LMWH) effect is more predictable than UFH, and routine laboratory monitoring is not required to assess its efficacy. LMWH also have a great specificity for factor Xa binding and are resistant to inhibition by activated platelets. In addition, LMWH cause less drug-induced thrombocytopenia.

Evidence-based Medicine: The ESSENCE trial

The Efficacy and Safety of Subcutaneous Enoxaparin in Non-Q-Wave Coronary Events investigators compared the LMWH enoxaparin to UFH in 3171 patients with UA or non-Q-wave MI. At 14 days the risk of death, MI, or recurrent angina was significantly lower in patients treated with enoxaparin and aspirin compared to those treated with UFH and aspirin (16.6% vs. 19.8%; $P = 0.019$). This benefit continued at 30 days (19.8% vs. 23.3%; $P = 0.016$). In addition, the need for revascularization procedures was also decreased (27.0% vs. 32.2%; $P = 0.001$). There was no difference in the rates of major bleeding [9].

These studies have demonstrated that LMWH are at least as good as (and probably better than) UFH in the treatment of ACS [9,10]. In addition, they are easier to administer owing to short intravenous (IV) infusion times, and because routine laboratory monitoring is not necessary.

Direct Thrombin Inhibitors

Working directly against free and clot-bound thrombin, direct thrombin inhibitors (DTIs) do not require antithrombin III as a cofactor. Thus, these agents can produce a stable and predictable level of anticoagulation. DTI was tested in the REPLACE trial in which the patients were randomly assigned to receive IV bivalirudin with provisional Gp 2b3a inhibition (GPI), or to receive heparin with planned GPI. The results showed that at 6 months there was no difference in mortality (1.4% vs. 1%; $P = 0.15$), MI, or repeat revascularization [11]. This is why the ACUITY trial was designed to test again the effects of DTI in ACS patients undergoing primary coronary intervention (PCI).

Evidence-based Medicine: The ACUITY trial

In the Acute Catheterization and Urgent Intervention Triage strategy trial, 13,800 patients with moderate- to high-risk ACS are being prospectively randomly assigned to UFH or enoxaparin + GPI, vs. bivalirudin + GPI, vs. bivalirudin + provisional GPI. All patients undergo cardiac catheterization within 72 hours, followed by percutaneous or surgical revascularization when appropriate. In a second random assignment, patients assigned to receive GPI are sub-randomized to upstream drug initiation vs. GPI (provisional) administration during angioplasty only. The results showed that the primary study end points (composite of death, MI, unplanned revascularization for ischemia, and major bleeding) at 30 days were similar between UFH, LMWH or DTI. However, DTI alone gave the best results because it caused the lowest level of bleeding. GPI did not improve the outcome on top of DTI [12].

Factor Xa Inhibitor

Heparin binds to antithrombin III and induces a conformational change, increasing its affinity to bind and inactivate thrombin (factor IIa), Xa, XIa, IXa, and other components of the coagulation cascade. The binding site of heparin to antithrombin consists of five sugar molecules which have become the basis for the creation of the synthetic pentasaccharides, of which fondaparinux is the first one to be extensively studied. Fondaparinux binds specifically to antithrombin, giving a very specific inhibition of Xa without interfering with other clotting factors.

EMERGING TREND

The OASIS 5 trial 20,078 ACS patients were randomized to either fondaparinux 2.5 mg ($n = 10,057$) or enoxaparin 1 mg/kg twice daily ($n = 10,021$). At 30 day follow-up, outcomes were significantly better for patients treated with fondaparinux, with a 17% reduction in 30-day mortality. Furthermore, major bleeding rates at 30 days remained significantly higher in patients treated with enoxaparin. These results were maintained at 6 months with a 9% reduction in the risk of death or MI, and a 13% reduction in the risk of death, MI, refractory ischemia, or major bleeding in patients who underwent percutaneous coronary intervention during the study period. Vascular-access-site complications were more frequent in the enoxaparin arm (8.1% vs. 3.3%, $P < 0.0001$). Death and/or MI following PCI were similar in both arms of the study [13].

β-Blockers

Competitive antagonists to catecholamines, β-blockers cause a decrease in heart rate and cardiac contractility, thus decreasing myocardial oxygen demand. Although these agents have not been shown to decrease mortality in patients with ACS, β-blockers have been shown to decrease mortality in STEMI and stable angina with silent ischemia. It therefore seems logical to extend these observations to patients with non-STEMI. A meta-analysis from Yusuf *et al.* has demonstrated a reduction in the risk of progression to acute MI (AMI) with the use of β-blockers in patients with ACS [14].

Nitroglycerin

Nitroglycerin (NTG) vasodilates coronary arteries, promotes coronary collateral flow, and decreases cardiac preload. Although these effects have not been shown to decrease death or MI, nitrates can clearly decrease the ischemic burden. Nitrate tolerance can, however, occur in as little as 24 hours, such that patients require a nitrate-free interval or increasing doses of IV NTG. Although NTG is an excellent antianginal agent and may be effective for acute management of ischemia, routine long-term nitrate therapy is not mandatory, since it has not been shown to be effective in the secondary prevention of coronary events.

Glycoprotein 2b3a Inhibitors

The benefits of aspirin in the treatment of ACS highlight the pivotal role of he platelet. The limitations of aspirin have also been recognized, given that it is effective against only one of the pathways leading to platelet aggregation. GPI such as abciximab, eptifibatide and tirofiban block circulating fibrinogen from binding to its receptor on activated platelets, and thus inhibit platelet aggregation. The first major randomized controlled trial (RCT) for PCI in ACS patients is the EPIC trial. It showed lower mortality with GPI, however, with an increase in major bleeding [15]. The problem was fixed in the EPILOG trial when UFH was given at lower dose (70 U/kg) without decreasing its effect but with less bleeding [16]. In this era of drug eluting stent (DES), more RCTs have been conducted to test the efficacy of GPI in different high-risk subsets of patients.

Evidence-based Medicine: The TACTICS-TIMI 18 trial

2220 patients with UA and MI without ST-segment elevation who had electrocardiographic evidence of changes in the ST segment or T wave, elevated levels of cardiac markers, a history of CAD, were enrolled. All patients were treated with aspirin, heparin, and the GPI tirofiban. They were randomly assigned to an early invasive strategy, which included routine catheterization within 4–48 hours and revascularization as appropriate, or to a more conservative (selectively invasive) strategy, in which catheterization was performed only if the patient had objective evidence of recurrent ischemia or an abnormal stress test. The primary end point was a composite of death, non-fatal MI, and rehospitalization for ACS at six months. At six months the results showed that the rate of the primary end point was 15.9% with use of GPI and the early invasive strategy, and 19.4% with use of the conservative strategy (OR, 0.78; 95% CI 0.62–0.97; $P = 0.025$). The rate of death or non-fatal MI at six months was similarly reduced (7.3% vs. 9.5%; OR, 0.74; 95% CI 0.54–1.00; $P < 0.05$) [17].

These trials have demonstrated the benefit of IV GPI in reducing recurrent ischemic events in patients with ACS. However, selective use of different levels of platelet inhibition gives the best protection to patients without causing further harm. Low risk patients in elective PCI benefit the most from high-loading dose of clopidogrel without the need of GPI [18]. The patients with chest pain from progression of a stable plaque without platelet activation would not benefit from GPI, and may even be harmed. Biomarkers such as troponin I (evidence of possible distal embolization), TIMI risk score, B-type natriuretic peptide, and ST-segment depressions, help in identifying the high-risk patients who benefit the most from GPI on top of the usual clopidogrel treatment [19].

Lipid-Lowering Drugs

Secondary prevention clearly begins with aspirin and β-blockers. More recently, the critical role of lipid-lowering therapy has been demonstrated. The "statin" drugs seem to stabilize coronary plaques, since the reduction in coronary events appears out of proportion to the degree of coronary artery disease regression.

Evidence-based Medicine: The PROVE IT-TIMI 22 trial

In the Pravastatin or Atorvastatin Evaluation and Infection Therapy – Thrombolysis In Myocardial Infarction 22 (PROVE IT-TIMI 22) trial, 4162 patients with ACS were randomized to intensive statin therapy (atorvastatin 80 mg) or standard therapy (pravastatin 40 mg). The results showed that the composite end point (death, MI, or rehospitalization for recurrent ACS) at 30 days occurred in 3.0% of patients receiving atorvastatin 80 mg vs. 4.2% of patients receiving pravastatin 40 mg ($P = 0.046$). In stable patients, atorvastatin 80 mg was associated with a composite event rate of 9.6% vs. 13.1% in the pravastatin 40 mg group ($P = 0.003$). Thus, ACS patients should be started in hospital and continued long term on intensive statin therapy [20].

Comprehensive Care

In order to overcome the acute phase of ACS, the patients need comprehensive care which includes medication, coronary revascularization, teaching on diet, life-style change, and exercise. Once the unstable condition of ACS is converted into more controlled and stable CAD, oral medication is the first line of long term medical intervention. Usually, these patients have to take many other medications either for ACS, diabetes, hypercholesterolemia, arthritis, congestive heart failure or chronic obstructive pulmonary disease. So many patients feel that they are overmedicated and/or many could not afford to pay for all these drugs. In these situations, many patients rebel by stopping all medications. This author tries to explain to the patients the importance of each cardiovascular drug and the reason why that particular drug should be taken; which medications the patients can omit, when, why, whether it can be exchanged, and with what. In order to emphasize the importance of each modality and its priority rank of a comprehensive care program, the patient is given a set of seven questions

Table 1.3 Importance rank of different medications or modalities of treatment.

Question	Answer
1. If you can afford to buy only one medication to take every day, which one do you have to buy?	ASA
2. If you can afford to buy a second medication to take every day, which one do you have to buy?	Thienopyridines
3. If you can afford to buy a third medication every day, which one do you have to buy?	β-blocker
4. Which is the next most important modality of treatment?	Low cholesterol diet
5. Which one is the next most important modality of treatment?	Exercise
6. Which one is the next most important modality of treatment?	Coronary revascularization
7. Which one is the next most important medication?	Cholesterol-lowering drug

ASA, acetylsalicyic acid.

asking the reason and the importance rank of the medications or modalities of treatment. The importance and priority (necessity) ranking is shown in Table 1.3.

The answer to question 1 is aspirin, because it is indicated for ACS and for stable CAD. It is also universally affordable. The unstable ACS patients are to be converted into stable CAD with medications or coronary revascularization (if not, it is a treatment failure). The indication for acetylsalicyic acid (ASA) is nearly absolute, except for rare contraindication or intolerance. The second most important medication for ACS is clopidogrel. It should be taken for 9 months as suggested in the CURE trial, or one month after bare metal stent (BMS) stenting, or one year after DES stenting. The indication for clopidogrel is absolute especially after DES stenting. The answer to question 3 is a β-blocker, because it prevents MI and hospital readmission. For patients in all phases of CAD, from stable to UA to non-Q MI and to STEMI, β-blockers are the main medication.

The answer to question 4 is low cholesterol diet. This author does not think a patient with CAD should take a cholesterol-lowering drug without trying a low cholesterol diet first. After failure to achieve an ideal low LDL level (which often happens), then the patient would be prescribed cholesterol-lowering medication. Adherence to a low salt and low cholesterol diet would help to curb obesity, another strong and stubborn risk factor for CAD.

CLINICAL PEARLS
Did you give comprehensive care to your ACS patients? In a comprehensive care plan, a patient with ACS should receive antiplatelet agents and β-blockers. Without ASA (and clopidogrel) and without β-blockers at optimal dosage, the patient did *not* receive basic medical care for ACS. With regard to risk factor modification, we never stop emphasizing and reinforcing the

instructions on exercise, stopping smoking, better control of diabetes, losing weight. Percutaneous or surgical coronary revascularization never works in the long term if the patient continues to smoke, is non-compliant with medications (specifically ASA, clopidogrel, β-blockers), does not exercise, does not try to diet, has high cholesterol level and does not lose weight.

Difficult Situations and Suggested Solutions

Real World Question How Should You Prevent a New MI?

Without compliance with medication, especially the antiplatelet drug, exercise, stopping smoking, diabetes control, and losing weight, the patient will experience ACS again in the near future. A very important question the patient should ask, or we have to teach the patient, is how to prevent a new MI. Measures to prevent AMI are listed in Table 1.4.

Table 1.4 Measures to prevent acute myocardial infarction.

1. ASA and/or clopidogrel (compliance with medications)
2. β-blockers every day (compliance with medications)
3. Cholesterol-lowering drug (compliance with medications)
4. Exercise every day
5. **No unaccustomed heavy activities**
6. Stop smoking
7. Control diabetes

ASA, acetylsalicyic acid.

What are unaccustomed heavy activities? Sudden, strenuous and prolonged activities that the patients are not used to on a daily basis e.g. shoveling snow, moving furniture, long and strenuous yard works, etc. What about sexual activity? Is it an unaccustomed heavy activity?

CRITICAL THINKING

The SHEEP study. The Stockholm Heart Epidemiology Programme (SHEEP) is to investigate sexual activity as a trigger of MI and the potential effect modification by physical fitness. 699 patients with a first non-fatal AMI participated in the study. The results showed that only 1.3% of the patients without premonitory symptoms of MI had sexual activity during two hours before the onset of MI. The relative risk of MI was 2.1 (95% CI 0.7–6.5) during one hour after sexual activity, and the risk among patients with a sedentary life was 4.4 (95% CI 1.5–12.9) [21].

So the data showed that there was an increased risk of MI after sexual activity and the further increase in risk among the less physically fit support the hypothesis of causal triggering by sexual activity. However, the absolute risk per hour is very low, and exposure is relatively infrequent [21].

CLINICAL PEARLS
Preventing a new MI In order to prevent new MI, ASA and β-blockers – cholesterol-lowering drugs – are the main medications. Stopping smoking is a must because smoking causes rupture of vulnerable plaques.
Lowering LDL cholesterol below 75 mg/dL is a goal to be attained. Counseling on low salt and low cholesterol diet should be reinforced regularly. Exercise is a must. Avoid all unaccustomed heavy activities. Sexual activities will not trigger MI if couples do not abstain, (or practice on a regular basis >2 times a week) [22].

Real World Question Early Invasive or Selective Invasive Strategies?

Even with recent improvements in the pharmacologic management of patients with ACS, the rates of death and MI remain quite high. As a result, early coronary angiography with an eye toward revascularization has been studied. No-one would argue the pivotal role of coronary angiography in UA patients who are refractory to medical therapy or who develop ischemia during a provocative test or patients with non-STEMI. However, routine early angiography is more controversial. The superiority of early invasive approach was evidenced through the RCTs showcased below.

Evidence-based Medicine: The FRISC II trial
In the FRISC II study, 2465 patients with UA or non-Q-wave MI were randomized either to an aggressive strategy or to a more conservative approach. The patients in the early interventional group underwent coronary angiogram followed by early revascularization, if needed, within the first 7 days. The patients in the conservative-approach group underwent invasive procedures only if they had severe symptoms or ischemia during exercise testing. The rate of death or MI in male patients at 6 months was reduced from 12% in the non-invasive arm to 9.5% in the early invasive arm. There was no clinical benefit seen in women because 30% were found to have a normal coronary angiogram [23].

A Dissenting View from Europe

Current US guidelines recommend an early invasive strategy for patients who have ACS without ST-segment elevation and with an elevated cardiac troponin T level. However, according the Dutch investigators, previous RCTs have not shown an overall reduction in mortality, and the reduction in the rate of MI in previous trials has varied depending on the definition of MI [24].

CRITICAL THINKING
The ICTUS trial. 1200 patients with ACS without ST-segment elevation who had chest pain, an elevated cardiac troponin T level ($\geqslant$0.03 μg/L), and either ECG evidence of ischemia at admission or a documented history of CAD were randomized to an early invasive strategy (EIS) or to a selectively

invasive strategy (SIS). Patients received ASA daily, enoxaparin for 48 hours, and abciximab at the time of PCI. The use of clopidogrel and intensive lipid-lowering therapy was recommended. After one year follow-up the results showed that the rate of primary end point was 22.7% in the group assigned to EIS and 21.2% in the group assigned to SIS ($P = 0.33$). The mortality rate was the same in the two groups (2.5%). MI was significantly more frequent in the group assigned to EIS (15% vs. 10%; $P = 0.005$), but rehospitalization was less frequent in that EIS group (7.4% vs. 10.9%; $P = 0.04$). The results could not demonstrate that, given optimized medical therapy, an EIS was superior to a SIS in patients with ACS without ST-segment elevation and with an elevated cardiac troponin T level [25].

The criticism of the ICTUS trial is that this is a low-risk patients population (i.e. <50% of patients older than 65 years of age), <15% have diabetes, <50% had ST-T change and 54% of the conservative strategy underwent early PCI. So if it is a low-risk group in the conservative strategy of whom many underwent early PCI, then there should be no difference in outcome between the two groups.

In general, coronary revascularization is indicated in patients with ACS who fail medical therapy or develop ischemia during a functional study. In addition, high risk patients should be considered for early catheterization (Table 1.5).

Table 1.5 High-risk features favoring an early invasive strategy [26].

1. Recurrent angina/ischemia at rest or with low-level activities despite intensive anti-ischemic therapy
2. Elevated troponin level
3. New or presumably new ST-segment depression
4. Recurrent angina/ischemia with symptoms of heart failure, an S_3 gallop, pulmonary edema, worsening rales, or new or worsening mitral regurgitation
5. High-risk findings on non-invasive stress testing
6. Left ventricular systolic dysfunction (ejection fraction <40% on a non-invasive study)
7. Hemodynamic instability
8. Sustained ventricular tachycardia
9. Percutaneous coronary intervention within 6 months
10. Prior coronary artery bypass graft surgery

In all other patients, a decision should be based on the patient's risk, available facilities, and the patient's preference. As the medical therapy improves with newer and stronger antiplatelet and anticoagulant drugs; and if there is a way to detect normal coronary arteries in ACS patients (30% in the FRISC II trial [23]; then a selective invasive approach is the best. This is a clinically-effective, cost-effective, intellectually satisfactory and common sense approach. It is hard for a cardiologist who tries to convince the referring physician, the patient, and the family that the best treatment is coronary angiogram with possible PCI (an invasive approach) in accordance with the guidelines, when the results of the angiogram shows patent coronary arteries. Did the cardiologist consultant over-diagnose and aggressively over-treat the patients with ACS?

However, is the prognosis benign and the future rosy for ACS patients with an angiogram-filled with non-significant lesions?

Real World Question Risks of MI and Stroke from Non-Significant Coronary Lesions

Coronary angiographies performed during ACS show different levels of coronary stenoses including widely patent coronary arteries. In a study by Germing *et al.*, out of a total of 897 coronary angiographies, 76 patients (8.5%) had no coronary artery stenosis. However, according to the pre-angiographic risk stratification, coronary artery disease (CAD) was strongly suspected in these patients. During a mean follow-up of 11.2 ± 6.4 months, one patient developed an AMI requiring coronary intervention [27].

In another study by Maurin, where the patient has moderate lesion (50% stenosis) the mortality rate was 13%; 20 patients (12%) had major cardiac event; 8 patients (5%) had stroke; and 10 patients (6%) underwent revascularization after 6 years follow-up. Multivariate analysis matched for age and ejection fraction showed that moderate disease (stenosis 40–59%) (OR = 2.713, $P <$ 0.024) was an independent predictive factor of major cardiac event [28].

CRITICAL THINKING

Prognostic value of positive troponin level and non-significant lesion?
The TACTICS-TIMI-18 trial The purpose of this study is to determine whether there is clinical significance to elevated troponin I in patients with suspected ACS with non-critical angiographic coronary stenosis. Patients with ACS enrolled in the Treat Angina With Aggrastat and Determine Cost of Therapy With Invasive or Conservative Strategy-Thrombolysis In Myocardial Infarction (TACTICS-TIMI)-18 were included. Of 2220 patients enrolled in the trial, 895 were eligible. Patients were divided into four groups according to troponin status on admission and presence of significant angiographic stenosis. Baseline brain natriuretic peptide (BNP) and C-reactive protein (CRP) were obtained on all patients.The results showed that median troponin I levels were 0.71 ng/mL in patients with CAD compared with 0.02 ng/mL in patients without CAD ($P <$ 0.0001). Troponin-positive patients with or without angiographic CAD had higher CRP and BNP levels compared with troponin-negative patients ($P <$ 0.01 for both). The rates of death or reinfarction at six months were 0% in troponin-negative patients with no CAD, 3.1% in troponin-positive patients with no CAD, 5.8% in troponin-negative patients with CAD, and 8.6% in troponin-positive patients with CAD ($P =$ 0.012) [29].

So an angiographically non-significant lesion is not equal to a clinically non-significant lesion. These benign-looking lesions can rupture any time and cause thrombus. They cannot be cured by PCI. These vulnerable plaques with a large pool of cholesterol can be become more stable under the effect of statin replacing the cholesterol pool with hardened scar tissue. Aggressive treatment of risk factors and life style modification in patients with non-significant lesion is strongly indicated.

Real World Question Non-Cardiac Causes of High Troponin and Discordance with CK-MB [30]

The troponin complex is located on the thin filament of striated and cardiac muscle and regulates the movement of calcium between actin and myosin. Cardiac troponin has three components, T, C, and I. cTnI is specific to cardiac tissue and is released into serum after myocardial necrosis [30]. However, elevated cTnI levels are also found in patients with pericarditis [31], congestive heart failure (CHF), pulmonary embolism, ventricular arrhythmias and renal insufficiency [32,33]. Aside from the myocardium, troponin T (cTnT) is also found in diseased or regenerating skeletal muscle, so its levels can be elevated in patients with muscular dystrophy or polymyositis [34].

Elevated troponin has been also observed in patients with various level of renal insufficiency. The explanation is that troponin is fragmented into molecules small enough to be cleared by the normal kidneys, however, impaired renal function causes accumulation of these fragments seen in patients with chronic kidney insufficiency (CKD) or severe renal failure, uremic pericarditis or myocarditis [35]. During the acute phase of ACS for patients with CKD, a troponin level rise above the individual baseline is diagnostic of acute myocardial injury [36].

Currently, there are two major commercial immunoassays that measure cTnI levels. The Access System (Beckman Coulter, Fullerton, Calif) uses monoclonal mouse antibodies as both the capture and the conjugate antibodies. The AxSYM system uses monoclonal mouse antibodies as the capture antibody and goat anti-cTnI as the conjugate antibody [37].

Heterophilic antibodies can cause false-positive cTnI results. The antibodies bind to the capture and the conjugate antibodies, simulating cTnI. Using antibodies from two different species, as in the AxSYM system, might decrease the false positivity due to heterophilic antibodies [38]. Persons with more frequent exposure to animal proteins (such as veterinarians, farmers, and pet owners) can also develop heterophilic antibodies. In a similar fashion, rheumatoid factor can interfere with the immunoassay. Five percent of healthy patients might have circulating rheumatoid factor, and about 1% of patients who have elevated cTnI levels have this elevation purely because of the rheumatoid factor [39]. The causes of non-MI-related elevation of cardiac biomarkers (troponin or CK-MB) are listed in Table 1.6.

When the troponin is elevated, regardless of the results of CK-MB, the prognosis is poorer. In ACS patients who had both CK-MB and cTn measured, the hospital mortality was 2.7% in patients with CK-MB–/cTn–; 3.0% in patients with CK-MB+/cTn–; 4.5% in patients with CK-MB–/cTn+; and 5.9% in patients with CK-MB+/cTn+. So an elevated troponin level identifies patients

Table 1.6 Non-MI cause of elevation of troponin.

1. Defibrillator discharge [40]
2. Renal insufficiency [41]
3. Left ventricular failure [42]
4. Tachy-arrhythmias [43,44]
5. Myocarditis [30]
6. Pericarditis [31]
7. Pulmonary embolism [33]
8. Assay interference (heterophile antibody [38], rheumatoid factor [39], excess fibrin [45]

at increased acute risk regardless of CK-MB status, but an isolated CK-MB+ status has limited prognostic value [46].

Real World Question How should you manage anti-platelet drug resistance?

For patients with ACS undergoing stenting with DES, the greatest concern is subacute stent thrombosis (SAT) due to suboptimal stent deployment or due to failure of protection from anti-platelet drug. This phenomenon is called antiplatelet drug resistance. However, another definition of aspirin and clopidogrel resistance is non-responsiveness after the antiplatelet treatment (<10% absolute change in platelet aggregation), and the high post-anti-platelet drug treatment aggregation (>75th percentile aggregation after 300 mg clopidogrel).The question becomes more complex because a variety of techniques used to measure platelet function resulting in different ways of defining drug resistance so conclusive data are lacking [47,48]. However, non-compliance should be the first suspicion in any case of antiplatelet drug resistance [49].

Three distinct types of antiplatelet drug resistance have been described [50]. Type I, or pharmacokinetic resistance (problem with absorption), occurs when neither thromboxane A_2 (TXA_2) nor collagen-induced platelet aggregation is inhibited *in vivo*, but the addition of aspirin *in vitro* inhibits platelet aggregation in response to both platelet agonists. Type II, or pharmacodynamic resistance, occurs when neither TXA_2 nor collagen-induced platelet aggregation is inhibited *in vivo* or after the addition of aspirin *in vitro* (real resistance). Type III, or pseudoresistance, occurs when TXA_2 production is inhibited, but platelet aggregation is not inhibited (no clinical effect) [51].

 Evidence-based Medicine: What is the optimal dose of clopidogrel for PCI?
Levels of platelet aggregation were measured in patients undergoing stenting (*n* = 190) randomly treated with either a 300 mg or a 600 mg clopidogrel load. Non-responsiveness (NR) was defined as <10% absolute change in platelet aggregation, and high post-PA was defined as >75th percentile aggregation after 300 mg clopidogrel. The results showed that non-responsiveness was lower after

600 mg compared to the 300 mg dose (8% vs. 28% and 8% vs. 32% with 5 and 20 μmol ADP, respectively, $P < 0.001$). Among the patients with high post-PA after 300 mg clopidogrel, 62–65% had NR, whereas after the 600 mg dose, all of the patients with high post-PA had NR. So a 600 mg clopidogrel loading dose reduces the incidence of NR and high post-PA as compared to a 300 mg dose [52].

CLINICAL PEARLS

How to prevent subacute thrombosis after stenting? At the end of PCI, an excellent angiographic result with TIMI 3 flow without mechanical problems (stent under-expansion, malapposition, dissections, inflow/outflow stenoses) is the best guarantee against SAT. Compliance with double platelet therapy is best. According to the data above, 600 mg clopidogrel loading dose would give the highest level of platelet inhibition. In case of need for quicker and stronger platelet inhibition (after 10 minutes of infusion), GP 2b3a inhibitors would do the job. At present, there is no quantitative measure of the effect of aspirin that can reliably predict the drug's ability to prevent ischemic vascular events [53].

Take Home Message

Most patients with UA should be admitted and placed on bed rest with continuous electrocardiographic monitoring. All patients should receive regular ASA (160–324 mg) and LMWH or UFH as soon as possible. If there are no contraindications, β-blockade (BB) and NTG should be administered. If angina is still present, NTG can given. LMWHs, especially enoxaparin, appear superior to UFH, and are easier to administer. The addition of GP 2b3a inhibitors to heparin and ASA also decreased clinical endpoints. In addition, they have markedly improved the safety and efficacy of patients with ACS undergoing PCI, especially in patients with troponin positive.

An early invasive strategy seems warranted in high risk patients, in patients who fail medical therapy or have a positive stress test. In intermediate risk patients, the choice of early conservative or early invasive strategies depends on the physician's experience and the patient's preference.

Finally, all patients should receive intensive counseling on risk factor modification. Most patients should continue long-term aspirin, β-blockers, and a "statin" drug. Angiotensin-converting enzyme inhibitors are indicated in patients with LV dysfunction. In patients receiving drug eluting stent, clopidogrel should be given longer from 1 year to 2 years, according to the new data presented at the American Heart Association 2006 Scientific Sessions in Chicago.

References

1 Antman EM, Cohen M, Bernink PJ *et al.* The TIMI risk score for unstable angina/non-ST elevation MI:A method for prognostication and therapeutic decision making. JAMA 2000;284:835–842.

2 Abela G, Aziz K. Cholestrol Crystals rupture biological membranes and human plaques during acute cardiovascular events. A novel insight of plaque rupture by scanning electron microscopy. Scanning 2006;28:1–10.

3 Abela G, Aziz K. Cholesterol crystals cause mechanical damage to biological membrane: A proposed mechanism of plaque rupture and erosion leading to arterial thrombosis. Clinical Cardiology 2005;28:413–420.

4 Lewis HDJ, Davis JW, Archibald DG *et al.* Protective effects of aspirin against acute myocardial infarction and death in men with unstable angina. Results of a Veterans Administration Cooperative Study. N Engl J Med 1983;309:396–403.

5 Wallentin LC. Aspirin (75 mg/day) after an episode of unstable coronary artery disease:Long-term effects on the risk for myocardial infarction, occurrence of severe angina and the need for revascularization. Research Group on Instability in Coronary Artery Disease in Southeast Sweden. J Am Coll Cardiol 1991;18:1587–1593.

6 Cairns JA, Gent M, Singer J *et al.* Aspirin, sulfinpyrazone, or both in unstable angina. Results of a Canadian multicenter trial. N Engl J Med 1985;313:1369–1375.

7 Peters RJ, Mehta SR, Fox KA, for the CURE investigators. Effects of aspirin dose when used alone or in combination with clopidogrel in patients with acute coronary syndromes: observations from the Clopidogrel in Unstable angina to prevent Recurrent Events (CURE) study. Circulation 2003 Oct 7;108(14):1682–7.

8 Oler A, Whooley MA, Oler J, Grady D. Adding heparin to aspirin reduces the incidence of myocardial infarction and death in patients with unstable angina. A meta analysis. JAMA 1996;276:811–815.

9 Goodman SG, Cohen M, Bigonzi F *et al.* Randomized trial of low molecular weight heparin (enoxaparin) versus unfractionated heparin for unstable coronary artery disease: One-year results of the ESSENCE study. J Am Coll Cardiol 2000;36:693–698.

10 Mahaffey KW, Cohen M, Garg J. High–risk patients with acute coronary syndromes treated with low-molecular-weight or unfractionated heparin:outcomes at 6 months and 1 year in the SYNERGY trial. JAMA 2005;294(20):2594–2600.

11 Lincoff AM, Kleiman NS, Kereiakes DJ. Long-term efficacy of bivalirudin and provisional glycoprotein IIb/IIIa blockade vs heparin and planned glycoprotein IIb/IIIa blockade during percutaneous coronary revascularization:REPLACE-2 randomized trial. JAMA 2004;292(6):696–703.

12 ACUITY trial results: Presented by G. Stone at the American College of Cardiology meeting 2006 in Atlanta.

13 The Fifth Organization to Assess Strategies in Acute Ischemic Syndromes Investigators Comparison of Fondaparinux and Enoxaparin in Acute Coronary Syndromes NEJM 2006;354:1464–1476.

14 Yusuf S, Wittes J, Friedman L. Overview of results of randomized clinical trials in heart disease. II. Unstable angina, heart failure, primary prevention with aspirin, and risk factor modification. JAMA 1988;260:2259–2263.

15 The EPIC Investigators. Use of a monoclonal antibody directed against the platelet glycoprotein IIb/IIIa receptor in high risk coronary angioplasty. N Engl J Med 1994;330: 956–961.

16 The EPILOG Investigators. Platelet glycoprotein IIb/IIIa receptor blockade and low-dose heparin during percutaneous coronary revascularization. N Engl J Med 1997;336:1689–1696.

17 Cannon CP, Weintraub WS, Demopoulos LA *et al.* for the TACTICS–Thrombolysis in Myocardial Infarction 18 Investigators. Comparison of Early Invasive and Conservative Strategies in Patients with Unstable Coronary Syndromes Treated with the Glycoprotein IIb/IIIa Inhibitor Tirofiban. NEJM 2001;344:1879–1887.

18 Kastrati A, Mehilli J, Schuhlen H *et al.* A clinical trial of abciximab in elective percutaneous coronary intervention after pretreatment with clopidogrel. N Engl J Med 2004;350: 232–238.

19 Dalby M, Montalescot G, Sollier C. Eptifibatide provides additional platelet inhibition in non-ST-elevation myocardial infarction patients already treated with aspirin and clopidogrelresults of the platelet activity extinction in non-Q-wave myocardial infarction with aspirin, clopidogrel, and eptifibatide (PEACE) study. J Am Coll Cardiol 2004; 43:162–168.

20 Ray KK, Cannon CP, McCabe CH *et al.* PROVE IT–TIMI 22 Investigators. Early and late benefits of high-dose atorvastatin in patients with acute coronary syndromes: results from the PROVE IT-TIMI 22 trial. J Am Coll Cardiol 2005 Oct 18;46(8):1405–1410.

21 Möller J, Ahlbom A, Hulting J. Sexual activity as a trigger of myocardial infarction. A case-crossover analysis in the Stockholm Heart Epidemiology Programme (SHEEP). Heart 2001;86(4):387–390.

22 Mueller JE. Triggering cardiac events by sexual activities: findings from a case-crossover analysis Am J Cardiol 2000;86(suppl):14F–18F.

23 Fragmin during Instability in Coronary Artery Disease (FRISC) study group. Low-molecular-weight heparin during instability in coronary artery disease. Lancet 1996;347: 561–568.

24 Fox KA, Poole-Wilson P, Clayton TC *et al.* 5-year outcome of an interventional strategy in non-ST-elevation acute coronary syndrome:the British Heart Foundation RITA 3 randomised trial. Lancet 2005;366:914–920.

25 de Winter RJ, and the Invasive versus Conservative Treatment in Unstable Coronary Syndromes (ICTUS) Investigators. Early invasive versus selectively invasive management for acute coronary syndromes. N Engl J Med 2005 Sep 15;353(11):1095–104. N Engl J Med. 2005 Dec 22;353(25):2714–18; author reply 2714–8; discussion 2714–8; N Engl J Med 2005 Sep 15;353(11):1159–61.

26 Braunwald E, Antman EM, Beasley JW *et al.* ACC/AHA 2002 Guideline Update for the Management of Patients With Unstable Angina and Non-ST-Segment Elevation Myocardial Infarction: A Report of the American College of Cardiology/American Heart Association Task Force on Practice Guidelines (Committee on the Management of Patients With Unstable Angina). J Am Coll Cardiol 2000;36:970–1062.

27 Germing A. Normal angiogram in acute coronary syndrome – preangiographic risk stratification, angiographic findings and follow-up. Int J Cardiol 2005;99(1):19–23.

28 Maurin T *et al.* Long-term prognosis of patients with acute coronary syndrome and moderate coronary artery stenosis. Cardiology 2003;99(2):90–95.

29 Dokainish H, Pillai M, Murphy SA *et al.* TACTICS-TIMI-18 Investigators. Prognostic implications of elevated troponin in patients with suspected acute coronary syndrome but no critical epicardial coronary diseasea TACTICS-TIMI-18 substudy. J Am Coll Cardiol 2005;45:19–24.

30 Coudrey L. The troponins. Arch Intern Med 1998;158:1173–1180.

31 Bonnefoy E, Godon P, Kirkorian G, Fatemi M, Chevalier P, Touboul P. Serum cardiac troponin I and ST-segment elevation in patients with acute pericarditis. Eur Heart J 2000; 21:832–1836.

32 Heeschen C, Goldmann BU, Moeller RH, Hamm CW. Analytical performance and clinical application of a new rapid bedside assay for the detection of serum cardiac troponin I. Clin Chem 1998;44:1925–1930.

33 Douketis JD, Crowther MA, Stanton EB, Ginsberg JS. Elevated cardiac troponin levels in patients with submassive pulmonary embolism. Arch Intern Med 2002;162:79–81.

34 Bodor GS, Survant L, Voss EM, Smith S, Porterfield D, Apple FS. Cardiac troponin T composition in normal and regenerating human skeletal muscle. Clin Chem 1997;43: 476–484.

35 Ringdahl EN, Stevermer JJ. False-Positive Troponin I in a Young Healthy Woman with Chest Pain. J Am Board Fam Pract 2002;15(3):242–245.

36 Hojs R. Cardiac troponin T in patients with kidney disease. Ther Apher Dial 2005; 9(3):205–207.

37 Volk AL, Hardy R, Robinson CA, Konrad RJ. False-positive cardiac troponin I results – Two case reports. Lab Med 1999;30:610–612.

38 Fitzmaurice TF, Brown C, Rifai N, Wu AH, Yeo KT. False increase of cardiac troponin I with heterophilic antibodies. Clin Chem 1998;44:2212–2214.

39 Krahn J, Parry DM, Leroux M, Dalton J. High percentage of false positive cardiac troponin I results in patients with rheumatoid factor. Clin Biochem 1999;32:477–480.

40 Allan JJ, Feld RD, Russell AA *et al.* Cardiac troponin I levels are normal or minimally elevated after transthoracic cardioversion. J Am Coll Cardiol 1997;30:1052–1056.

41 Apple FS, Sharkey SW, Hoeft P *et al.* Prognostic value of serum cardiac troponin I and T in chronic dialysis patients:a 1-year outcomes analysis. Am J Kidney Dis 1997;29:399–403.

42 Del Carlo CH, O'Connor CM. Cardiac troponins in congestive heart failure (review). Am Heart J 1999;138:646–653.

43 Luna C, Adie MA, Tessler I, Acherman R. Troponin I elevation after supraventricular tachycardia in a child with hypertrophic cardiomyopathy. Paediat Cardiol 2002;22:147–149.

44 Vikenes K, Omvik P, Farstad M, Nordrehaug JE. Cardiac biochemical markers after cardioversion of atrial fibrillation or atrial flutter. Am Heart J 2000;140:690–696.

45 Abbott A. xSYM system. Package insert: troponin-I. List No. 3C29. Abbott Park, Ill: Abbott Laboratories, 1997.

46 Newby LK, Roe MT, Chen AY for the CRUSADE Investigators. Frequency and Clinical Implications of Discordant Creatine Kinase-MB and Troponin Measurements in Acute Coronary Syndromes. J Am Coll Cardiol 2006;47:312–318.

47 Gum PA, Kottke-Marchant K, Welsh PA, White J, Topol EJ. A prospective, blinded determination of the natural history of aspirin resistance among stable patients with cardiovascular disease. J Am Coll Cardiol 2003;41(6):961–965.

48 Andersen K, Hurlen M, Arnesen H, Seljeflot I. Aspirin non-responsiveness as measured by the PFA-100 in patients with coronary artery disease. Thromb Res 2003;108:37–42.

49 Schwartz KA, Schwartz DE, Ghosheh K, Reeves MJ, Barber K, DeFranco A. Compliance as a critical consideration in patients who appear to be resistant to aspirin after healing of myocardial infarction. Am J Cardiol 2005 Apr 15;95(8):973–975.

50 Weber AA, Przytulski B, Schanz A, Hohlfeld T, Schror K. Towards a definition of aspirin resistance:a typological approach. Platelets 2002;13:37–40.

51 Burns TL, Mooss AN, Hilleman DE. Antiplatelet drug resistance: not ready for prime time. Pharmacotherapy 2005;25(11):1621–1628.

52 Gurbel PA, Bliden KP, Hayes KM *et al.* The Relation of Dosing to Clopidogrel Responsiveness and the Incidence of High Post-Treatment Platelet Aggregation in Patients Undergoing Coronary Stenting. JACC 2005;49:1392–1396.

53 Steinhubl SR, Charnigo R, Moliterno DJ. Resistance to Antiplatelet Resistance Is it Justified? J Am Coll Cardiol 2005;45:1757–1758.

CHAPTER 2

ST-Elevation Acute Myocardial Infarction

Thach N. Nguyen, C. Michael Gibson, Borce Petrovski, Prakash Makam, Nguyen Duc Cong and Pham Gia Khai

Introduction

Every year in the United States more than 700,000 patients arrive at the emergency room with ST-segment elevation acute myocardial infarction (STEMI). Their in-hospital, 1-month, and 1-year mortality is high. For a cardiologist standing at the bedside of a critical patient with STEMI, the ultimate goal is to open, as quickly as possible, the acute infarct-related artery (IRA) and to turn the clinically volatile situation into controlled recovery without ventricular remodeling. With the advent of thrombolytic therapy (TT) and primary coronary interventions (PCIs), there came a great opportunity to open acutely occluded IRA and restore antegrade flow to the ischemic myocardium. The strategies which guide the cardiologist from the first encounter with the patient in the emergency room through the discharge day and the office follow-up ten years later, are listed in Table 2.1.

From the angiographic point of view, successful reperfusion is defined as early and complete restoration of coronary blood flow to a thrombolysis in acute myocardial infarction (TIMI) 3 flow [1]. This brisk flow allows sufficient microvascular perfusion to result in significant reduction in mortality.

Table 2.1 Management strategies for patients with ST elevation myocardial infarction.

1. Quickly screen patients for indication and risks
2. Start TT or send the patient quickly to the cardiac catheterization laboratories for emergency angioplasty and stenting
3. Open the IRA and its distal microvasculature with minimal incidence of stroke (<1%) by the fastest (<90 mins: door-to-balloon time) and most effective way (<3% 30-day mortality, <4% reinfarction, <2% restenosis in 1 year)
4. Prevent left ventricular remodeling (no left ventricular dilation)
5. Prevent another MI in the future (secondary prevention)

IRA, infarct-related artery; MI, myocardial infarction; TT, thrombolytic therapy.

Even the in-hospital and 30-day mortality can be improved greatly by the ability of interrupting the process of infarction, this short-term outcome still depends strongly on age, gender, Killip class, ejection fraction, number of diseased arteries and co-morbidities. The long-term outcome (6-month and more than one year morbidity and mortality) depends mainly on the magnitude of the disease state and the systemic factors that predispose the patient to the progression of the disease as well as restenosis [2]. Clinical signs or symptoms differentiating the high risk vs. the low risk STEMI patients are listed in Table 2.2.

Table 2.2 Factors suggestive of high risk patients.

1. Hypotension (blood pressure <100 mmHg)
2. Congestive heart failure
3. Sinus tachycardia (heart rate >100)
4. Advanced age
5. Female sex
6. Diabetes mellitus
7. Persistent ST segment elevation
8. Persistent chest pain
9. High BNP level
10. Anemia
11. High white blood cell count
12. Chronic kidney disease

BNP, brain natriuretic peptide.

In this chapter, from the above perspectives, the benefits, deficiencies, and technical considerations of standard of care for STEMI patients as recommended by the American College of Cardiology, American Heart Association and Society of Cardiovascular Angiography and Interventions task force on STEMI are presented [3]. Real world problems encountered when applying these guidelines, and suggested solutions, are discussed.

Thrombolytic Therapy

The indications for TT are for patients presenting with chest discomfort within 12 hours of onset and with ST-segment elevation (1 mm in at least two limb leads and 2 mm in two or more contiguous precordial leads suggestive of STEMI) or new left bundle branch block. To achieve optimal benefit from TT, the lytic drugs should be started as early as possible based on the electrocardiogram (ECG) criteria, without waiting for the creatinine kinase (CK) or troponin enzyme result. A 30-day overall 7% mortality rate achieved by TT is well proven in large randomized trials.

CLINICAL PEARLS

Which STEMI patient will not die in the next 24 hours? In patients with STEMI, if the heart rate is below 100 and the blood pressure is above 100, then the chance that the patient will die in the near future is low. These patients may develop ischemia, reinfarction etc., however, the mortality is still minimal in the next 24 hours [4]. A very low heart rate (<50 BPM (beats per minute)) is also detrimental because it can represent advanced atrio-ventricular block [5].

The current lytic agents are divided into two groups: the fibrin-selective and the less fibrin-selective agents. The drugs that lack or have less fibrin specificity, such as streptokinase (SK), urokinase, and lanoteplase (n-PA), activate plasminogen indiscriminately whether it is physically bound with fibrin inside the thrombus or free in the circulation. So they induce a systemic lytic state, evidenced by depletion of circulating plasminogen, degradation of fibrinogen, which causes a high level of fibrinogen degradation products (FDPs), and a decreased level of α-antiplasmin. This low level of fibrinogen and high level of FDPs with anticoagulant properties helps to sustain the process of thrombotic dissolution so there is no need for unfractionated heparin (UFH). The fibrin-selective agents are tissue plasminogen activators (t-PAs) such as alteplase, duteplase or saruplase (single-chain urokinase), tenecplase (TNK-tPA) and staphylokinase. They activate fibrin-associated plasminogen preferentially at the clot surface, cleaving plasminogen to plasmin. Since this plasmin is already bound to fibrin at the lysine-binding sites, this opens up new binding sites that can bind more of the fibrinolytic and more plasminogen, thus facilitating continued lysis of the clot [6]. By this mechanism, the fibrin-selective agents induce thrombolysis without causing a systemic lytic state or depletion of fibrinogen in the circulation so they need UFH and cause fewer intracranial hemorrhages (ICH).

The biochemical characteristics of any ideal lytic drug are to have slow plasma clearance, to be more fibrin-specific, and to be resistant to plasminogen activator inhibitor I. As the plasma clearance is slower, the half-life of the drug is longer. Then it can be given as a simple intravenous bolus which can decrease substantially the delay in the process of administration. If the drug is more fibrin-binding, its efficacy should be improved and it can be given in a smaller dose. To be effective, TT requires dissolution of the fibrin network of a thrombotic clot, complete suppression of further thrombin generation and platelet aggregation.

With current results, the advantage of TT is by earliest restoration of flow due to its quick and simple intravenous administration. It does not restore full epicardial or microvascular flow to the majority of patients, nor sustain its patency thereafter. The contraindications of TT are listed in Table 2.3 [7].

Table 2.3 Contraindications of thrombolytic therapy.

Absolute contraindications
1. Any prior intracranial bleeding
2. Known structural cerebral vascular lesion (e.g. arterio–venous malformations)
3. Known malignant intracranial neoplasm (primary or metastatic)
4. Ischemic stroke within 3 months, *except* ischemic stroke within 3 hours
5. Suspected aortic dissection
6. Active bleeding or bleeding diathesis (excluding menses)
7. Significant closed head or facial trauma within 3 months

Relative contraindications
1. History of chronic, severe, or poorly controlled hypertension
2. Severe uncontrolled HTN on presentation (systolic blood pressure >180 mmHg, diastolic blood pressure >110 mmHg)
3. History of prior ischemic stroke >3 months, dementia, or known intracranial pathology (not covered in absolute contraindications)
4. Traumatic (greater than 10 minutes) cardio-pulmonary resuscitation or major surgery (<3 weeks)
5. Non-compressive vascular puncture
6. For streptokinase/anistrepplase: prior exposure (more than 5 days ago) or prior allergic reaction to these agents
7. Pregnancy
8. Active peptic ulcer
9. Current use of anticoagulants: the higher the INR, the higher the risk of bleeding

HTN, hypertension; INR, international normalized ratio.

Primary Coronary Intervention

Because of the incomplete results of TT and inegilibility of many patients, at first balloon angioplasty (POBA) was performed on patients with STEMI. In the Primary Coronary Angioplasty vs. Thrombolysis (PCAT) study, the results showed clearly the short- and long-term mortality reduction of POBA over TT. The overall success rate of primary POBA was reported to be around 97%. However, the efficacy of POBA was limited with recurrent ischemia in 10–15%, early reocclusion and late restenosis in 31–45% of patients [8]. Not every STEMI patient was eligible for stenting because the artery could be too small, or the lumen of the IRA was wide open with TIMI 3 flow after POBA. The angiographic criteria for excluding PCI in STEMI are listed in Table 2.4 [9].

Table 2.4 Angiographic exclusions precluding performance of primary coronary interventions in ST elevation myocardial infarction.

1. Unprotected LM lesion >60%
2. IRA with TIMI 3 flow and lesion morphology extremely high risk for abrupt closure (extremely long lesion or severe angulated lesion)
3. Multivessel disease with TIMI-3 flow in the IRA, now stable and pain free
4. IRA supplies a small or secondary vessels supplying a small amount of myocardium, in which the risk of PCI may outweigh the benefit
5. Inability to clearly identify the IRA

IRA, infarct-related artery; LM, left main; TIMI, thrombolysis in acute myocardial infarction.

PCI techniques have evolved greatly since these trials were reported. Bare metal stent (BMS) was deployed in order to improve the angiographic achievements of POBA and sustain its long term clinical results. With the development of drug eluting stent (DES) and its track record of low in-stent-restenosis for elective stenting, DES was tried in STEMI patients with hope for long term patency. The safety, short- and long-term efficacy of DES in STEMI patients was impartially tested in the randomized clinical trial (RCT) described below.

Evidence-based Medicine: DES for STEMI – The TYPHOON trial
712 patients with STEMI randomized between Cypher stents, and balloon angioplasty and bare metal stent (BMS). The results showed that at 1 year, the rate of mortality was 2.2% for both groups. The overall rate of target-vessel failure was 7.3% for the Cypher stent and 14.3% among those treated with balloon angioplasty and a BMS (a 49% relative reduction). In a sub-study with 210 patients, there was 83% reduction in the rate of re-stenosis and an 83% reduction in tissue proliferation. The stent thrombosis rate was 3.4% for DES and 3.6% for POBA or BMS. These results met the expectations of low mortality and excellent long term major adverse cardio-vascular events (MACE) [10].

However, the results of PCI in STEMI are operator-dependent and institution-related. The indicators of excellent interventional service of a cardiac catheterization laboratory are listed in Table 2.5. If an institution's results are sub-optimal compared with the national levels, then the focus of treatment for patients with STEMI in that particular hospital should be the use of TT, with further referral to PCI when indicated [3]. Patients with STEMI should be referred for primary PCI once the cardiac catheterization laboratories provide better services which are translated into better patient outcomes.

The indications for PCI, as described by the American College of Cardiology/American Heart Association/Society of Cardiovascular Angiography and Interventions guidelines for PCI [3], each with its corresponding level of evidence (LOE) are listed in Table 2.6.

Table 2.5 Indicators of excellence in providing interventional services for ST elevation myocardial infarction.

1. Door-to-balloon time <90 mins
2. TIMI 2 or 3 flow attained in >90% of patients
3. Emergency CABG <2%
4. Actual performance of PCI in >85% of patients brought to the laboratory
5. Risk-adjusted in-hospital mortality rate 3% in patients without cardiogenic shock

CABG, coronary artery bypass grafting; PCI, primary coronary interventions; TIMI, thrombolysis in acute myocardial infarction.

Table 2.6 Indications for Primary Interventions in ST elevation myocardial infarction.

Guidelines	
Class I	If immediately available, primary PCI should be performed in patients with STEMI (including true posterior MI) or MI with new, or presumably new, LBBB who can undergo PCI of the IRA within 12 hours of symptoms onset, if performed in a timely fashion (balloon inflation goal within 90 mins of presentation) (LOE: B)
Class I	Primary PCI should be performed in patients with severe CHF and/or pulmonary edema (Killip class 3) and onset of symptoms within 12 hours (LOE: B)
Class IIa	It is reasonable to perform primary PCI in patients with onset of symptoms within the prior 12–24 hours and one or more of the following: (a) severe CHF; (b) hemodynamic or electrical instability; (c) evidence of persistent ischemia (LOE:C)

CHF, congestive heart failure; IRA, infarct-related artery; LBBB, left bundle branch block; LOE, level of evidence; MI, myocardial infarction; PCI, primary coronary interventions; Level of evidence A: Data derived from multiple RCTs; Level of evidence B: Data derived from single RCT or non-RCT; Level of evidence C: Only consensus opinion of experts, case studies or standard of care.

Acetylsalicyic Acid

Aspirin, or acetylsalicyic acid (ASA), is a weak platelet inhibitor; it works by irreversibly acetylating cyclooxygenase. ASA suppresses the production of the pro-aggregatory arachidonic-acid-mediated effect of thromboxane A2. Its *in vivo* inhibition occurs within 15–30 minutes of the ingestion of non-enteric-coated aspirin. Because platelets are primitive cells, this production cannot be restored until new platelets are formed 5–7 days later. Aspirin (100–300 mg) should be given as early as possible, preferably in the emergency room. Intravenous, chewable, or high-dose (>500 mg) oral administration of aspirin can more rapidly induce its therapeutic effects.

Thienopyridine

Clopidogrel is a thienopyridine derivative that inhibits the binding of adenosine diphosphate to its platelet receptors. It begins to exert its effectiveness 24 hours after a loading dose of 300–600 mg when >80% of platelets are inhibited. It has been effective in preventing the formation of thrombus after elective stenting for stable angina and improves outcomes in patients with acute coronary syndrome (ACS) [11]. The efficacy of thienopyridine in STEMI was tested in the CLARITY-TIMI 28 trial.

Evidence-based Medicine: The CLARITY-TIMI 28 trial

The Clopidogrel as Adjunctive Reperfusion Therapy-TIMI 28 trial enrolled 3491 patients with STEMI and randomized them to receive either clopidogrel (300 mg loading dose, then 75 mg once daily) or placebo. 53.4% underwent PCI and received open label clopidogrel. The results demonstrated that pre-treatment with clopidogrel resulted in a highly significant reduction in cardiovascular death, MI, or stroke from randomization through 30 days (7.5% vs. 12.0%). There was no significant excess in the rates of TIMI, major or minor bleeding (2.0% vs. 1.9%), between clopidogrel- and placebo-treatment groups [12].

Glycoprotein 2B3A Inhibitors

The platelet glycoprotein (GP) 2b3a receptor mediates the final pathway of platelet aggregation. This receptor becomes activated by a variety of soluble and adhesive agonists, and binds fibrinogen molecules between platelets in the aggregation process. The linkage of these fibrins provides a strong network to trap red cells, and subsequently form a firm thrombus. The GP 2b3a inhibitors (GPI) inhibit the cross-linking of platelets by fibrinogen, thus effectively prevent formation of new clot. The efficacy of abciximab in patients with STEMI was tested in the ADMIRAL and the CADILLAC trials.

CRITICAL THINKING

The ADMIRAL trial. In the Abciximab before Direct angioplasty and stenting in Myocardial Infarction Regarding Acute and Long term follow-up trial, 300 patients were randomized to have abciximab or placebo in the ambulance, in the emergency room (ER) or the cardiac catheterization laboratory. The composite end-point for death, reinfarction and urgent target vessel revascularization was 7.7% in the stent plus abxicimab group, and 14.6% in the stent plus placebo group ($P = 0.004$). This benefit was maintained at 6 months (8.0% vs. 15.9% respectively, $P = 0.02$). The better outcomes were related to improvements of TIMI-3 flow before the procedure (16% vs. 5.4%, $P = 0.012$), and a better left ventricular ejection fraction at 24 hours (57% vs. 53.9, $P = 0.046$) [13].

CRITICAL THINKING

The CADILLAC trial. To confirm the above findings, the Controlled Abciximab and Device Investigation to Lower Late Angioplasty Complications (CADILLAC) trial randomized 2082 STEMI patients in four treatment strategies between balloon angioplasty, stenting with and without abciximab. A composite of death, reinfarction, disabling stroke, and ischemia-driven TVR was similar in patients treated with stents with or without abciximab (9.5% vs. 10.4%, $P =$ NS) [14].

The results of the CADILLAC trial were different when compared with the results from the ADMIRAL study. Some observers speculate that the strategy of GPI randomization after angiography, the late administration of abciximab in the CADILLAC trial may have blunted the effect of GPI on stented patients [13]. Other investigators believe that the open design of the CADILLAC trial has nothing to do with the difference between the CADILLAC and ADMIRAL trials, because GPI did not statistically make a difference on TIMI flow or left ventricular (LV) function when measured by blinded core laboratories [15].

Unfractionated Heparin

Once the IRA is opened, to prevent further reocclusion it is imperative to completely suppress the generation of thrombin which is the most powerful agonist for activating platelets. The mechanism of UFH is to bind with antithrombin III, and together bind to the catalytic site on the thrombin molecule. The new antithrombin III–heparin complex will inhibit the cleavage of fibrinogen to fibrin and factor Xa.

So, in clinical practice UFH is used to prevent the propagation of the thrombus, formation of new mural thrombosis, systemic embolism, and coronary reocclusion. It also prevents the formation of a stable fibrin clot by inhibiting the activation of the fibrin stabilizing factor. It is indicated when the STEMI patients receive relatively fibrin-specific agents, such as alteplase or reteplase, which produce a variable effect on the systemic coagulation system, and in many patients very little breakdown of fibrinogen or depletion of coagulation factors. The aPTT is maintained at 1.5–2 times control (50–70 seconds).

In patients undergoing primary interventions with the concommitant use of GPI, it is now common to give 70 U/kg of heparin to achieve an activated clotting time (ACT) of 200–250 seconds. If GPI is not used, high dose heparin to achieve ACT > 350 seconds has been associated with reduced subacute thrombosis. Heparin is not continued after the procedure because it has not been proven to decrease the rate of reocclusion or ischemia, unless there are a lot of residual thrombi.

Low Molecular Weight Heparin

A smaller fraction of UFH, low molecular weight heparin (LMWH) has a more predictable anticoagulant effect. Routine laboratory monitoring is not required. The efficacy of LMWH was tested in the ASSENT-3 plus trial, in which 1639 patients with STEMI were randomly assigned to treatment with tenecteplase and either: (1) intravenous bolus of 30 mg enoxaparin followed by 1 mg/kg subcutaneously BID for a maximum of 7 days; or (2) weight-adjusted UFH for 48 hours. The results showed that enoxaparin tended to reduce the composite of 30-day mortality or in-hospital reinfarction, or in-hospital refractory ischemia to 14.2% vs. 17.4% for UFH ($P = 0.080$). However, there were increases in total stroke (2.9% vs. 1.3%, $P = 0.026$) and intracranial hemorrhage (2.20% vs. 0.97%, $P = 0.047$) seen in patients >75 years of age [16]. Since then, a new trial testing LMWH in STEMI is being conducted. As part of this new trial, reduced doses of enoxaparin were given to elderly patients to determine whether a more carefully defined dose of enoxaparin can maintain the thrombolytic results while avoiding the excess bleeding.

Evidence-based Medicine: The EXTRACT-TIMI 25 trial

In the Enoxaparin and Thrombolysis Reperfusion for Acute Myocardial Infarction-Study TIMI 25 trial, 20,506 patients with STEMI, who were scheduled to undergo fibrinolysis, received enoxaparin throughout the index hospitalization or UFH for at least 48 hours. At 30 days, the results showed that the primary efficacy end point (death or non-fatal recurrent MI) occurred in 12% of patients in the UFH group and 9.9% of those in the enoxaparin group (17% reduction in relative risk, $P < 0.001$). Non-fatal reinfarction occurred in 4.5% of the patients receiving UFH and 3% of those receiving enoxaparin (33% reduction in relative risk, $P < 0.001$); 7.5% of patients given UFH died, as did 6.9% of those given enoxaparin ($P = 0.11$). The composite of death, non-fatal reinfarction, or urgent revascularization occurred in 14.5% of patients given UFH and 11.7% of those given enoxaparin ($P < 0.001$); major bleeding occurred in 1.4% and 2.1%, respectively ($P < 0.001$). The composite of death, non-fatal reinfarction, or non-fatal intracranial hemorrhage (a measure of net clinical benefit) occurred in 12.2% of patients given UFH and 10.1% of those given enoxaparin ($P < 0.001$) [17].

Direct Thrombin Inhibitor

In a meta-analysis of patients with STEMI in the Direct Thrombin Inhibitor Trialists' collaboration, direct thrombin inhibitors (DTIs) were found to reduce the rate of reinfarction at 30 days (3.9% vs. 4.8% with UFH, $P < 0.001$), but did not reduce mortality (9.1% vs. 9.0%, $P = 0.68$) or the combined incidence of death/reinfarction at 30 days (11.8% vs. 12.4, $P = 0.18$) [18]. DTIs are not given for STEMI.

Factor X Inhibitor

Fondaparinux, a synthetic pentasaccharide, is a factor Xa inhibitor that selectively binds antithrombin and rapidly inhibits factor Xa. The Organization for the Assessment of Strategies for Ischemic Syndromes (OASIS)-5 trial reported superior efficacy of fondaparinux compared with enoxaparin in preventing ischemic events in ACS patients, with a large reduction in bleeding [19]. This resulted in significant reductions in mortality, MI, and strokes at 3–6 months. The OASIS-6 trial evaluated the impact of fondaparinux in STEMI patients in preventing the primary and composite outcome of death or reinfarction at 30 days.

EMERGING TREND

The OASIS 6 trial 12,092 patients with STEMI were randomized in a double-blind comparison of fondaparinux 2.5 mg once daily, or control. The results showed that the rates of death or reinfarction at 30 days was significantly reduced from 11.2% in the control group to 9.7% in the fondaparinux group ($P = 0.008$); mortality was significantly reduced throughout the study. However, there was no benefit in those undergoing PCI (7% vs. 6% mortality in both groups). Significant benefits were observed in those receiving TT (HR (hazard ratio), 0.79; $P = 0.003$) and those not receiving any reperfusion therapy (HR, 0.80; $P = 0.03$). There was a tendency to fewer severe bleeds and tamponade with fondaparinux at 9 days. How can the data to be applied in the US when the majority of STEMI patients go for PCI? According to this study, fondaparinux did not provide any advantage to them [20].

β-Blockers

Systemic review of RCTs of β-blockers in STEMI has found that β-blockers given within hours of infarction reduce both mortality and reinfarction. β-blockers may reduce the rates of cardiac rupture and ventricular fibrillation. This may explain why people older than 65 years of age and those with large infarcts benefit the most, as they also have higher rate of complications. In patients with moderate heart failure (NYHA class II or III), β-blockers were found to decrease re-admission, mortality and sudden death [21]. The benefits of β-blockers was evidenced in patients with STEMI after TT or before PCI. However, in the CADILLAC trial, β-blockers were beneficial to the patients who were not on prior β-blocker therapy [22]. The optimal dose of β-blockers used in RCTs are listed in Table 2.7.

Evidence-based Medicine: The CAPRICORN trial

In the Carvedilol Post-Infarct Survival Control in Left Ventricular Dysfunction Study, 1959 patients with an acute MI and an LV ejection fraction (EF) ≤ 0.40– were enrolled and treated with a maximum dose of 25 mg carvedilol bid. The results showed that the all-cause mortality alone was lower in the carvedilol group than in the placebo group (12% vs. 15%; $P = 0.03$). Cardiovascular mortality, non-fatal MIs, and all-cause mortality or non-fatal MI were also lower on carvedilol + ACEI than on placebo [23].

Angiotensin Converting Enzyme Inhibitors

The benefits of counteracting the mechanism of dilatory LV remodeling by inhibition of the angiotensin converting enzyme (ACE) are well evidenced in many trials of patients with chronic heart failure. Applying the same strategy to patients with STEMI receiving TT, a meta-analysis of the FAMIS, CPTIN and CATS trials showed the beneficial effect of ACE inhibitors (ACEI) on LV dilation for patient with failed TT without any improvement in mortality.

Evidence-based Medicine: Meta-analysis of ACEI on LV dilation after MI

The data on 845 patients with three-month echocardiographic follow-up after MI were combined from three randomized, double-blind, placebo-controlled studies. The criteria for these studies included: (1) TT; (2) ACE inhibition within 6–9 hours; and (3) evaluation of LV dilation as the primary objective. The results showed that after 3 months, LV dilation was not significantly attenuated by very early treatment with ACEI. The diastolic volume index was attenuated by 0.5 mL/m^2 (95% CI: 1.5–2.5; $P = 0.61$), and the systolic volume index by 0.5 mL/m^2 (95% CI: 1.0–1.9; $P = 0.50$). Subgroup analysis demonstrated that LV dilation was significantly attenuated by ACEI treatment for patients in whom reperfusion failed. In contrast, LV dilation was almost unaffected by ACEI treatment in successfully reperfused patients.

The attenuation of LV dilation in patients receiving TT by ACEI treatment within 6–9 h after MI could not be demonstrated. Very early treatment with an ACEI only has a beneficial effect on LV remodeling for patients in whom reperfusion failed. Other mechanisms may be responsible for the beneficial effects of ACEI in successfully reperfused patients after MI [24].

Angiotensin II Receptor Blockers

Angiotensin II receptor blockers (ARB) are a new blocker acting on the angiotensin receptor. It has been tried on patients with chronic congestive heart failure (CHF). In the Losartan Heart Failure Survival Study (ELITE) II trial [25], the results showed that losartan caused fewer side effects than captopril, but losartan was not superior in reducing morbidity and mortality. In order to clarify these beneficial effects, ARBs were compared with ACEI in patients with STEMI complicated by LV dysfunction.

Evidence-based Medicine: The VALIANT trial

In the Valsartan in Acute Myocardial Infarction Trial, 14,703 patients were randomized for captopril, valsartan, or their combination. The results showed that the number of individuals adjudicated as having a fatal or non-fatal MI in the captopril group was 559 (total investigator reported events 798), 587 (796) in the valsartan group, and 554 (756) in the combination group; valsartan vs. captopril, $P = 0.651$ (0.965); combination vs. captopril, $P = 0.187$ (0.350). Overall, all atherosclerotic events examined occurred at a similar frequency in the captopril and valsartan groups [26].

Since then, the guidelines allowed the use of ARBs for LV dysfunction after MI in case of intolerance of ACEI [3]. However, the concrete evidence for correcting or preventing heart failure is by reversing the dilated LV size (or LV remodeling). It was proved after β-blockers, ACEI or ARB or any modality of treatment for MI (PCI or stem cell infusion). Between ACEI and ARB, which one showed concrete shrinking of the LV in patient with STEMI receiving ACEI or ARB?

CRITICAL THINKING

Which is better at reversing LV remodeling – ARB or ACEI? In a small study of Onodera *et al.* with 203 patients treated with either ARB or ACEI after PCI for AMI, the results showed that the changes in LV end-diastolic index (18 ± 25 vs. 8 ± 24 mL/m^2) and LV end-systolic volume index (10 ± 20 vs. 2 ± 18 mL/m^2) from acute phase to 6 months and the EF, were significantly better in the enalapril group than in the losartan group. This indicates that enalapril suppresses ventricular remodeling after AMI more effectively than losartan [27]. Can these results withstand the test of time and large RCTs?

Lipid Lowering Drugs

Statin therapy is known to decrease mortality in patients with stable angina, ACS or prior MI. RCTs with statin were conducted in order to clarify the benefits of statins on patients in the acute phase of STEMI.

Evidence-based Medicine: The National Registry of Myocardial Infarction 4 analysis

Data were collected on 300,823 patients who had AMI in the National Registry of Myocardial Infarction 4. In-hospital events were compared between patients who continued statin therapy received before the index AMI hospitalization ($n = 17,118$), or newly started statin therapy within the first 24 hours of hospitalization ($n = 21,978$), and patients who did not receive early statin treatment ($n = 126,128$) or whose statin therapy was discontinued ($n = 9,411$). New or continued treatment with a statin in the first 24 hours was associated with a decreased risk of mortality compared with no statin use (4.0% and 5.3% compared with 15.4% no statin, respectively). Discontinuation of statin treatment was associated with a slightly increased risk of mortality (16.5%). Early statin use was also associated with a lower incidence of cardiogenic shock, arrhythmias, cardiac arrest, rupture, but not recurrent MI [28].

With the results of analysis of data from the National Registry of Myocardial Infarction 4, the use of statin therapy within the first 24 hours of hospitalization for AMI was suggested because it is associated with a significantly lower rate of early complications and in-hospital mortality.

Comprehensive Management

In the assessment of quality care, identification of factors associated with failure to use proven treatments, including in high-risk groups that would derive particular benefit from effective therapies, provides an opportunity to focus on quality-improvement interventions [29]. Applying that principle, hospitals are under increasing pressure to measure and improve quality of care, and to implement evidence-proven modalities of therapy. The success depends on organizational support for quality-improvement efforts and physician leadership.

For patients with STEMI, the comprehensive management requires early administration of oral or intravenous antiplatelet agents, early β-blockade, early medical or mechanical reperfusion, ACE inhibition (if there is LV dysfunction), early cardiac rehabilitation, stop-smoking teaching and AMI-prevention teaching to patients and family. In real life, besides the above measures, the comprehensive management of STEMI patients requires: (1) the prescription of same dose of benefit-proven drug as used in randomized clinical trial; (2) explanation of the absolute- or relative-necessity of a particular drug or modality of treatment to improve compliance. The optimal dosage as used in RCTs are listed in Table 2.7.

Table 2.7 Optimal dosage of medications in randomized clinical trials.

Drug	First dose	Maximal dose	RCT
Carvedilol	3.125 mg po bid	25 mg po bid	CAPRICORN [23]
Atenolol	25 mg po bid	200 mg po qd	ISIS-1 [30]
	5 mg IV	10 mg IV	
Metoprolol tartrate	up to 15 mg IV	200 mg po qd	COMMIT [31]
Valsartan	20 mg po bid	160 mg po bid	VALIANT [26]
Captopril	6.25 mg po tid	50 mg po tid	VALIANT [26]
Lisinopril	2.5 mg po qd	5–10 mg po qd	Meta-analysis [24]
Ramipril	1.25 mg po bid	5 mg po bid	AIRE [32]
Trandolapril	1 mg po qd	4 mg po qd	TRACE [33]

Table 2.8 Performance indicators of comprehensive care for ST elevation myocardial infarction patients.

Indicator	Average US Hospital	
	Benchmark	(4th quarter of 2005)
ASA administration within 24 hours after arrival	94.45%	95.65%
ASA prescribed at discharge (if no contra-indications)	95%	82.5%
β-blocker administration within 24 hours after arrival	90.86%	77.78%
β-blocker prescribed at discharge	94%	81.92%
Documentation of LDL in patient record	%	%
Patients with high LDL-c are prescribed drug at discharge	%	%
ACEI or ARB prescribed at discharge in patients with EF < 40%	83%	66.67%
Door-to-needle time (for TT) <30 mins	36.41%	%
Door-to-balloon time <90 mins	64.33%	33.33%
Reperfusion therapy for STEMI	%	%
Adult smokers receive smoking cessation advice and counseling	88.74%	100%
AMI mortality	7.34%	6.9%

ACEI, ACE inhibitors; AMI, acute MI; ARB, angiotensin II receptor blockers; EF, ejection fraction; LDL, low density lipoprotein; LDL-c, low density lipoprotein cholestrol; STEMI, ST elevation myocardial infarction; TT, thrombolytic therapy.

In order to evaluate the completeness in the management of the patients with STEMI, a checklist for excellent performance indicators is shown in Table 2.8. All the benchmarks are set by the Center of Medicare and Medicaid Services.

Difficult Situations and Suggested Solutions

Real World Question What to Do After Failed Thrombolysis?

Despite the beneficial effects of TT, unfortunately less than 33% of AMI patients are candidates for this treatment. Once the drug is infused, less than 50% of the IRAs have TIMI grade 3 flow, which is decisive for lowering mortality. Then, more than one third of these just-opened arteries with high grade residual obstructive lesion are prone, and in fact many were observed, to be reoccluded (silently) over time [34]. The reason is that the current fibrinolytic agents are mainly effective in dissolving the fibrin network of an occlusive clot without dismantling the platelet-rich core. They cannot reverse the ongoing process of platelet aggregation, which in turn sustains the fibrin complicity of an ultimately occlusive clot. They have no effect on thrombin, which is the most potent activator of platelets. Their lytic effects are blocked by platelet activator inhibitor I (PAI-I), which is an inhibitor of fibrinolysis [6], and of which high level predicts future reocclusion. The accurate identification of patient who fails TT is limited. The clinical markers of reperfusion, such as relief of chest pain, partial resolution of ST-segment elevation, and reperfusion arrhythmias, have limited predictive value [35]. The appropriate treatment for patients in whom reperfusion fails to occur after TT for STEMI remains unclear. The advantages and disadvantages of each modality – rescue PCI, repeat TT or conservative treatment – were evaluated in the REACT trial described below.

Evidence-based Medicine: The REACT trial

In the Rescue Angioplasty after Failed TT for AMI (REACT) trial, 427 patients with STEMI in whom reperfusion failed to occur (less than 50% ST-segment resolution) within 90 minutes after TT, were randomly assigned to repeated TT (142 patients), conservative treatment (141 patients), or rescue PCI (144 patients). The results showed that the rate of event-free survival among patients treated with rescue PCI was 84.6%, as compared with 70.1% among those receiving conservative therapy and 68.7% among those undergoing repeated TT (overall $P = 0.004$). There were no significant differences in mortality from all causes [36].

According to the results of the REACT trial, repeat PCI is the best strategy. High level of suspicion for failed TT is needed. Prompt transfer for PCI is strongly suggested. There was no difference in mortality between the three strategies because the window of myocardial salvage and decreased mortality has passed. However, with PCI, the patients has less morbidity (open artery is better than a closed artery).

Real World Question Who Should Stay for TT or be Transferred for PCI?

The technical success rate of stenting after STEMI has been remarkably high while the procedural complication rate was extremely low, even when more high risk patients were included. In the large National Registry of Myocardial Infarction 2 and 3 Investigators (NRMI 2 and 3) registry of more than 300,000 patients, the result of PCI was excellent if performed by experienced operators in high volume interventional laboratories, while there was no difference in mortality between TT or mechanical interventions in low-volume hospitals [37]. As more patients with STEMI prefer mechanical interventions, the problem now is the availability of this modality of treatment. Only 20% of US hospitals have cardiac catheterization laboratories and even less have the capability of performing emergency PCI. Although transfer of the MI patient to a facility that can perform PCI is possible, 87% of transferred patients had more than 2 hours delay which may theoretically outweigh any added benefit. In the case of PCI performed in hospitals without on-site surgical capability, the results from the Atlantic Cardiovascular Patient Outcomes Research Team (C-PORT) trial of primary PCI vs. thombolysis in STEMI trials showed that the transferred patients had better outcome than the patients who received TT locally [38]. An excellent mortality result is dependent on short door-to-balloon time, optimally less than 90 minutes, which is not attainable in every US cardiac catheterization laboratory.

CRITICAL THINKING

Was long door-to-balloon time detrimental for everybody? 2322 consecutive patients treated with primary PCI were prospectively identified and followed up for a median of 83 months. The results showed that prolonged door-to-balloon times (0–1.4 hours vs. 1.5–1.9 hours vs. 2.0–2.9 hours vs. ⩾3.0 hours) were associated with higher in-hospital mortality (4.9% vs. 6.1% vs. 8.0% vs. 12.2; $P < 0.0001$) and late mortality (12.6% vs. 16.4% vs. 20.4% vs. 27.1% at 7 years; $P < 0.0001$) and were an independent predictor of late mortality by Cox regression ($P = 0.0004$). Prolonged door-to-balloon times (⩾2 hours vs. <2 hours) were associated with higher late mortality in high-risk patients (32.5% vs. 21.5%; $P = 0.0002$) but not in low-risk patients (10.8% vs. 9.2%; $P = 0.53$) and in patients presenting early (less than 3 hours, 24.7% vs. 15.0%; $P = 0.0001$) but not in late presentation (>3 hours, 21.1% vs. 18.5%; $P = 0.80$) [39].

CLINICAL PEARLS

Who will benefit the most, or not benefit, from an expediate PCI? The patients who need an expedited process for PCI are the ones with high risks and with short interval from symptom onset to presentation. The physicians can make a difference in mortality of these patients by focusing on, and making a real effort to shorten, the door-to-balloon time. While the patients with low risk and long interval between symptom onset to presentation also need to have a short door-to-balloon time, they do not benefit from an expedited PCI because the window of myocardial salvage is passed or the MI is too small to be benefited from invasive interventions. To understand this is to rationalize the fairness in triage and to give priority to patient who should receive PCI first, or be transferred first when two patients arrive at the same time, in the same ER, or are transferred at the same time from different hospitals.

Real World Question How to Shorten Door-To-Balloon Time in Transferred Patients?

Because time is myocardium, a rapid plan must be determined and implemented upon recognizing a patient with STEMI who needs rapid transfer [40]. Besides strong involvement of the medical and administrative team, there is a problem with logistics. The transport system requires significant individualization based on hospital location and transport availability. Variables include distance between two hospitals, availability of ambulance and helicopters, weather and road conditions. Each hospital should develop a preferred system for transport with specific backup for weather and availability issues [39]. The patient should be transferred directly to the cardiac catheterization laboratories. The ER of the receiving hospital is used for back-up in case of emergencies such as two simultaneous patients with MI arriving at the same time. The cardiac catherterization laboratory (CCL) team and the interventional cardiologist should be waiting for the patient in the CCL. The goal is CCL-arrival-to-balloon time is < 15 minutes. Education of the health care providers involved in all levels of the transfer process is crucial for a successful D2B program [40].

CRITICAL THINKING

How to trigger the transfer process with one phone call? A standardized protocol is a critical factor in the initial evaluation and treatment of STEMI arriving at the ER. An algorithm is used to facilitate a smooth and quick transfer process [40]. In the transfer protocol, it takes only *one* phone call to activate the emergency team alerting the arrival of a STEMI patient (emergency MD, laboratories), *one* phone call to dispatch the transport team (helicopter or ground ambulance), *one* phone call to contact the tertiary hospital for a bed and then transfer the patients with a goal of in–out-door time less than 30 minutes [41].

Real World Question How to Perform PCI in Patients with STEMI and Complex Bleeding and Thrombotic Problems?

Bleeding or intra-arterial thrombosis before, during, or after PCI of STEMI could be a major (or possibly fatal) problem triggering a small- to full-scale crisis situation. Different problems and solutions with bleeding or thrombosis are discussed below.

STEMI in >400 lb patients

The problem is that there are no tables in the cardiac catheterization laboratories which can tolerate a weight >400 lbs. While using TT there are no guidelines for dosage because in the RCTs all overweight patients were excluded.

CRITICAL THINKING

PCI in patients with current bleeding. In general, the principle is if the bleeding can be stopped by mechanical means (compressing or ligating the artery), then the patient could tolerate 4 hours of anticoagulant during PCI. The favorite anticoagulant is UFH owing to its short half life, and because it can be reversed by protamine.

Patients with bleeding

If the patient has gastric bleeding and is hemodynamically stable, a gastroenterologist could do a gastroscope and stop the bleeding by stapling the culprit artery. After that, the patient can be treated with H2 antagonist and should tolerate short term anticoagulant and oral antiplatelet (Clopidogrel and ASA) for stenting of the IRA. GP 2b3a inhibitors are to be avoided. If the patient has fracture in the extremities and AMI at the same time, the orthopedic surgeons may put splints and stabilize the extremities. Then the patient may undergo the diagnostic coronary angiogram and bilateral femoral angiogram to check extravasion of contrast due to injury in the arterial system. If there is no arterial bleed in the extremities, the patient could undergo PCI of the IRA under coverage with low dose UFH (5000 U) and clopidogrel. At this present time, intracranial, bleedings, or bleeding from the esophageal varices are the real contraindications for PCI for AMI.

AMI in patients following recent surgery

Less than 4 hours after removal of the right kidney because of cancer, a patient developed ST elevation in leads 2,3 AVF. So the patient was brought to the CCL, had balloon angioplasty of the RCA with standard dose of heparin, and an ACT of 250–300 seconds. No stent was used and no heparin given after the procedure. Because of the short term of heparin use, not much bleeding in the surgical area was noted and no there was no impact on the surgical results. If the patient has a clean and limited surgery, then they can undergo DES stenting because there is no problem with long-term antiplatelet therapy with ASA and clopidogrel.

AMI in patients with concurrent stroke

If the patient has ischemic stroke, then with the agreement of the neurologist consultant, the patient could be given short term anticoagulant (UFH or DTI) and long term oral antiplatelet drug. Then the patient could undergo PCI and stenting. The two concerns are: (1) the risk of hemorrhagic conversion of the ischemic stroke with anticoagulant therapy; and (2) risk of cerebral emboli from the protruding plaques in the aortic arch if they were the cause of emboli stroke in the first place. The patient needs to have strong indication for PCI and the family and patient need to understand the benefits and the risks. If the benefits outweigh the risks, then the patient should have PCI.

PCI for patients with STEMI right after coronary artery bypass surgery

Sometimes, shortly after returning from the operating room (OR) after coronary artery bypass (CABG), the patient was found to have ST segment elevation in one of the areas just bypassed. There is strong suspicion of acute occlusion of one of the bypass grafts. The patient could be brought back to the OR to recheck the patency of the bypass grafts, or the patient could go to the CCL for emergency angiography. If there is a need for PCI, a full dose of UFH could be given. The reason is that during CABG surgery, with the chest open, the patient was fully heparinized without extra bleeding. After the chest was closed, anticoagulation was reversed with protamine. Now, when there is a need for short term anticoagulant therapy during PCI, the patient could tolerate, without problem, DES stenting with subsequent clopidogrel therapy. The risk of returning to the OR is higher due to bleeding caused by clopidogrel.

STEMI in patients with atrial fibrillation on coumadin, INR >2

Because coumadin does not have any effect on platelet, so patients with therapeutic level of international normalized ratio (INR) still have STEMI. During PCI, the patient can be given oral loading and maintenance dose of antiplatet drug as usual. If the patient has high INR, no UFH is needed. If the INR is less than 2, then patient can be given UFH (as in the treatment of pulmonary embolism).

STEMI in patients with heparin induced thrombocytopenia

Heparin-induced thrombocytopenia (HIT) is an immune-mediated complication of heparin. It involves a decrease in circulating platelets (thrombocytopenia) and an increased tendency to form blood clots, which can have devastating clinical consequences such as limb ischemia requiring amputation (10–20%), MI, stroke, pulmonary embolism and even death (20–30%). In patients with HIT, LMWH cannot be used because they have cross-reactivity. Either bivalirudin or argatroban should be used during PCI [3]. However, there is a problem with argatroban administration. In a report of Reichert with four patients receiving argatroban; even after argatroban was initiated at the recommended starting dose of 2 μg/kg/min or at a lower dose, 1 μg/kg/min. All patients had relatively normal hepatic function. The resulting activated partial thromboplastin time was super-therapeutic and exceeded 100 seconds in three patients. Additionally, argatroban clearance appeared to be prolonged upon discontinuation [42].

How to perform PCI in patients with hemophilia

Hemophilia B is a severe inherited coagulopathy caused by mutations in the gene that encodes factor IX. Surgical and invasive procedures in patients suffering from this congenital disease are to be considered as being at high risk of hemorrhage. Regularly, the patient with hemophilia was administered recombinant factor VIII pre- and post-procedure to maintain activity levels between

60–80% in order to prevent bleeding. Anticoagulation during the PCI procedure for STEMI was maintained with a direct thrombin inhibitor, bivalirudin: a thrombin-specific anticoagulant. There were no complications. Bivalirudin can be safely used in patients with a very high risk of bleeding (hemophilia) undergoing PCI [43].

Real World Question When to Perform PCI After TT?

Previous studies of PCIs performed in the early POBA era, have shown no advantage of immediate intervention compared with delayed intervention, or with a conservative approach after full dose TT for STEMI [43].Then later, combined low-dose TT and immediate PCI as needed was thought to increase the rate of IRA-opening and reduce the need for rescue PCI [34]. With better interventional technique and equipment, the availability of stent, safer anticoagulant- and antiplatelet-drugs, and effective bleeding prevention at the arterial access site, PCI after TT showed less bleeding complications [44]. So the ASSENT 4 trial was conducted to clarify the role of PCI after TT.

CRITICAL THINKING

The ASSENT-4 PCI trial. In the ASSENT-4 trial, thrombolytic agent TNK was given at full dose to STEMI patients who were being referred for primary PCI.The results showed that mortality, recurrent MI, stroke, intracranial hemorrhage, and major bleeding, as well as stent thrombosis, were all significantly increased in patients who had received full-dose TT prior to PCI. The overall 30-day mortality was quite low, just 3.8% for primary PCI; and quite high, 6.0%, for the TT + PCI patients [45].

The implications are quite clear: any patient who is being referred for primary PCI, with an estimated door-to-balloon time of 1–3 hours, should not receive full-dose TT prior to PCI. If the patient receives TT and is stable, the patient should wait for more than 24 hours before going for angiogram and PCI.

Real World Question Is the Management of STEMI in Elderly Patients Different?

Less than one third of elderly STEMI patients present with typical angina. The most common complaint is dyspnea. Others complain of dizziness, vertigo, weakness, confusion, abdominal pain, delirium, or syncope [46]. In the management of STEMI in elderly patients, TT alone showed high mortality and morbidity. However, for the elderly patients in the ASSENT-3 trial, the use of TT with intravenous GPI provides no clear advantage over TT alone, and may adversely affect outcomes [47]. Is primary PCI is the preferred strategy in the treatment of elderly patients with STEMI?

Evidence-based Medicine: The Senior-PAMI trial

In the Senior-PAMI: a multicenter, randomized trial comparing primary PCI to TT, 483 patients aged 70 and above were randomized for primary PCI or TT. At 30 days, for patients aged from 70–80, the mortality rate was 7% for PCI and 11% for TT. The rate of stroke was 1.2–2.2%, ICH was 0% vs. 1.3%, respectively. However, there was no difference in mortality (19% vs. 16%), mortality + CVA + reinfarction (both 22%) in patients aged >80. Therefore the conclusions showed that PCI was superior to TT at reducing combined death, disabling stroke, and reinfarction but not the primary endpoints of death or disabling stroke. The advantage of PCI is to avoid ICH and reduce reinfarction and recurrent ischemia. The results only benefit the 70–80 years of age and not the >80, (from the statistical point of view the >80 years of age has a small sample size: $n = 130$) [48].

Regarding optimal medical therapy with β-blockers, the outcome for the elderly patient was worse if they could not take β-blockers because of contraindications (e.g. chronic obstructive pulmonary disease [COPD]) [49]. However, even when the patient was given ACEI, ARB or both according to the guidelines, was the outcome much better?

CRITICAL THINKING

The VALIANT trial. The Valsartan in Acute Myocardial Infarction Trial randomized 14,703 patients with heart failure and/or LV ejection fraction <40% to receive captopril, valsartan, or both. Mortality and a composite end point, including cardiovascular mortality, readmission for heart failure, reinfarction, stroke, and resuscitated cardiac arrest, were compared for the age groups of <65 ($n = 6988$), 65–74 ($n = 4555$), 75–84 ($n = 2777$), and ≥85 ($n = 383$) years. With increasing age, 3-year mortality almost quadrupled (13.4%, 26.3%, 36.0%, and 52.1%, respectively), composite end-point events more than doubled (25.2%, 41.0%, 52.3%, and 66.8%), and hospital admissions for heart failure almost tripled (12.0%, 23.1%, 31.3%, and 35.4%). Outcomes did not differ between the three study treatments in any age group. Adverse events associated with captopril and valsartan were more common in the elderly and patients receiving combination therapy [50].

So, in the care of elderly patients physicians must recognize that age *per se* does not cause positive or negative outcomes of TT, but rather that it is a marker for underlying pathophysiologic factors and comorbid illnesses that may influence treatment effects [51]. Their outcomes were better when undergoing PCI if they were less than 80 years old. For the patients above 80 years, neither TT nor PCI help them to live longer. TT caused more ICH. Other managements include β-blockers, full antiplatelet drug coverage, ACEI and cholesterol lowering drugs, complete revascularization, meticulous bleeding prevention at the arterial access site and in the gastro-intestinal tract (due to antiplatelet drugs). Even after everything is done according to the guidelines, the outcomes of the elderly patients are still poor.

Real World Question Is the Management of STEMI in Women Still Unsuccessful?

Women with STEMI have higher morbidity and mortality rates than men. When receiving TT they have higher unadjusted rates of mortality compared with men (9.2% vs. 5.4%), reinfarction (6.4% vs. 2.6%), and hemorrhagic stroke (2.0% vs. 0.55%) [52]. One explanation for this is that female patients experience MI at a more advanced age and with more comorbidities. To clarify the role of catheter-based interventions in women, stenting was performed in 227 women in the PAMI trial [53]. The results showed no improvement in mortality or overall adverse events. The mortality of female patients was five times higher than in men (10% vs. 2.4%, respectively). The overall adverse events were doubled, with 21% vs. 10%, respectively. Even with all of the sophisticated technologies and higher operator experiences in this stent era, women with STEMI remain at higher risk of death, reinfarction, and TVR [53].

Real World Question How to Improve the Outcomes of Diabetic Patients with STEMI?

When having STEMI, diabetic patients frequently present with atypical symptoms. Only 77% of these patients complain of chest pain compared with 84% in patients without diabetes. Even when the diabetic patients had recurrent angina prior to acute occlusion, they do not benefit from ischemic preconditioning, which decrease the mortality and LV dysfunction in non-diabetic patients, because the ability to develop collaterals may be impaired. Diabetic patients also complain more of dyspnea, as they incur more acute LV dysfunction compared with non-diabetic patients (26% vs. 13.5%). The in-hospital mortality has been reported to be 8.7% vs. 5.8% for male diabetic and non-diabetic patients respectively; the mortality of female diabetic patients was 24% compared with 13% in female non-diabetic patients [54]. In a prospective study comparing diabetic patients with non-diabetic patients, even when both groups were treated with the same medications (β-blockade, ACE inhibitors, statins) and achieved the same rate of patency after TT, mortality of diabetic patients was still three-times the rate of non-diabetics [55].

CRITICAL THINKING

The CADILLAC trial. Reperfusion success in those with and without diabetes mellitus was determined by measuring myocardial blush grade (MBG) (*n* = 1301) and ST-segment elevation resolution (STR) analysis (*n* = 700) in two substudies of the Controlled Abciximab and Device Investigation to Lower Late Angioplasty Complications trial among patients undergoing primary PCI for AMI. The results showed no differences between those with or without diabetes with regard to postprocedural TIMI flow grade 3 (>95%), distribution of infarct-related artery, and the frequency of stent deployment or abciximab administration. Patients with diabetes mellitus were more likely to have absent myocardial perfusion (MBG 0/1, 56.0% vs. 47.1%, *P* = 0.01) and absent STR (20.3% vs. 8.1%, *P* = 0.002) [56].

Despite similar high rates of TIMI flow grade 3 after primary PCI in patients with and without diabetes, patients with diabetes are more likely to have abnormal myocardial perfusion as assessed by both incomplete STR and reduced MBG. Diminished microvascular perfusion in diabetics after primary PCI may contribute to adverse outcomes [56].

Real World Question What is the Best Strategy for Patients with Reinfarction?

In patients with STEMI, after the IRA is opened by reperfusion therapy, reocclusion of the IRA increased the rate of death, LV dysfunction or clinical CHF. The incidence of reinfarction after TT was 4%. It is hard to predict which patient will reinfarct after TT. Once there is reinfarction, the three available options are: readministration of TT, PCI or conservative treatment [57].

Evidence-based Medicine: The TIMI data

20,101 patients were enrolled in the Thrombolysis In Myocardial Infarction (TIMI) 4, 9, and 10 B and Intravenous nPA for the Treatment of Infarcting Myocardium Early (InTIME-II) acute MI trials. Recurrent MI during the index hospital period was associated with increased 30-day mortality (16.4% vs. 6.2%, $P < 0.001$). Likewise, recurrent MI was associated with a sustained increase in mortality up to two years, even after adjustments were made for covariates known to be associated with mortality and recurrent MI (hazard ratio 2.11, $P < 0.001$). However, this higher mortality at 2 years was due to an early divergence in mortality by 30 days and was not due to a significant increase in late mortality between 30 days and 2 years (4.38% vs. 3.76%, P = NS) [58].

So in practice, for the patient with reinfarction after STEMI, PCI is the best choice. PCI during the index hospitalization was associated with a lower rate of in-hospital recurrent MI (1.6% vs. 4.5%, p < 0.001) and lower two-year mortality (5.6% vs. 11.6%, p < 0.001) [58].

Real World Question How to Improve the Prognosis of STEMI Patients with Renal Dysfunction?

Renal impairment is a strong independent indicator of increased mortality in patients who are admitted with STEMI. In patients with mild or moderate renal dysfunction and having primary interventions, the early or late outcome depends on the creatinine clearance (less than 75 mL/min) and not on the serum creatinine level [59]. The patients with creatinine clearance <75 mL/min, have more hypotension in the catheterization laboratories (10% vs. 6.5%), intubation (1.3% vs. 0%), in-hospital mortality (5.1% vs. 0.8%), or 6-month mortality 7.4% vs. 1.1%. However, the overall mortality in STEMI patients on long-term dialysis was much worse at 59% in 1 year, 73% in 2 years, and 89% in 5 years [60].

CLINICAL PEARLS

Diagnosis of fluid overload and ischemia in ESRD patients The patient with end-stage renal disease (ESRD) used to present with atypical symptoms and the non-specific ST-T changes of LV hypertrophy can make the diagnosis of STEMI more difficult. Among dialysis patients who experience one day of increased volume stress after a long weekend interval between dialysis sessions, the volume overload associated with elevation of LV diastolic pressure may produce anginal symptoms or shortness of breath. Thus symptoms of ischemia, particularly on a monday morning or after eating a large meal, may be indistinguished from symptoms of volume overload [61]. In this immediate peri-infarction period, echocardiography can provide useful information about the LV, RV systolic function and volume status. Non-invasive measurement of the right atrial pressure can be estimated through information from the inferior vena cava [62]. Dialysis is better deferred in the first 24 hours of STEMI, unless dictated by acute metabolic derangement or volume overload. PCI can be performed with low-osmolar contrast agents in order to decrease acute volume stress. Modification of dialysis runs may be required in low-output states [61].

Real World Question How to Prevent Slow Flow in PCI for Lesions with Heavy Thrombotic Burden?

Small red thrombi are frequently seen by the angioscope before intervention and after stenting or rotoblation. Massive thrombus is more often seen when the culprit lesion is in the right coronary artery and in patients who present late to the ER. The presence of a moderate size thrombus is not considered a contraindication for primary stenting, however, vessels with huge thrombi were excluded from randomization in stent trials. When an angiographic filling defect consistent with the presence of a thrombus after stenting is observed, repeat balloon dilatation with higher pressure should be tried first, since the most powerful antithrombotic maneuver is to maintain a brisk non-turbulent flow inside the stented lumen. If a large thrombus persists, even after repeating balloon dilatation, mechanical thrombectomy with the Angiojet catheter (Possis Medical, Inc., Minneapolis, MN) or TEC atherectomy (aspiration without turning on the cutter) or a transport catheter with large lumen (the Pronto catheter) have been found to be effective in removing thrombus from native arteries [63] and to improve the IRA flow as measured by the corrected frame count.

Management of distal microembolization can be evidenced by distal filling defect with an abrupt cut-off in any of the peripheral branches of the IRA. The use of distal protection devices which can filter or trap embolic debris offsets the delay in perfusion on the recovery of angiographic parameters in primary interventions. By reversing the detrimental effects of microemboli and vaso-constricting factors in the distal vasculature, the use of distal protection devices may keep the microvascular flow open.

CRITICAL THINKING

The EMERALD trial. The Enhanced Myocardial Efficacy and Recovery by Aspiration of Liberated Debris trial is a prospective randomized controlled trial which enrolled 501 patients with STEMI undergoing primary PCI or rescue intervention after failed thrombolysis. Patients were randomized to receive PCI with a balloon occlusion and aspiration distal microcirculatory protection system vs. angioplasty without distal protection. The results showed that among 252 patients assigned to distal protection, aspiration was performed in 97%, all angioplasty balloon inflations were fully protected in 79%, and visible debris was retrieved from 73%. Complete ST segment resolution was achieved in a similar proportion reperfused with vs. without distal protection (63.3% vs. 61.9%, respectively; absolute difference, 1.4% ($P = 0.78$), and LV infarct size was similar in both groups (median, 12.0% vs. 9.5%, respectively; $P = 0.15$). Major adverse cardiac events at 6 months occurred with similar frequency in the distal protection and control groups (10.0% vs. 11.0%, respectively; $P = 0.66$). A distal balloon occlusion and aspiration system effectively retrieves embolic debris in most patients with acute STEMI undergoing emergent PCI without resulting in improved microvascular flow, greater reperfusion success, reduced infarct size, or enhanced event-free survival [64].

As the EMERALD trial failed to prove the benefit of distal protection devices in *all* STEMI patients with or without visible thrombi, common sense and good medical judgement dictates distal protection and thrombectomy in patients with large thrombotic burden, in order to prevent slow flow and maintain good myocardial perfusion.

Real World Question Should We Perform PCI in the Non-IRA in STEMI Patients with Multivessel Disease?

If the patients have lesions in other arteries besides the IRA, intervention in the non-IRA is not indicated. It should be planned on a later date. However, if the patient is still symptomatic or unstable, the intervention of the non-IRA should be carried out probably under the protection of an intra-aortic balloon pump (IABP), if needed. The ACC/AHA/SCAI guidelines suggest no PCI of the non-IRA, however, the meta-analysis of New York state showed a different result.

CRITICAL THINKING

The Multivessel Disease PCI of the New York State Angioplasty Registry Analysis. In a retrospective study of multi-vessel disease (MVD) PCI using the 2000–2001 New York State Angioplasty Registry database, the in-hospital clinical outcomes of patients with multi-vessel disease (>70% stenosis in at least two major coronary arteries), who underwent either multi-vessel angioplasty ($n = 632$) or infarct-related vessel angioplasty ($n = 1350$) within 24 hours of AMI were compared. The results showed that the patients in the multi-vessel angioplasty group were less likely to be female, to have peripheral vascular disease or diabetes. They had more complex lesions and were more likely to receive stents. In-hospital mortality was three-fold lower (0.8% in the multi-vessel angioplasty group vs. 2.3%, (P = 0.018) in the IRA-only angioplasty group. No differences were observed in other ischemic complications, renal failure, or length of stay. After multivariate analysis, multi-vessel angioplasty remained a significant predictor of lower in-hospital death (OR = 0.27, 95% CI = 0.08–0.90, P = 0.03) [65].

The latest recommendations of the ACC/AHA guidelines do not support PCI in the non-IRA unless the patient is still symptomatic (chest pain or hypotension) after PCI of the IRA [3]. However, a strategy of PCI of MVD during STEMI may be applied in experienced laboratories [66].

Real World Question Is it Worth Opening the IRA After Symptom Onset of >48 hours?

Is there a place for the late opening of the IRA, beyond the 12-hour window for myocardial salvage? The rationale included the prevention of infarct expansion and ventricular remodeling leading to ventricular dilatation, the provision of electrophysiologic stability lessening the likelihood of malignant ventricular arrhythmias, and the ability of collaterals emanating from the recanalized artery to perfuse the ischemic, but still viable, myocardium [67]. There were also reasons that late reperfusion might be harmful, including the risk of inducing myocardial stunning, microvascular damage, and intramyocardial hemorrhage leading to an increased likelihood of myocardial rupture. However, in reality, is the patency of the late opened IRA translated into better mortality and morbidity?

CRITICAL THINKING

The TAMI-6 trial. The Thrombolysis and Angioplasty in Myocardial Infarction-6 Study Group randomized 197 patients within 6–24 hours of symptom onset, to t-PAs or placebo. Coronary angiography within 24 hours was used to determine IRA patency status. Patients with infarct-related occluded arteries were then eligible for a second randomization to either angioplasty (n = 34) or no angioplasty (n = 37). The results showed that the primary end point, infarct vessel patency, was 65% for t-PA patients compared with 27% in the placebo group (P < 0.0001). There were no differences between these groups in ejection fraction or infarct zone regional wall motion at 1 or 6 months. At 6 months, infarct vessel patency was 59% in both groups. In the placebo group there was a significant increase in end-diastolic volume, from acute phase of 127 mL to 159 mL at 6-month follow-up (P = 0.006) but no increase in cavity size for the t-PA group patients. Coronary angioplasty was associated with an initial 81% recanalization success and improved ventricular function at 1 month, but by late follow-up no advantage could be demonstrated for this procedure, and there was a 38% spontaneous recanalization rate in the patients assigned to no angioplasty [68].

The same negative results were confirmed again in the Open Artery (OAT) trial where patients underwent stenting 3 weeks after the index MI [69]. There were no reduced rates of death, reinfarction, or heart failure compared with optimal medical therapy in ASYMPTOMATIC myocardial infarction survivors who do not receive PCI within the first 12 hours.

Take Home Message

Based on worldwide availability of facilities, logistics, and resource affordability (especially in developing countries), the benchmark reperfusion strategy remains TT. However, given the availability of catheterization laboratories, interventional expertise, rapid restoration of patency by catheter-based reperfusion can result in excellent outcomes. This is certainly the case in institutions with large volume interventional laboratories and experienced operators [70].

Because of the universal access to TT, certain clinical issues must be underscored. More important than pursuing the ideal thrombolytic agent is the need to administer TT at the earliest possible juncture after the onset of symptoms heralding MI. It is important to use those agents that the practitioner knows best. The earliest administration of any agent is better than the delayed administration of the best agent.

Primary mechanical intervention is an emergency procedure that may reduce mortality, reinfarction, and stroke as primary objectives, and prevention of recurrent ischemia and early discharge as secondary objectives. If experienced operators are available and if the interval between door and balloon is less than 120 minutes, it is suggested that the patients undergo primary intervention. Early subacute stent thrombosis still needs to be monitored, especially in patients with initial TIMI-0 to TIMI-1 flow. Adjunctive therapies, especially ACEI, β-blockers, and statins are needed to improve short- and long-term outcomes. In addition to the clinical indications, accessibility and costs are obviously relevant variables to be taken into account. The choice of any reperfusion strategy is therefore not only related to scientific rationale, but also depends on affordability of available resources.

References

1 Gibson CM. The time dependent open vascular hypothesis. Cardiol Rounds 2000;4:10.
2 King SB. Acute myocardial infarction: Are diabetics different? J Am Coll Cardiol 2000;35:1513–1515.
3 Smith SS et al. ACC/AHA/SCAI 2005 Guideline update for percutaneous coronary intervention. Cath and Cardiovasc Intervent 2006;67:87–112.
4 Lee K, Woodlief LH, Topol E et al. for the GUSTO-I investigator Predictor of 30-day mortality inthe era of reperfusion for AMI. Circulation 1995;91:1659–1668.
5 Crimm A, Severance HW, Coffey K et al. Prognostic significance of isolated sinus tachycardia during the first three days of AMI. Am J Med 1984;73:983–988.

6 Califf R, Gibler WB, Gibson M *et al*. Myocardial reperfusion:New strategies for the new century. Clinician 2000;18:4–23.

7 Antman EM, Anbe DT, Armstrong PW *et al*. ACC/AHA guidelines for the management of patients with ST-elevation myocardial infarction: A report of the American College of Cardiology/American Heart Association Task Force on Practice Guidelines (Committee to Revise the 1999 Guidelines for the Management of Patients with Acute Myocardial Infarction). J Am Coll Cardiol 2004;44:E1–E211.

8 Weaver D, Simes J, Betriu A *et al*. Comparison of primary PTCA versus intravenous TT for AMI: A quantative review. JAMA 1997;278:2093–2098.

9 Wharton TP Jr, McNamara NS, Fedele FA *et al*. Primary angioplasty for the treatment of acute myocardial infarction: experience at two community hospitals without cardiac surgery. JACC 1999;33:1257–1265.

10 Spaulding C. Final results of the TYPHOON study, a multi-center randomized trial comparing the use of sirolimus-elutin stents to bare metal stents in primary angioplasty for acute myocardial infarction. Presented at the American College of Cardiology Scientific Session 2006. March 11–14, 2006, Atlanta.

11 Peters RJ, Mehta SR, Fox KA; for the CURE investigators. Effects of aspirin dose when used alone or in combination with clopidogrel in patients with acute coronary syndromes: observations from the Clopidogrel in Unstable angina to prevent Recurrent Events (CURE) study. Circulation 2003;108(14):1682–1687.

12 Sabatine M, Morrow D, Montalescot G *et al*. Clopidogrel as Adjunctive Reperfusion Therapy (CLARITY) TIMI 28 trial. Circulation 2005;112:3846–3854.

13 Montelescot G, Barragan P *et al*. Platelet glycoprotein 2b3a inhibition with coronary stenting for acute myocardial infarction N Engl J Med 2001;344:1895–1903.

14 Tcheng JE, Kandzari DE, Grines CL *et al*. Benefits and risks of abciximab use in primary angioplasty for acute myocardial infarction: The Controlled Abciximab and Device Investigation to Lower Late Angioplasty Complications (CADILLAC) trial. Circulation 2003;108:1316–1323.

15 Personal communication with Cindy Grines.

16 Wallentin L, Goldstein P, Armstrong PW *et al*. Efficacy and safety of tenecteplase in combination with the low-molecular-weight heparin enoxaparin or unfractionated heparin in the prehospital setting: The Assessment of the Safety and Efficacy of a New Thrombolytic Regimen (ASSENT)-3 PLUS randomized trial in acute myocardial infarction. Circulation 2003;108(2):135–142.

17 Antman EM, Morrow DA, McCabe C; and the ExTRACT-TIMI 25 Investigators. Enoxaparin versus Unfractionated Heparin with Fibrinolysis for ST-Elevation Myocardial Infarction. N Engl J Med 2006;354:1477–1488.

18 French JK, Edmond JJ, Gao W, White HD, Eikelboom JW. Adjunctive use of direct thrombin inhibitors in patients receiving fibrinolytic therapy for acute myocardial infarction. Am J Cardiovasc Drugs 2004;4(2):107–115.

19 The Fifth Organization to Assess Strategies in Acute Ischemic Syndromes Investigators Comparison of Fondaparinux and Enoxaparin in Acute Coronary Syndromes. NEJM 2006;354:1464–1476.

20 The OASIS-6 Trial Group. Effects of Fondaparinux on Mortality and Reinfarction in Patients With Acute ST-Segment Elevation Myocardial Infarction: The OASIS-6 Randomized Trial. JAMA 2006;295(13):1519–1530.

21 MERIT-HF study group. Effect of metoprolol CR/XL in chronic heart failure:metoprolol CR/Xl randomized trial in CHF. Lancet 1999;353:2001–2007.

22 Halkin A, Grines CL, Cox DA *et al.* Impact of intravenous beta–blockade before primary angioplasty on survival in patients undergoing mechanical reperfusion therapy for acute myocardial infarction. J Am Coll Cardiol 2004;43(10):1780–1787.

23 Dargie HJ. Effect of carvedilol on outcome after myocardial infarction in patients with left–ventricular dysfunction: The CAPRICORN randomised trial. Lancet 2001;358: 1457– 1458.

24 de Kam PJ, Voors AA, van den Berg MP *et al.*, on behalf of the FAMIS CAPTIN and CATS Investigators Effect of very early angiotensin-converting enzyme inhibition on LV dilation after myocardial infarction in patients receiving thrombolysis Results of a meta-analysis of 845 patients. J Am Coll Cardiol 2000;36:2047–2053.

25 Pitt B, Poole-Wilson PA, Segal R *et al.* Effect of Losartan compared with captopril on mortality inpatients with symptoms of heart failure randomized trial: The Losartan Heart Failure Survival Study ELITE II. Lancet 2000;255:1582–1587.

26 McMurray J, Solomon S, Pieper K *et al.* The Effect of Valsartan, Captopril, or Both on Atherosclerotic Events After Acute Myocardial Infarction An Analysis of the Valsartan in Acute Myocardial Infarction Trial (VALIANT). J Am Coll Cardiol 2006;47:726–733.

27 Onodera H, Matsunaga T, Tamura Y *et al.* Enalapril suppresses ventricular remodeling more effectively than losartan in patients with acute myocardial infarction. Am Heart J 2005;150(4):689.

28 Fonarow GC, Wright RS, Spencer FA *et al.* Effect of statin use within the first 24 hours of admission for acute myocardial infarction on early morbidity and mortality. Am J Cardiol 2005;96(5):611–616.

29 Granger CB, Steg PG, Peterson E, and the GRACE Investigators. Medication performance measures and mortality following acute coronary syndromes. Am J Med 2005;118(8):858–865.

30 First international study of infarct survival (ISIS-1). Randomized trial of intravenous atenolol among 16,027 cases of suspected acute myocardial infarction. Lancet 1986; 2(8498):57–66.

31 Chen ZM, Pan HC, Chen YP, for the COMMIT (ClOpidogrel and Metoprolol in Myocardial Infarction Trial) collaborative group. Early intravenous then oral metoprolol in 45,852 patients with acute myocardial infarction:randomised placebo-controlled trial. Lancet 2005;366(9497):1587–1589.

32 The Acute Infarction Ramipiril Efficacy (AIRE) Study Investigators. Effect of ramipiril on mortality and morbidity of survivors of AMI with clinical evidence of HF. Lancet 1993;342:821–828.

33 Kober L, Torp-Pedersen C, Carlsen JE *et al.* A clinical trial of the angiotensin-converting-enzyme inhibitor trandolapril in patients with left ventricular dysfunction after myocardial infarction. N Engl J Med 1995;333:1670–1676.

34 Ross AM, Coyne KS, Reiner JS *et al.* A randomized trial comparing primary angioplasty with a strategy of short-acting thombolysis and immediate planned rescue angioplasty in acute myocardial infarction: The PACT trial. J Am Coll Cardiol 1999;34:1954–1962.

35 Goldman LE, Eisenberg MJ. Identification and management of patients with failed thrombolysis after AMI Ann Intern Med 2000;132:556–565.

36 Gershlick AH, and the REACT Trial Investigators. Rescue angioplasty after failed thrombolytic therapy for acute myocardial infarction. N Engl J Med 2005;353(26):2758–2768.

37 Magid DJ, Calonge BN, Rumfeld JS *et al.* for the National Registry of Myocardial Infarction 2 and 3 Investigators. Relations between hospital primary angioplasty volume and mortality for patients with AMI treated with primary angioplasty vs. thrombolytic therapy. JAMA 2000;284:3131–3138.

38 Aversano T, Aversano LT, Passamani E *et al.* Thrombolytic therapy vs. primary percutaneous coronary intervention for myocardial infarction in patients presenting to hospitals
without on-site cardiac surgery: a randomized controlled trial. JAMA 2002;287:1943–1951.

39 Bruce R, Brodie BR, Hansen C *et al.* Door-to-Balloon Time With Primary Percutaneous
Coronary Intervention for Acute Myocardial Infarction Impacts Late Cardiac Mortality
in High-Risk Patients and Patients Presenting Early After the Onset of Symptoms. J Am
Coll Cardiol 2006;47:289–295.

40 Henry TD, Unger BT, Sharkey SW *et al.* Design of a standardized system for transfer of
patients with ST-elevation myocardial infarction for percutaneous coronary intervention.
Am Heart J 2005;150(3):373–384.

41 Bradley EH, Roumanis SA, Radford MJ *et al.* Achieving Door-to-Balloon Times That Meet
Quality Guidelines: How Do Successful Hospitals Do It? J Am Coll Cardiol 2005;46:
1236–1241.

42 Reichert MG, MacGregor DA, Kincaid EH, Dolinski SY. Excessive argatroban anticoagulation for heparin-induced thrombocytopenia. Ann Pharmacother 2003;37(5): 652–654.

43 Virtanen R, Kauppila M, Itala M Percutaneous coronary intervention with stenting in a
patient with haemophilia A and an acute myocardial infarction following a single dose of
desmopressin. Thromb Haemost 2004 Nov;92(5):1154–1156.

44 ADVANCE MI Investigators. Facilitated percutaneous coronary intervention for acute
ST-segment elevation myocardial infarction: results from the prematurely terminated
ADdressing the Value of facilitated ANgioplasty after Combination therapy or Eptifibatide
monotherapy in acute Myocardial Infarction (ADVANCE MI) trial. Am Heart J 2005;150:
116–122.

45 Assessment of the Safety and Efficacy of a New Treatment Strategy with Percutaneous
Coronary Intervention (ASSENT-4 PCI) Investigators. Primary versus tenecteplase-
facilitated percutaneous coronary intervention in patients with ST-segment elevation acute
myocardial infarction (ASSENT-4 PCI): randomised trial. Lancet 2006;367(9510):569–578.

46 Yang XS, Willems JL, Pardeans J *et al.* Acute myocardial infarction in the very elderly. A
comparison with younger age groups. Acta Cardiol 1987;42:59–68.

47 Assessment of the Safety and Efficacy of a New Thrombolytic Regimen (ASSENT-3)
Investigators. Efficacy and safety of tenecteplase in combination with enoxaparin, abciximab, or unfractionated heparin: The ASSENT-3 randomised trial in acute myocardial
infarction. Lancet 2001;358(9282):605–613.

48 SENIOR-PAMI trial: Presented by Cindy Grines at the American College of Cardiology
meeting in Atlanta 2006.

49 Guagliumi G, Stone GW, Cox DA. Outcome in elderly patients undergoing primary coronary intervention for acute myocardial infarction: results from the Controlled Abciximab
and Device Investigation to Lower Late Angioplasty Complications (CADILLAC) trial.
Circulation 2004;110(12):1598–1604.

50 White HD, Aylward PE, Huang Z *et al.*; for the VALIANT Investigators Heart Failure
Mortality and Morbidity Remain High Despite Captopril and/or Valsartan Therapy in
Elderly Patients With Left Ventricular Systolic Dysfunction, Heart Failure, or Both After
Acute Myocardial Infarction Results From the Valsartan in Acute Myocardial Infarction
Trial (VALIANT) Circulation 2005;112:3391–3399.

51 Ayanian JZ, Braunwald E. Thrombolytic therapy for patients with MI who are older than
75 years of age. Do the risks outweigh the benefits? Circulation 2000;101:2224–2226.

52 Lincoff M, Califf RM, Ellis SG *et al.* Thrombolytic therapy for women with myocardial
infarction: Is there a gender gap? Thrombolysis and Angioplasty in Myocardial Infarction
Study Group. J Am Coll Cardiol 1993;22:1780–1787.

53 Stone G, Marcovitz P, Lansky A *et al.* Differential effects of stenting and angioplasty in women versus men undergoing a primary mechanical reperfusion strategy in AMI: The PAMI Stent randomized trial. J Am Coll Cardiol 1999;33(2 suppl A):557A.

54 Stone PH, Muller J, Hartwell T *et al.* The effects of diabetes mellitus on prognosis and seria left ventricular function after acute myocardial infarction: Contribution of both coronary disease and left ventricular dysfunction to the adverse prognosis. The MILIS study group. J Am Coll Cardiol 1989;14:49–57.

55 Lindsay M, Kelly C, Goodfield N *et al.* Increased poST-infarct mortality in diabetics persists despite delivery of optimal care. J Am Coll Cardiol 1999;33(2 suppl A):331A.

56 Prasad A, Stone GW, Stuckey TD *et al.* Impact of diabetes mellitus on myocardial perfusion after primary angioplasty in patients with acute myocardial infarction. J Am Coll Cardiol 2005;45(4):508–514.

57 Barbash G, Birnbaum Y, Bogearts K *et al.* Treatment of reinfarction after thrombolytic therapy for AMI: An analysis of outcome and treatment choices in the GUSTO-I and ASSENT-2 trial. Circulation 2001;103:954–960.

58 Gibson CM, Karha J, Murphy SA *et al.* Early and long-term clinical outcomes associated with reinfarction following fibrinolytic administration in the Thrombolysis in Myocardial Infarction trials. J Am Coll Cardiol 2003;42(1):7–16.

59 Dixon SR, Grines C, Cox D *et al.* Creatinine clearance but not the serum creatinine on admission predicts early and late death after primary angioplasty. J Am Coll Cardiol 2001;37:361A.

60 Herzog C, Ma J, Collins A. Poor long term survival after acute myocardial infarction among patients on long term dialysis. N Engl J Med 1998;339:799–805.

61 Herzog C. Acute MI in dialysis patients: How can we improve the outlook? J Crit Illness 1999;14:613–621.

62 Simonson JS, Schiller NB. Sonorespirometry: A new method for non-invasive estimation of mean right atrial pressure based on 2-D echocardiographic measurements of the inferior vena cava during measured inspiration. J Am Coll Cardiol 1988;11:557–564.

63 Nobuyoshi M, Nakagawa Y. Update on extractional thrombectomy catheter, AngioJet. J Intervent Cardiol 1998;11(5 suppl II):S77–S79.

64 Stone GW, Webb J, Cox DA, and the Enhanced Myocardial Efficacy and Recovery by Aspiration of Liberated Debris (EMERALD) Investigators. Distal microcirculatory protection during percutaneous coronary intervention in acute ST-segment elevation myocardial infarction: a randomized controlled trial. JAMA 2005;293(9):1116–1118.

65 Kong JA, Chou ET, Minutello RM *et al.* Safety of single versus multi-vessel angioplasty for patients with acute myocardial infarction and multi-vessel coronary artery disease: report from the New York State Angioplasty Registry. Coron Artery Dis 2006;17(1):71–75.

66 Schuhlen H, Kastrati A, Dirschinger J *et al.* Primary angioplasty in patients with AMI and multivessel disease. One year outcome after single vessel versus multivessel angioplasty. J Am Coll Cardiol 2001;37(2):306A.

67 Rapaport E. Early vs. late opening of coronary arteries: The effect of timing. Clin Cardiol 1990;13:VIII18–VIII22.

68 Topol EJ, Califf RM, Vandormael M *et al.* A randomized trial of late reperfusion therapy for acute myocardial infarction. Thrombolysis and Angioplasty in Myocardial Infarction-6 Study Group. Circulation 1992;85:2090–2099.

69 The results of the Occluded Artery Trial (OAT) presented by Judith Hochman at the American Heart Association 2006 Scientific Sessions, in Chicago November 2006.

70 Timmis G, Timmis S. The restoration of coronary blood flow in acute myocardial infarction. J Intervent Cardiol 1998;11(5 suppl II):S9–S17.

CHAPTER 3

Hypotension and Cardiogenic Shock in Acute Myocardial Infarction

Thach N. Nguyen, Sim Kui Hian, Nikola Bakraceski, Haiyun Wu and Shiwen Wang

Introduction

In the setting of acute myocardial infarction (MI), cardiogenic shock (CS) is defined as systolic blood pressure (SBP or BP) less than 90 mmHg, or a decrease of >30 mmHg in mean pressure, compared with prior normal baseline values, lasting for more than 30 minutes and associated with peripheral hypoperfusion. The diagnostic criteria for CS are listed in Table 3.1 [1].

The majority of patients with CS had no hypotension on arrival. Less than 1% of patients with acute MI (AMI) presented to the hospital with shock. 6.4% developed shock during hospitalization while being observed and treated [2].

This raises speculation that the diagnosis of severe pump failure or pre-shock may be missed at presentation or by suboptimal early therapy, including use of agents that may induce hypotension or may aggravate iatrogenic shock in marginally compensated patients [3]. By 48 hours, almost three quarter (59%) of those who would eventually develop shock had done so. Surprisingly, the patients with early shock development (days 1–2) had a significantly lower 30-day mortality (45%) than those with intermediate or late shock development (>80%) ($P < 0.05$) [4]. How these patients could develop CS while under intensive medical care? Did we undertreat the patients who are going to develop CS? In this chapter, specific characteristics, clinical identifications of different subsets of patients are presented, management plans discussed, and practical implementation suggested. The management strategies are listed in Table 3.2.

Table 3.1 Diagnostic criteria for cardiogenic shock.

1. BP <90 mmHg for at least >30 minutes, not improved with fluid administration
2. Signs of hypoperfusion (cold extremities), altered mental status: restlessness, agitation
3. Reduced urine output (<20 cc/hour)
4. Cardiac index of <2.2 L/min/m^2

BP, blood pressure.

Table 3.2 Management strategies for cardiogenic shock.

1. Identify the patient with early cardiogenic shock, even if the blood pressure is not yet low
2. Revascularize the patient with a percutaneous or surgical approach
3. Close follow-up and correct all non-cardiac problems such as respiratory, liver, kidney failure

Management in the Emergency Room

When any patient with AMI arrives in the emergency room (ER), the heart rate (HR) and systolic BP are very strong prognostic factors. When there is sinus tachycardia, a BP less than 100 mmHg, or the SBP begins to decrease 20–30 mmHg from the patient's known baseline BP, then the patient should be investigated thoroughly for any cause of hypotension and for possible CS. In order to correct the problem effectively, patients with shock are classified according to the mechanism of low BP and degree of tissue hypoperfusion (Table 3.3).

Any patient with AMI should have a comprehensive examination at the time of arrival to the ER. The presence of sinus tachycardia and borderline low BP (<100 mmHg but >90 mmHg) should trigger the process of investigating carefully the causes of declining BP. The four main questions are:

1 Does the patient still have ongoing ischemia as evidenced by chest pain or angina-equivalent?

Table 3.3 Classification of acute myocardial infarction patients with hypotension and shock.

Class	Blood pressure	Hypoperfusion	Mortality
		CI < 2.2 PCWP > 22	
The pre-shock patients			
1. Hypovolemic hypotension	Low	−	
2. Clinical shock (hypotension without hypoperfusion)	Low	−	23%
3. Compensatory shock (hypoperfusion without hypotension)	Normal	+ +	43%
The patient with shock			
4. Classic cardiogenic shock (hypotension and hypoperfusion)	Low	+ +	66%

AMI, acute myocardial infarction; BP, blood pressure; CI, cardiac index (L/min/m^2); PCWP, pulmonary capillary wedge pressure.

2 Are there any rales in the lung auscultation, suggestive of LV failure with pulmonary congestion?

3 Does the patients have signs of peripheral hypoperfusion (cold extremities, agitation, restlessness or low urine output <20 mL/h)?

4 Are there signs of mechanical complication from AMI – new (possibly very soft) murmur of mitral regurgitation (MR), muffled heart sounds of pericardial effusion, ventricular septal defect (VSD), etc?

Work-up in the Pre-shock Period

Pre-emptive aggressive measures should be started once the BP is detected to be declining, in order to reverse the process of imminent CS. The optimal strategies for work-up during the pre-shock period are listed in Table 3.4.

Table 3.4 Work-up during the pre-shock period.

1. Frequent monitoring of HR and BP
2. Generous IV fluid challenge
3. Reassessment with ECG
4. STAT echocardiography
5. Comprehensive physical examination
6. Right heart catheterization

BP, blood pressure; ECG, electrocardiogram; HR, heart rate; IV, intravenous; STAT, emergency.

Electrocardiogram

An electrocardiogram (ECG) with extensive change in the anterior leads or other sites (multi-site MI) would point to possible CS in > 50% of patients. If the patient showed change in the inferior leads, the most common cause of hypotension is increased vagal tone. The inferior wall MI rarely caused shock, unless associated with prior MI or presence of lesion in other arteries [4], or other mechanical complications. It caused only 2.8% isolated RV infarction and subsequent shock [5]. Therefore a decreasing BP in the presence of anterior wall MI, multi-site MI, or previous MI would alert the cardiologist for imminent CS. The ECG features which trigger the suspicion for CS are summarized in Table 3.5.

Table 3.5 Suspicion of early cardiogenic shock by electrocardiogram.

1. Anterior wall MI or multisite MI with decreasing SBP (most common)
2. >20 mmHg decrease of BP in patient with history of prior MI
3. >20 mmHg decrease of BP in patient with inferior wall MI
4. Decreasing BP with clear lungs due to right ventricular infarction

BP, blood pressure; MI, myocardial infarction; SBP, systolic blood pressure.

To evaluate the ECG parameters as predictors of 1-year mortality in patients developing CS, and to document associations between these ECG parameters and the survival benefit of emergency revascularization vs. initial medical stabilization, a substudy of the SHOCK trial was performed.

CRITICAL THINKING

The electrocardiographic pointers. In a prospective substudy of 198 SHOCK trial patients, the baseline HR was higher in non-survivors than in survivors (106 ± 20 vs. 95 ± 24 BPM, $P = 0.001$). There was a significant association between the QRS duration and 1-year mortality in medically stabilized patients (115 mins in non-survivors vs. 99 mins in survivors, $P = 0.012$), but not in emergently revascularized patients (110 ± 3 mins vs. 116 ± 27 mins respectively, $P = 0.343$). Among patients with inferior AMI, a greater sum of ST depression was associated with higher 1-year mortality in medically stabilized patients ($P = 0.029$), but not in emergently revascularized patients ($P = 0.613$, treatment interaction $P = 0.0250$ [6]).

STAT Echocardiography

An emergency bedside echocardiograph will give instant information about the LV function and any mechanical complications (Table 3.6).

CLINICAL PEARLS

Can a patient with EF = 50% have CS? A 50% ejection fraction (EF) does not rule out imminent CS because the EF is the combination of decreased segmental wall motion from the damaged area with a hyperdynamic compensatory response from the other non-injured wall areas. If there is no hyperdynamic compensatory contraction from the previously un-identified non-infarct related artery (IRA) territory, then there are possible significant lesions in the non-IRA or the presence of multivessel disease which can trigger CS. The ventricle should contract vigorously, especially under the influence of positive inotropic agents such as dopamine.

Table 3.6 Echocardiographic features in patients with acute myocardial infarction.

1. Hypokinesis or akinesis in the IRA territory
2. Compensatory increased contractility of the non-IRA segments
3. Hyperdynamic contraction under the effect of IV inotropic agents
4. Hyperdynamic contraction of the RV if there is hypovolemia
5. Pericardial effusion
6. Right atrial and ventricular collapse in diastole suggestive of tamponade
7. Mechanical complications: VSR, MR, Free-wall rupture or pseudoaneurysm

IRA, infarct-related artery; IV, intravenous; MI, myocardial infarction; MR, mitral regurgitation; RV, right ventricle; VSR, ventricular septal rupture.

The mechanical causes of shock requiring repair (acute MR, ventricular septal rupture (VSR), free wall rupture/tamponade) can be evidenced clearly by echo. However, they are rare and account for only 12% of CS [1].

Pre-emptive Measures

When there is decreasing SBP without sign of pulmonary congestion, generous intravenous (IV) normal saline (NS) fluid challenge should be started to maintain a decent BP. If there is sign of left ventricular (LV) failure by auscultation or by echocardiography, then the IV fluid has to be adjusted accordingly. Vasodilators can begin to be given in order to improve the cardiac output without increasing oxygen demand. However, if the BP is still low and there is doubt about the cause of hypotension, or the response to empiric IV fluid is suboptimal, then a right heart catheterization (RHC) should be performed. The reason is that the finding of cold peripheries was subjective and clinical exam can under-diagnose 15% of patients with low cardiac index or high PCWP [8]. An RHC would also give comprehensive information about the hemodynamic status and the results of the intrinsic neurohormonal compensatory mechanisms. The PCWP would reflect the volume status and the ventricular compliance (Table 3.7).

Coronary Angiography

If there is sign of ongoing ischemia, then left heart catheterization and coronary angiography should be performed quickly to assess the severity of the

Table 3.7 Volume status according to right heart catheterization.

Volume status	Cardiac index	Pulmonary Capillary Wedge pressure
	(L/min/m²)	(mmHg)
Normal	>2.2	<18
Cardiogenic shock	<2.2	>18
Hypovolemia	<2.2	<18
Fluid overload	>2.2	>18
Sepsis	>2.2	<18, low SVR

SVR: systemic vascular resistance.

coronary artery disease (CAD), its extent and damage. Reversal of on-going ischemia by percutaneous or surgical intervention should be performed as soon as possible. The management plan is shown in Table 3.8.

Table 3.8 Pre-emptive measures in patients with decreasing blood pressure.

1. Early recognition of decreasing BP, borderline BP with possible CS
2. Generous IV fluid intake
3. Stabilization of patient by correction of arrhythmia, electrolyte imbalance, acid–base abnormality
4. Readjust the fluid intake according to result of RHC
5. If there is declining BP, insertion of an IABP in the left femoral artery, for possible access for PCI via the right femoral artery
6. Identification of ideal or high risk patients
7. Early percutaneous or surgical coronary revascularizations

BP, blood pressure; CS, cardiogenic shock; IABP, intra-aortic balloon pump; IV, intravenous; PCI, primary coronary interventions; RHC, right heart catheterization.

Management of Hypovolemic Hypotension

Hypotension is defined as SBP less than 90 mmHg or a decrease of 30 mmHg from the baseline or known SBP of the patient. Many patients can tolerate a BP of 80 mmHg for many hours [9]. The causes include increased vagal tone, stunned RV, RV infarction or intravascular contraction secondary to excessive diuresis, or medications such as morphine or nitrate which provoke venodilation and pre-load reduction. They can have hypotension without sign of hypoperfusion unless the hypovolemia is quite severe.

These patients often have low LV-filling pressure and their hypotension usually resolves with the administration of IV fluid. The treatment of bradycardia and hypotension is with atropine and 250 cc IV fluid challenge. Dehydration from excessive diuretic is reversed with IV fluid resuscitation. However, caution must be exercised in older patients, patients with prior MI, prior congestive heart failure (CHF), hypertensive heart disease, diabetes and small size body [10]. Elderly patients are sensitive to excessive administration of fluids due to reduced LV compliance.

Management of Clinical Shock

Many patients with AMI can have hypotension and significant peripheral hypoperfusion even when they have a fairly decent cardiac index: >2.2 L/min/m^2 [1]. In the SHOCK registry, the RHC results of all the hypotensive patients with clinical signs of poor peripheral perfusion showed a majority of patients with frank CS and a sizable minority with acceptable cardiac index: >2.2 L/min/m^2. The latter also had high PCWP (>22 mmHg), even though only half had pulmonary congestion. They received aggressive treatment, however their in-hospital mortality was low at 20% which is a tremendous improvement from the average 60% mortality of classic CS patients: an absolute 40% mortality decrease [1]. Even so, this 20% mortality is still high compared with 3% mortality of patients without shock. These patients with normal CI are those who fail the first line of compensatory mechanism for hypotension, in the pre-shock period. Now they develop clinical shock without evidence of hypoperfusion by invasive parameters. If the cause of hypotension was not reversed, these patients would have deteriorated into classic CS. In the SHOCK trial registry, these patients underwent the highest number of invasive (75–85%) and interventional procedures (45–85%) which were translated into a best mortality rate of 20% [1].

Management of Compensatory Shock

Patients with this syndrome maintained BP above 90 mmHg [3]. However, the lack of low BP can be deceptive. The signs of peripheral hypoperfusion (oliguria, cold and clammy skin) were more strongly associated with the 30-day mortality than was baseline systolic BP [11]. These patients experienced decreased tissue perfusion associated with decreased cardiac output and high PCWP. Their systemic vascular resistance (SVR) tended to be greater, even it was not statistically significant. The hemodynamic differences between the three groups are highlighted in Table 3.9.

With the occlusion of a major IRA, the cardiac output decreases. In order to maintain an adequate BP and to preserve tissue perfusion, several

Table 3.9 Hemodynamic data of the 3 classes of shock [3].

Measurements	Normotension hypoperfusion (compensatory)	Hypotension normal perfusion (clinical)	Hypotension hypoperfusion (classic)	
Heart rate	94	100	95	($P = 0.28$)
Systolic BP	104	97	86	($P \leqslant 0.001$)
PCWP	25	22	23	($P = 0.25$)
Cardiac index*	1.9	2.5	2.0	($P = 0.48$)
SVR	1753	1378	1389	($P = 0.19$)

*(L/min/m^2).
BP, blood pressure; PCWP, pulmonary capillary wedge pressure; SVR, systemic vascular resistance.

neurohormonal compensatory mechanisms are activated resulting in increased HR, and peripheral vasoconstriction [3]. This results in a decent BP even if the patients has low cardiac index, high PCWP and high SVR. It is seen similarly under the effect of exogenous catecholamines such as dopamine, epinephrine, etc.

It is not clear whether all patients with classic CS go through a stage of non-hypotensive CS. The similar time frame between the two groups suggests that it is not always the case. However, the subsequent requirement of vasopressor or intra-aortic balloon pump (IABP) support during the hospital stay suggests that normotensive CS is often followed by hypotension and circulatory collapse [3]. Their mortality rate was 43% compared with 66% in patients with classic CS [3].

In the management of patients with compensatory CS, it is important to avoid hypoperfusion or low BP. The main strategies are as always: (1) to keep a decent BP; (2) to detect the early signs of hypoperfusion; and (3) to reverse any cause of CS as early as possible, including ongoing ischemia, in order to prevent the patient advancing into CS.

Management of Classic CS

The management of CS includes the treatment of its causes, by opening of the IRA with thrombolytic therapy (TT) or mechanical interventions, surgical repair for the mechanical complications, and maintaining a decent BP with good peripheral perfusion, compatible with life. The causes of CS, its prevalence and mortality are listed in Table 3.10 [1].

Table 3.10 Etiologies, prevalence and mortality [1].

Causes	Incidence	Mortality
Predominant LV failure	78%	59%
Severe MR	6.9%	55%
VSR	3.9%	87%
Isolated RV shock	2.8%	55%
Free wall rupture and tamponade	1.4%	55%
Average		*60%*

LV, left ventricular; MR, mitral regurgitation; RV, right ventricular; VSR, ventricular septal rupture.

Evidence-based Medicine: The SHOCK registry

At 30 days, the mortality was 46% in the revascularized group (angioplasty or stenting PTCA or coronary artery bypass (CABG) surgery); and 56% for those given medical therapy ($P = 0.11$). At 6 months, however, the corresponding figures were 50% vs. 63% ($P = 0.027$) [12]. These beneficial results from the aggressive approach were not seen in the group over 75 years-of-age; on the contrary, they were worse (Table 3.10). Their one-year survival from medical therapy was 46.7% vs. 33.6% with revascularized ($P < 0.03$).

In order to clarify the different strategies in the management of AMI patients complicated by CS, in the SHOCK registry the patients with CS due to AMI were randomized for a direct invasive strategy with early revascularization comparing with initial medical stabilization, including thrombolysis, IABP, and possible revascularization after 48 hours.

There was, however, a bias in the comparison. The patients who underwent angiography had lower baseline risk and better hemodynamic profile [12]. The more stable patients had primary interventions and the very sick ones died before having a chance trying the procedure. This is why the patients who underwent angiogram had a mortality of 47% while the patients who were too sick to tolerate an angiogram had a mortality of 86% [13].

In this presentation of CS, aggressive catheter-based intervention by experienced operators is suggested. Rapid transfer of CS patients, particularly those younger than 75 years, to medical centers capable of providing early angiography and revascularizations is recommended [14]. The management strategies are shown in Table 3.11.

Table 3.11 Management of cardiogenic shock.

1. Early recognition of CS
2. Stabilization of patient by correction of arrhythmia, electrolyte imbalance, acid–base abnormality.
3. Insertion of IABP in the left femoral artery, for possible angioplasty via the right femoral artery access
4. Early intubation and mechanical ventilation to decrease the work of the respiratory muscles and myocardial oxygen consumption
5. Right, left heart catheterization and coronary angiography
6. Early percutaneous intervention or CABG

CABG, coronary artery bypass grafting; CS, cardiogenic shock; IABP, intra-aortic balloon pump.

Benefits of Pharmacologic or Mechanical Revascularizations

In patients with CS, TT opened only 40% of arteries to the thrombolysis for myocardial infarction (TIMI) flow grade 2 or 3. Without thrombolysis, 91% of patients had the arteries virtually closed at TIMI 0 or 1. TT lowered the mortality rate to 54% vs. 64% in patients without reperfusion [15]. They still have high in-hospital mortality even after successful PTCA, stenting, and IABP. However, revascularization at any time during hospitalization was associated with a lower mortality (39% vs. 78% in patients without revascularization). Among the SHOCK trial patients randomized to emergency revascularization, those treated with CABG had a greater prevalence of diabetes and worse coronary anatomy than those treated with PCI, but both groups had similar survival rates [16]. Consequently emergency CABG is an important component of an optimal treatment strategy in patients with CS, and should be considered for patients with diabetes and extensive coronary disease [17].

Technical Aspects of Percutaneous Revascularization

As the patients survive the ischemic injury with BP maintained artificially by intravenous inotropic agents and IABP, they are barely stable enough to be transported into the cardiac catheterization laboratories for a diagnostic angiogram. The factors associated with shock and/or mortality are mostly patient-based, reflecting poor ventricular function and the extent of coronary disease (Table 3.12).

Table 3.12 Angiographic mechanism of shock.

LV dysfunction (EF <30%)
IRA supplying more than 50% viable myocardium
Circulation to both papillary muscles compromised
Significant disease in non-IRA

EF, ejection fraction; IRA, infarct-related artery; LV, left ventricle.

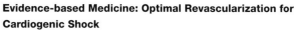

Evidence-based Medicine: Optimal Revascularization for Cardiogenic Shock

In the SHOCK trial, angiographic films of the 82 patients randomized to a strategy of early PCI or CABG were analyzed. The one-year mortality in PCI patients was 50%. Mortality was 39% if PCI was successful but 85% if unsuccessful ($P < 0.001$). Mortality was 38% if TIMI flow grade 3 was achieved, 55% with TIMI grade 2 flow, and 100% with TIMI grade 0 or 1 flow ($P < 0.001$). Mortality was 67% if severe MR was documented. Independent correlates of mortality were as follows: increasing age ($P < 0.001$), lower systolic BP ($P < 0.009$), increasing time from randomization to PCI ($P = 0.019$), lower post-PCI TIMI flow (0/1 vs. 2/3) ($P < 0.001$), and multivessel PCI ($P = 0.040$) [18].

Benefit appeared to extend beyond the generally accepted 12-h post-infarction window. Surgery should be considered in shock patients with severe mitral insufficiency or multivessel disease not amenable to relatively complete revascularization by PCI [18].

CLINICAL PEARLS

Which CS patient will recover best from PCI? Quite a few patients have hypotension and subsequent CS due to severe myocardial stunning from abrupt occlusion of a major artery. These patients may recover very quickly if the IRA is opened early. The characteristics of the patients ideal for PCI are listed in Table 3.13.

Table 3.13 Best candidates for primary intervention in cardiogenic shock.

Age less than 65
No prior myocardial infarction
No triple vessel disease
Early presentation
Stunned myocardium

Overall, 15% of patients had left main lesion, 41% had lesions in the left anterior descending artery (LAD) and 53% had triple vessel disease [13]. The culprit lesion of left-ventricular failure (LVF) was more often in the patient with LAD lesion while the patients with mechanical complication had more often lesion in the left circumflex artery [13].

In patients with multivessel disease, shock may be related not only to the culprit lesion, but also to other severe lesions in the non-IRA. PCI of other major non-IRAs does not seem to increase the risk when performed by experienced operators. The mortality was 35% (in patients with the non-IRA and IRA opened) compared with 51% in patients who had only the IRA opened [15]. In patients with slow flow after opening of the IRA, vasodilators for the distal microvasculature, such as adenosine, nicorandil or nitroprusside can improve the flow distally and speed up the reversal of myocardial hypokinesis. In other non-IRAs with slow flow, the above medications should be given to improve the microvascular perfusion at these vascular beds too.

CLINICAL PEARLS

Cardiogenic shock from acute papillary dysfunction   Many patients developed CS triggered by acute MR secondary to ischemia or infarction of the papillary muscles. When there is suspicion of MR due to lesion in the artery supplying the papillary muscles, angioplasty of these specific branches is strongly suggested. The blood supply to the papillary muscles is summarized in Table 3.14.

Table 3.14 Blood supply to the papillary muscles.

1. The diagonal branches to the anterolateral papillary muscle
2. The obtuse marginal branch to the posterior medial papillary muscle
3. In the case of right dominance, the LV branch of the RCA to the posterior medial papillary muscle
4. In the case of dual supply, the distal PDA and the posterolateral branch of the LCX to the posterior medial papillary muscle

LCX, left circumflex artery; LV, left ventricular; RCA, right coronary artery; PDA, posterior descending artery.

The example of severe ischemic MR due to acute papillary muscle dysfunction causing reversible CS is illustrated in a case report of complication during PCI of the circumflex from no-reflow. Baseline echocardiography before PCI showed only mild MR. As no-reflow occurred after stenting, the patient developed acute hypotension, hypoxia, pulmonary edema, increase in pulmonary mean wedge pressure to 42 mmHg with very high V-wave during pulmonary wedge tracing, and CS requiring IABP insertion. Urgent echocardiography revealed severe MR. With the establishment of normal flow in the circumflex artery after IABP insertion and intracoronary adenosine, severe MR, hypoxia and all hemodynamic instability were resolved [19].

Although survival in patients with CS due to mechanical complications remains poor, an aggressive approach including a combination of platelet receptor inhibitors, IABP, and early surgical or percutaneous coronary revascularization may help to improve mortality [13].

Management of Specific Patients

Acute Septal Rupture

Patients with ventricular septal rupture present with sudden, severe LVF in association with a pansystolic murmur, (sometimes too soft to be heard or no murmur at all) often accompanied by a parasternal thrill or they die suddenly [20]. It is often impossible to differentiate this condition from rupture of a papillary muscle with resulting MR by RHC, because the presence in both conditions of a tall "V" wave in the capillary wedge pressure further complicates the differentiation. The diagnosis of ventricular septal rupture is made by color flow Doppler echocardiography [21].

Usually the patients are older, more often female, and less often had previous infarction. Their average in-hospital mortality was very high at 87%. 20% of patients who underwent surgery survived, however, only 5% patients on medical treatment survived. The patients with anterior wall MI and apical VSR do better than those with inferior wall MI [22]. RCA occlusion may lead to rupture of the lower ventricular septum, with development of VSD [23].

Delaying surgery to permit infarct-healing risks the development of shock, which is unpredictable and associated with poor surgical prognosis. Despite the poor outcome, surgery in this setting remains the best therapeutic option. However, in the patient population of the SHOCK trial, surgery was near futile for elderly patients with inferior wall MI complicated by shock, VSR and other comorbidity.

Cardiac Free Wall Rupture and Tamponade

Rupture of the LV free wall after AMI is a catastrophic event [24]. The clinical presentation typically is a sudden loss of pulse, BP and consciousness, while the electrogram continues to show sinus rhythm (apparent electromechanical dissociation). This condition is almost universally fatal [21].

In the SHOCK registry, the incidence of free-wall rupture was 2.7%, but it is impossible to know the true prevalence because many patients died immediately and the cause of death is not confirmed [24]. Tamponade alone may represent instances of spontaneously sealed or unrecognized rupture. The presence of pericardial effusion >5 mm was 100% sensitive for the diagnosis of subacute ventricular free-wall rupture [25].

Real World Question How to Predict which Patients will Die?

Although PCI in the setting of CS still has a high in-hospital mortality rate, it has been shown to decrease the mortality rate in certain subgroups. The identity and relative importance of variables that are predictive of in-hospital mortality rate after PCI for CS are uncertain. There are many ways to make an educated guess about the mortality of a particular patient. It is either by conventional clinical data, calculated hemodynamic data (cardiac power), or by ECG criteria. In identifying the sicker patient, early revascularization will help to reduce mortality and increase survival.

CRITICAL THINKING

The American College of Cardiology – National Cardiovascular Data Registry (ACC-NCDR) Analysis. Data from >300,000 patients in the ACC-NCDR were evaluated. The outcomes of 483 patients who underwent emergency PCI for CS were studied. Patients' mean age was 65 ± 13 years, with men predominating (61%). Mean LV EF was 30 ± 16%. Stents were placed in 64% of patients, and thrombolytic agents were administered in 26%. Although PCI was angiographically successful in 79% of patients, the in-hospital mortality rate was 59.4%. Logistic regression using all available variables identified six multivariate predictors of death: age ($P < 0.001$ for each 10-year increment, female gender (OR 1.55; 95%CI 1.00–2.41; $P < 0.001$), baseline renal insufficiency (creatinine > 2.0 mg/dL; OR 4.69; 95%CI 1.96–11.23; $P < 0.001$), total occlusion in the LAD (OR 1.99; 95%CI 1.28–3.09; $P < 0.01$), no stent used (OR 2.55; 95%CI 1.63–3.96; $P < 0.01$), and no glycoprotein IIb/IIIa inhibitor used during PCI (OR 1.96; 95%CI 1.30–2.98; $P < 0.01$). In a second analysis using only variables known to the clinician at the time of initial presentation, gender, age, renal insufficiency, and total occlusion of the LAD were significant [26].

Real World Question Acute Mitral Regurgitation: When Should We Perform Surgery?

The reported incidence of apical systolic murmurs of MR during the first few days after the onset of AMI varies widely (from 10–50%) depending on the population studied and the acumen of the observers [27]. The most common cause of MR following AMI is dysfunction of the mitral valve. LV dilatation or alteration in the size or shape of the LV due to impaired contractility or to aneurysm formation causes disordered contraction of the papillary muscles. The most dramatic scenario occurs when a papillary muscle, or more commonly the head of a papillary muscle, ruptures causing severe acute MR leading to CS. This is a medical catastrophe portending very poor prognosis [28].

Shock due to acute MR (AMR) developed late at a median of 12 hours while it was 6 hours for LVF. More of the patients were women, had less STEMI at presentation, and more frequently inferior or posterior MI. Consistent with the mechanism of acute MR, the MR cohort had higher median EF (37% vs. 30% $P = 0.001$) and more pulmonary edema. However, the 37% EF represents marked impairment of LV systolic function performance in the presence of MR. In the past, thrombolysis or angioplasty did not reverse MR in a group of patients with moderately severe or severe MR [29]. At that time, no stent or effective antiplatetet medications were available. The patients who had mitral valve surgery had a mortality rate of 40% while the patients who did not go for surgery had a mortality rate of 71%. The reason for not undertaking mitral valve surgery were: (1) the patient could not be stabilized or died awaiting surgery (half of patients); and (2) the presence of co-morbidities related to current illness or secondary to shock (one-third of patients). As the aortic pressure is lowered by IABP, a greater fraction of the LV output will be ejected antegradely, thus lessening the regurgitant fraction. To this end, both IABP (which lowers the aortic pressure mechanically), and the infusion of nitroglycerin or sodium nitroprusside (which reduce systemic vascular resistance), have been used with success in the interim management of patients with severe AMR from MI. Ideally, definitive operative treatment should be postponed until pulmonary congestion has cleared and the infarct has had time to heal. However, if the patient's hemodynamic and/or clinical condition does not improve or stabilize, surgical treatment should be undertaken, even in the acute stage [21].

Real World Question How to Avoid Mortality in Cardiogenic Shock?

Not every patient with CS died from heart failure. If many died from ventricular arrhythmias, did the cardioverter defibrillator (ICD) prevent these deaths? The DINAMIT trial did not show improved mortality after ICD implantation. How did these patients die?

Data regarding 62 patients who died in the SHOCK trial were reviewed. 65% did not survive. 20% died from fatal arrhythmia, 35% died with low CI [i.e., $<2.2\,L/min/m^2$], and 45% died with normalized CI (i.e., $>2.2\,L/min/m^2$) and a higher CI/oxygen extraction ratio. The patients with normalized CI were younger and stayed longer in the intensive care unit (ICU) than patients with low CI. So a substantial number of patients with CS died with a normalized CI, suggesting a distributive defect, in the absence of obvious infection. The release of mediators may be secondary to gut hypoperfusion [30]. This is why a clinical trial is randomizing patients for L-NAME (a nitric oxide synthase inhibitor) in the setting of CS. The results will not be available for the next 2 years. Preliminary data on the small group are highlighted below.

CRITICAL THINKING

L-NAME for Cardiogenic Shock. To evaluate the effect of L-NAME (a nitric oxide synthase inhibitor) in the treatment of refractory CS, 30 patients were randomized to supportive care alone ($n = 15$, control group) or to supportive care in addition to L-NAME (1 mg/Kg bolus and 1 mg/Kg/h continuous IV drip for 5 h $n = 15$). Death at one month was 27% in the L-NAME group vs. 67% in the control group ($P = 0.008$). Unaugmented mean arterial BP at 24 h from randomization was 86 ± 20 mmHg in the L-NAME group vs. 66 ± 13 mmHg in the control group ($P = 0.004$). Urine output increased at 24 h by 135 ± 78 cc/h in the L-NAME group vs. a decrease of 12 ± 87 cc/h in the control group ($P < 0.001$). Time on IABP and time on mechanical ventilation were significantly shorter in the L-NAME group [31].

Real World Question Why is the Mortality in Shock from RV Infarction High?

In the case of hypotension secondary to RV infarction, usually the patient has an occluded RCA proximal to the major RV branches and presents with an inferior MI with or without recognized RV failure [32,33]. The clinical presentation ranges from asymptomatic mild RV dysfunction, through CS. Most patients demonstrate a return of normal RV function over a period of weeks to months, suggesting RV stunning has occurred rather than irreversible necrosis [34].

CRITICAL THINKING

Right ventricular infarction in the SHOCK trial. Investigators at the SHOCK registry evaluated 49 patients with CS predominantly due to RV infarction, and compared them with 884 patients with CS and predominantly LV failure. Their in-hospital mortality of patients with RV shock was similar to patients with LV shock (53% vs. 61%, $P = 0.296$), despite the fact that patients with RV shock were younger, with a lower prevalence of previous infarctions, fewer anterior infarct locations, and less multivessel disease. There was a shorter median time between index infarction and diagnosis of shock in patients with RV shock. In multivariate analysis, RV shock was not an independent predictor of lower in-hospital mortality [35].

The severity of the hemodynamic derangements associated with RV ischemia is related to factors listed in Table 3.15 [33].

Table 3.15 Factors influencing the hemodynamic status of RV infarction.

1. The extent of ischemia and subsequent RV dysfunction
2. The restraining effect of the surrounding pericardium
3. The interventricular dependence related to the shared interventricular septum

RV, right ventricle.

When the RV becomes ischemic, it acutely dilates, resulting in an increased intrapericardial pressure caused by the restraining forces of the pericardium. As a consequence, there is a reduction in RV systolic pressure and output, decreased LV preload, a reduction in LV end-diastolic dimension and stroke volume, and a shifting of the interventricular septum toward the LV [36]. Because of this RV systolic and diastolic dysfunction, the pressure gradient between the right and left atria becomes an important driving force for pulmonary perfusion. Factors that reduce preload (volume depletion, diuretics, nitrates) or diminish augmented right atrial contraction (concomitant atrial infarction, loss of AV synchrony), as well as factors that increase RV afterload (concomitant LV dysfunction), are likely to have profoundly adverse hemodynamic effects [37]. The importance of a paradoxical interventricular septal motion that bulges in piston like fashion into the RV, is important in generating systolic force, which allows pulmonary perfusion. The loss of this compensatory mechanism with concomitant septal infarction may result in further deterioration in patients with RV ischemia [38].

A right atrial pressure of 10 mmHg or greater and greater than 80% of pulmonary wedge pressure is a relatively sensitive and specific finding in patients with RV infarction [39]. The waveform of the right atrium shows a steep right atrial Y descent and an early diastolic dip and plateau in the RV waveform.

Demonstration of 1 mm ST-segment elevation in the right precordial lead V4R is the single most predictive electrocardiographic finding in patients with RV infarction [40]. The finding may be transient; half of patients show resolution of ST elevation within 10 hours of onset of symptoms [41]. Echocardiography can be helpful in patients with suspicious but non-diagnostic findings. It can show RV dilation and asynergy, abnormal interventricular and interatrial septal motion, and even right to left shunting through a patent foramen ovale [42]. The treatment of RV infarction is highlighted in Table 3.16.

Table 3.16 Management of right ventricular infarction [43].

1. Early maintenance of RV preload
2. Reduction of RV afterload
3. Inotropic support of the dysfunctional right ventricle
4. Early pharmacological and percutaneous mechanical reperfusion

RV, right ventricular.

Because of their influence on preload, drugs routinely used in management of LV infarctions, such as nitrates and diuretics, may reduce cardiac output and produce severe hypotension when the RV is ischemic. Indeed, a common clinical presentation for RV infarction is profound hypotension following administration of sublingual nitroglycerin, with the degree of hypotension often out of proportion to the ECG-severity of the infarct. Volume loading with normal saline alone often resolves accompanying hypotension and improves cardiac output [44]. In other cases, volume loading further elevates the right-sided filling pressure and RV dilatation, resulting in decreased LV output [45]. Although volume loading is a critical first step in the management of hypotension associated with RV ischemia, inotropic support (in particular, dobutamine) should be initiated promptly if cardiac output fails to improve after 0.5–1 L of fluid has been given. Another important factor for sustaining adequate RV preload is maintenance of AV synchrony. High-degree heart block is common, occurring in as many as half of these patients [46]. Atrioventricular sequential pacing leads to a significant increase in cardiac output and reversal of shock, even when ventricular pacing alone has not been of benefit [47]. Atrial fibrillation may occur in up to one-third of patients with RV ischemia [48] and has profound hemodynamic effects. Prompt cardioversion from atrial fibrillation should be considered at the earliest sign of hemodynamic compromise. When LV dysfunction accompanies RV ischemia, the RV is further compromised because of increased RV afterload and reduction in stroke volume [49]. In such circumstances, the use of afterload-reducing agents such as sodium nitroprusside or an intra-aortic counterpulsation device is often necessary to "unload" the left and subsequently the RV.

Take Home Message

While treating a patient with AMI, the main principle is to avoid hypotension leading to tissue hypoperfusion. It is easier for the auxiliary and nursing staff to detect a declining BP at earliest by setting and monitoring the frequent BP measurements with the automatic cuffs which can give false results because of peripheral vasoconstriction. The patient should be observed carefully to detect early signs of declining BP and raising HR, all harbingers of possible and imminent CS. However, they can sound false alarms too. In a sizable minority of patients, there is no hypotension at all even they have signs of peripheral hypoperfusion which is a more sensitive and prognostic marker for imminent hemodynamic collapse or death. Once there is sign of declining BP and raising HR, pre-emptive measures should be put in place to avoid the spiraling effect of further hypotension. If these measures fail, then clinical shock without invasive evidence of tissue hypoperfusion will follow. At this juncture there is still time and opportunity to aggressively reverse the declining BP by PCI or CABG so the patient does not deteriorate into tissue hypoperfusion. Once hypoperfusion is evident, frank CS will be fully developed. Then it is too late because with the best intentions, efforts and interventions, only a lowest mortality of 66% can be achieved.

References

1 Hochman JS, Buller C, Sleeper L et al. for the SHOCK Investigators. Cardiogenic shock complicating AMI-Etiologies, management and outcome: A report from the SHOCK trial registry. J Am Coll Cardiol 2000;36:1063–1070.
2 Holmes D, Bates E, Kleiman N et al. Contemporary reperfusion therapy for cardiogenic shock: The GUSTO-I trial experience. J Am Coll Cardiol 1995;26:668–674.
3 Menon V, Slater J, White H et al. AMI complicated by systemic hypoperfusion without hypotension. A report from the SHOCK trial registry. Am J Med 2000;108:374–380.
4 Lindholm MG, Køber L, Boesgaard S et al. Cardiogenic shock complicating acute myocardial infarction; prognostic impact of early and late shock development. Eur Heart J 2003;24(3):258–265.
5 Kosuge M, Kimura K. Ishikawa T et al. Implications of the absence of ST-segment elevation in lead V4R in patients who have inferior wall AMI with right ventricular involvement. Clin Cardiol 2001;24:225–230.
6 White HD, Palmeri ST, Sleeper LA et al. Electrocardiographic Findings in Cardiogenic Shock, Risk Prediction, and the Effects of Emergency Revascularization: Results From the SHOCK Trial. Am Heart J 2004;148(5):810–817.
7 Picard MH, Davidoff R, Sleeper LA et al. Echocardiographic predictors of survival and response to early revascularization in cardiogenic shock. Circulation 2003;107(2):279–284.

8 Forrester JS, Diamond GA, Swan JS. Correlative classification of clinical and hemo-dynamic function after AMI. Am J Cardiol 1977;39:137–145.

9 Antman E. Braunwald E. Acute Myocardial Infarction, pp. 1184–1288. In: Braunwald E, Editor, Heart Disease, a textbook of cardiovascular medicine, 5th edition. WB Saunders Philadephia; 1997.

10 Sanford CF, Corbett J, Nicod P *et al.* Value of radionuclide ventriculography in the imme-diate characterization of patients with AMI. Am J Cardiol 1982;49:637–644.

11 Hasdai D, Holmes DR Jr, Califf RM *et al.* Cardiogenic shock complicating AMI: Predictors of death. Am Heart J 1999;138:21–31.

12 Hochman JS, Sleeper LA, Webb JG *et al.* Early revascularization in acute myocardial infarc-tion complicated by cardiogenic shock. SHOCK Investigators. Should We Emergently Revascularize Occluded Coronaries for Cardiogenic Shock. NEJM 1999;341:625–634.

13 Wong SC, Sanborn T, Sleeper LA *et al.* Angiographic findings and clinical correlates in patients with cardiogenic shock complicating AMI: A report from the SHOCK trial reg-istry. J Am Coll Cardiol 2000;36:1077–1083.

14 Calvo FE, Figueras J, Cortadellas J *et al.* Severe mitral regurgitation complicating AMI. Clinical and angiographic differences between patients with and without papillary mus-cle rupture. Eur Heart J 1997;18(10):1606–1610.

15 Sanborn T, Sleeper LA, Bates E *et al.* Impact of thrombolysis, intra-aortic balloon pump counterpulsation and their combination in cardiogenic shock complicating AMI: A report from the SHOCK trial registry. J Am Coll Cardiol 2000;36:1123–1129.

16 Hochman JS, Sleeper LA, Godfrey E *et al.* for the SHOCK trial study group. Should we revascularize occluded coronaries for cardiogenic shock: An international randomized trial of emergency PTCA/CABG trial design. Am Heart J 1999;137:313–321.

17 White HD;Assmann SF;Sanborn TA *et al.* Comparison of percutaneous coronary interven-tion and coronary artery bypass grafting after acute myocardial infarction complicated by cardiogenic shock:results from the Should We Emergently Revascularize Occluded Coronaries for Cardiogenic Shock (SHOCK) trial. Circulation 2005;112(13):1992–2001.

18 Webb JG, Lowe AM, Sanborn TA *et al.* Percutaneous coronary intervention for cardio-genic shock in the SHOCK trial. J Am Coll Cardiol 2003;42(8):1380–1386.

19 Movahed MR, Balian H, Moraghebi P. Reversible severe ischemic MR and cardiogenic shock as a complication of percutaneous coronary intervention. J Invasive Cardiol 2005; 17(2):104–107.

20 Menon V, Webb J, Hillis D *et al.* Outcome and profile of ventricular septal rupture with cardiogenic shock after MI: A report from the SHOCK trial registry. J Am Coll Cardiol 2000;36:1110–1116.

21 Braunwald E. Acute myocardial infarction, pp. 19–42. In: Nguyen T, Hu D, Editors, Advances and challenges in today's cardiology. Griffith Publishing, Caldwell ID, 1997.

22 Moore CA, Nygaard TW, Kaiser DL *et al.* Postinfarction ventricular septal rupture: The importance of location of infarction and right ventricular function in determining sur-vival. Circulation 1986;74:45–55.

23 Oliva PB, Hammill SC, Edwards WD. Cardiac rupture, a clinically predictable compli-cation of AMI:report of 70 cases with clinicapathologic correlations. J Am Coll Cardiol 1993;22:72–76.

24 Slater J, Brown RJ, Antonelli TA *et al.* Cardiogenic shock due to cardiac free-wall rupture and tamponade after AMI: A report from the SHOCK trial registry. J Am Coll Cardiol 2000;36:1117–1122.

25 Lopez-Sendon J, Gonzalez A, Lopez de Sa E *et al.* Diagnosis of subacute ventricular wall rupture after AMI: Sensitivity and specificity of clinical, hemodynamic, and echocardio-graphic criteria. J Am Coll Cardiol 1992;19:1145–1153.

26 Klein LW, Shaw RE, Krone RJ *et al*. Mortality after emergent percutaneous coronary intervention in cardiogenic shock secondary to acute myocardial infarction and usefulness of a mortality prediction model. Am J Cardiol 2005;96(1):35–41.

27 Jacobs A, French JK, Col J *et al*. Cardiogenic shock with non-ST segment elevation MI: A report from the SHOCK trial registry. J Am Coll Cardiol 2000:36:1091–1096.

28 Hochman JS, Sleeper LA, White H *et al*. One-year survival following early revascularization for cardiogenic shock. JAMA 2001;285:190–192.

29 Tcheng JE, Jackman JD Jr, Nelson CL *et al*. Outcome of patients sustaining acute ischemic mitral regurgitation during AMI. Ann Intern Med 1992;117(1):18–24.

30 Lim N, Dubois MJ, De Backer D. Do all nonsurvivors of cardiogenic shock die with a low cardiac index? Chest 2003;124(5):1885–1891.

31 Cotter G, Kaluski E, Milo O *et al*. LINCS:L-NAME (a NO synthase inhibitor) in the treatment of refractory cardiogenic shock: A prospective randomized study. Eur Heart J 2003; 24(14):1287–1295.

32 Eagle K, Guyton G *et al*. ACC/AHA Guidelines for Coronary Artery Bypass Graft Surgery. JACC 1999;34(4):1262–1347. Recommendations of the ACC/AHA Task Force in order to decrease morbidity and mortality in patients undergoing CABG. Circulation 1999;100: 1464–1480.

33 Roberts N, Harisson DG, Reimer KA *et al*. Right ventricular infarction with shock without significant LV infarction: A new clinical syndrome. Am Heart J 1985;110: 1047–1053.

34 Bowers TR, O'Neill WW, Grines C *et al*. Effect of reperfusion on biventricular function and survival after right ventricular infarction. N Engl J Med 1998;338:933–940.

35 Jacobs A *et al*. J Am Coll Cardiol 2003;341:1273–1279. *And* Pfisterer M. Right ventricular involvement in myocardial infarction and cardiogenic shock. Lancet 2003;362(9381): 392–394.

36 Goldstein JA, Vlahakes GJ, Verrier ED *et al*. The role of right ventricular systolic dysfunction and elevated intrapericardial pressure in the genesis of low output in experimental right ventricular infarction. Circulation 1982;65:513–522.

37 Goldstein JA, Tweddell JS, Barzilai B, Yagi Y, Jaffe AS, Cox JL. Importance of left ventricular function and systolic ventricular interaction to right ventricular performance during acute right heart ischemia. J Am Coll Cardiol 1992;19:704–711.

38 Goldstein JA, Barzilai B, Rosamond TL, Eisenberg PR, Jaffe AS. Determinants of hemodynamic compromise with severe right ventricular infarction. Circulation 1990;82:359–368.

39 Cohn JN, Guiha NH, Broder MI, Limas CJ. Right ventricular infarction:clinical and hemodynamic features. Am J Cardiol 1974;33:209–214.

40 Robalino BD, Whitlow PL, Underwood DA, Salcedo EE. Electrocardiographic manifestations of right ventricular infarction. Am Heart J 1989;118:138–144.

41 Braat SH, Brugada P, De Zwaan C, Coenegracht JM, Wellens HJ. Value of electrocardiogram in diagnosing right ventricular involvement in patients with an acute inferior wall myocardial infarction. Br Heart J 1983;49:368–372.

42 Sharkey SW, Shelley W, Carlyle PF, Rysavy J, Cohn JN. M-mode and two-dimensional echocardiographic analysis of the septum in experimental right ventricular infarction:correlation with hemodynamic alterations. Am Heart J 1985;110:1210–1218.

43 Kinch JW, Ryan TJ. Right ventricular infarction. N Engl J Med 1994;330:1211–1217.

44 Goldstein JA, Vlahakes GJ, Verrier ED *et al*. Volume loading improves low cardiac output in experimental right ventricular infarction. J Am Coll Cardiol 1983;2:270–278.

45 Dell'Italia LJ, Starling MR, Blumhardt R, Lasher JC, O'Rourke RA. Comparative effects of volume loading, dobutamine, and nitroprusside in patients with predominant right ventricular infarction. Circulation 1985;72:1327–1335.

46 Braat SH, De Zwaan C, Brugada P, Coenegracht JM, Wellens HJ. Right ventricular involvement with acute inferior wall myocardial infarction identifies high risk of developing atrioventricular nodal conduction disturbances. Am Heart J 1984;107:1183–1187.

47 Love JC, Haffajee CI, Gore JM, Alpert JS. Reversibility of hypotension and shock by atrial or atrioventricular sequential pacing in patients with right ventricular infarction. Am Heart J 1984;108:5–13.

48 Sugiura T, Iwasaka T, Takahashi N *et al.* Atrial fibrillation in inferior wall Q-wave acute myocardial infarction. Am J Cardiol 1991;67:1135–1136.

49 Fantidis P, Castejon R, Fernandez Ruiz A, Madero-Jarabo R, Cordovilla G, Sanz Galeote E. Does a critical hemodynamic situation develop from right ventriculotomy and free wall infarct or from small changes in dysfunctional right ventricle afterload? J Cardiovasc Surg (Torino) 1992;33:229–234.

CHAPTER 4

Coronary Artery Bypass Graft Surgery

Thach N. Nguyen, David Jayakar, Felix Gozo and Vijay Dave

Introduction: Scope of the Problems

In 2005, there were more than 250,000 patients undergoing coronary artery bypass (CABG) surgery in the US. Their mortality rate is supposed to be low, their length of stay short, and their outcomes rosy. According to the standards set by economists and printed as a financial transaction on the Federal Register [1], these patients are to be programmed to ambulate cheerfully 24 hours after surgery and to walk out of the hospital three days later. This sequence of engineered events becomes the mantra of third party payers, government, health administration bureaucrats, Wall Street movers and shakers. However, these ideal standards can be applied only to simple and non-complicated cases. The high risk patients have higher morbidities, mortalities and length of stay (LOS) even with the ideal management by the best surgical team [2]. The economists and statisticians just ignore them as they do not exist in their lexicon. These CABG programs are to be marketed as financially robust, profitably managed, and surgically competitive so that the network administrator can eagerly negotiate and grasp for more contracts to service more covered lives covered by the insurance companies, health maintenance organizations, preferred provider organization, point-per-service providers, or traditional service payors etc [3]. The end results is that many doctors and hospitals concentrate their efforts only on low risk patients who constitute a minority of patients undergoing CABG. The trial lawyers also claim they are the only one who show concern, however retrospectively, about the lives and well-being of these patients. In the middle of the deafening cacophony of claims and counterclaims, between the shoutings or whisperings of the open or secret bargainings, in the midst of the frantic tradings on the big board or small screen; only the physicians (cardiologists, cardiac surgeons, family physicians, internists, anesthesiologists, pulmonologists, neurologists, physiatrists, etc.) and the operating room (OR) and intensive care unit (ICU) technical and nursing staff labor from dawn to dusk, to create conduits, direct blood flows, revitalize hibernating myocardium, re-energize the heart and restore physical activities to each individual patient. The quality assurance committee of the cardiology section and the surgery department of the local hospital has to monitor the case individually and prospectively, in order to assure that the outcomes are best by its circumstances; that preventable errors are indeed prevented; and that the statistical results are accurate and acceptable to federal regulators, hospital, and third-party monitors as they are reported on the internet (not to the Interpol) and printed on the medical or lay press, (rather on the Congress mandated Data Bank report). The four problems encountered and to be overcome by physicians during and after CABG are: higher than expected mortality, stroke, renal dysfunction and mediastinitis (Table 4.1).

Table 4.1 Management strategies for patients undergoing coronary artery bypass surgery.

1. Screen patients so the high risk patients can be focused for better preparation before CABG
2. Stabilize the patients with maximal medical therapy prior to CABG
3. Over-utilize myocardial protection measures during surgery
4. Lower the rate of stroke due to aortic manipulation
5. Early extubation, early physical ambulation and rehabilitation

CABG, coronary artery bypass (surgery).

Mortality

According to the data from the Society of Thoracic Surgeons (STS), for a mixed group of patients undergoing CABG, the overall 30-day mortality is 3%, which is the average from much higher mortality of high risk patients and nearly zero mortality of very low risk patients [4]. The clinical outcomes documented by the STS are listed in Table 4.2 [5]. However, these rates are meaningful only if the levels of severity are taken into account, so they are readjusted as risk-adjusted mortality rates. The most common cause of death is left ventricular (LV) failure (80%) while the most common complications with subsequent high fatality are stroke, mediastinitis or postoperative renal dysfunction (PRD).

Table 4.2 Clinical outcomes of coronary artery bypass surgery.

Mortality (%)	2.8
Deep sternal wound infection (%)	0.6
Re-operation (%)	4.9
Permanent stroke (%)	1.6
Prolonged ventilation (%)	5.4
Renal failure (%)	3.3
Post-operative length of stay	6.3 days
Re-admission rate <30 days (%)	8.9

Source: RH Jones [6], and www.cms.hhs.gov/regulations/ecomments

Stroke

The social and emotional impact of stroke on the CABG patient, family, medical and surgical team is devastating. In the post-CABG patients, the neurological deficits are divided into 2 types: type 1 deficits with major, focal neurological deficits, stupor, or coma; and type 2 deficits with cognitive decline [7]. The incidence of type 1 deficit is 3.1% with an in-hospital mortality of 24% [8]. The incidence of type 2 deficits was 50% at discharge, and 24% at 6 months [9]. The predictors of neurological deficit type 1 are listed in Table 4.3 [10]. The main culprit is the mobile plaque in the ascending aorta which is manipulated during surgery.

Table 4.3 Predictors of type 1 neurologic deficits.

1. Proximal aortic atherosclerosis (OR 4.52)
2. Prior CVA (OR 3.19)
3. IABP (OR 2.60)
4. Diabetes (OR 2.59)
5. History of hypertension (OR 2.31)
6. History of unstable angina (OR 1.83)
7. Age (OR 1.75 per decade)
8. Perioperative hypotension
9. Use of ventricular venting

CVA, cerebro-vascular accident; IABP, intra-aortic balloon pump.

Renal Dysfunction

Postoperative renal dysfunction (PRD) is defined as a postoperative serum creatinine level = 2.0 mg/dL or an increase in the serum creatinine level of 0.7 mg/dL from the preoperative to maximum postoperative values [11]. PRD occurred in 7.7% of all patients, of whom 1.4% will eventually require dialysis. The in-hospital mortality rates were low in patients with normal renal function and extremely high in patients with PRD (Table 4.4) [12].

Table 4.4 Mortality rate of patients with renal dysfunction.

Renal function	*Mortality rate*
Normal renal function	0.9%
PRD without dialysis	19%
PRD with dialysis	63%

PRD, postoperative renal dysfunction.

Measurement of serum creatinine alone should not be used to assess the level of preoperative kidney function. The glomerular filtration rate (GFR) is more accurate in reflecting the risk of postoperative complications. The National Kidney Foundation recommends using either the MDRD (Modification of Diet in Renal Disease) or the Cockcroft–Gault equation to calculate the GFR. The MDRD equation performs better than the Cockcroft–Gault equation. It can be calculated according to the instructions from the website www.kidney.org/professionals/kdoqi/gfr_calculator.cfm

This calculator takes into consideration the plasma creatinine level, age of the patient, race of the patient, and gender. Knowing the GFR before surgery could help the physicians to better plan the operative and postoperative strategy.

Several preoperative risk factors for PRD were identified and included advanced age, moderate to severe congestive heart failure (CHF), prior CABG, type 1 diabetes mellitus, and pre-existing renal disease (preoperative creatinine levels between 1.4–2.0 mg/dL).

Elderly patients are more prone for PRD, because their kidneys have a greater reduction in functioning nephrons, so they are more vulnerable to the maldistribution of renal blood flow, the increase in renal vascular resistance, and the decrease in total renal blood flow and glomerular filtration rate during CABG [13].

Mediastinitis

Deep sternal wound infection has been reported to occur in 1–4% of patients and carries a mortality rate of nearly 25% [4,14]. Obesity is a strong correlate of mediastinitis after CABG [15]. In these obese patients, the causes of easy infection are frequent: antibiotics may be poorly distributed in adipose tissue; it is difficult to maintain sterility in the multiple skin folds; large regions of adipose tissue serve as an ideal substrate for bacteria multiplication and represent a clinical challenge for early detection if infected.

Diabetic patients are more vulnerable to infection due to microvascular changes, and slow wound healing from elevated blood glucose levels [16]. Higher risk of infection is also due to re-operation which requires additional dissection, longer perfusion times, more bleeding, and greater need for transfusion [17]. The use of both internal mammary arteries (IMA) and excessive use of electrocautery for hemostasis may predispose to devascularization of the sternum and promotes infection, especially when combined with other risk factors such as diabetes and/or obesity [18].

Strategies to Decrease Morbidity and Mortality

Identify the High Risk Patients

In order to identify the factors influencing mortality and morbidity, many cardiac surgery databases developed in the 1970's were analyzed for variables [19,20]. The most common use of large cardiovascular databases has been to compare risk-adjusted expected with observed mortality, to monitor the quality of care of institutions and their providers [7].

A few core variables were found to contain larger amount of prognostic information with the greatest predictive power [21]. They relate to the urgency of operation, advanced age, and prior coronary bypass surgery, while the variables describing coronary anatomy had the least predictive power (Table 4.5).

Table 4.5 Core variables and relative risks.

1. Urgency of operation (2.0–7.4)
2. Older age (2.1–3.9)
3. Prior CABG (1.7–3.6)
4. Female gender (1.2–1.63)
5. LV ejection fraction less than 30% (2.89)
6. Left main artery disease (1.3–1.43)
7. Number of diseased vessels with greater than 70% stenosis (1.6)

CABG, coronary artery bypass surgery; LV, left ventricular.

The EuroSCORE

The EuroSCORE (European System for Cardiac Operative Risk Evaluation) involved the greatest possible number of patients in its development – more than 19,000 consecutive patients were studied in 128 centers in eight European countries [22]. The database was subjected to multiple regression analysis to decide which risk factors were associated with operative mortality, and weights were allocated to each risk factor. Selected for availability and measurability, all but four of the risk factors are derived from the patient's clinical status. While developed as a risk model for European adult cardiac surgery, investigators considered whether EuroSCORE also was applicable in North American cardiac surgical patients. Using the STS database, EuroSCORE was applied to predictive mortality in 188,913 surgical patients in 1995, and 401,684 patients undergoing coronary or valve surgery in 1998 and 1999 [22]. Despite some significant differences in risk factor prevalence between the EuroSCORE and STS databases, EuroSCORE predicted mortality was virtually identical to observed mortality. This predictive power was maintained when patients were divided into quintiles of equal risk [22]. By the EuroSCORE, the variables which predict best outcomes are listed in Table 4.6. The logistic regression model of EuroSCORE showed these to be the core variables. It is evident that ventricular septal rupture (post myocardial infarction (MI)), thoracic aortic surgery, active endocarditis, low ejection fraction (EF) $<30\%$, and previous surgery top the list (Table 4.6).

Table 4.6 Logistic regression model of EuroSCORE.

Ventricular septal rupture	1.4620090
Thoracic aortic surgery	1.1597870
Active endocarditis	1.1012650
LVEF $<30\%$	1.0944430
Previous cardiac surgery	1.0026250
Critical preoperative state	0.9058132
Neurological dysfunction	0.8416260
Systolic PAP >60 mmHg	0.7676924
Emergency operation	0.7127953
Extracardiac arteriopathy	0.6558917
Serum creatinine >200 Mol/L	0.6521653
Unstable angina	0.5677075
Recent MI	0.5460218
Other than isolated coronary surgery	0.5420364
Pulmonary disease	0.4931341
LVEF 30–50%	0.4191643
Female	0.3304052
Age (continuous)	0.0666354

Constant $=$ 0–4.789594.
LVEF, left ventricular ejection fraction; PAP, pulmonary artery pressure
Full definition of these variables are published and can be seen online at www.euroscore.org

Applying this important information to real world practice, the patients with high risk were identified preoperatively and received more focused perioperative and intra-operative management. Subsequently, their mortality rates have decreased although their expected mortality increased. Therefore, the ability to predict outcome with traditional risk factors has diminished, as the results of the outcomes were subjectively altered and statistically changed.

Identification of the Local Risk Factors

In general, in order to decrease morbidities, mortality and LOS of a CABG program, the first task is to identify the high risk factors derived from predicted probability models of the surgical and medical databases. They are classified according to their degree of importance and priority reflecting the magnitude of morbidities and mortality affecting a local CABG program [23]. They should be identified as concrete and correctable abnormal laboratory numbers and clinical conditions. The cardiologists, cardiac surgeons and anesthesiologists can stay focused on screening these exact abnormal, clinical situations and allocate more time and resources in correcting them before, during and after surgery. These risk factors vary from one hospital to another and from year to year, as one risk factor is controlled and another rises more prominently. Continued efforts are required for better understanding and detection of these ever changing risk factors [24].

Estimate of the Mortality Risk of Each Individual Patient

If the overall risk for an institution or region is known, then a general estimate for the individual patient can be rendered preoperatively by using mathematical models or the EUROScore. This concrete application may help the patients and their physicians in weighing the potential vs. risks of proceeding with isolated CABG and to correct any abnormalities prior to surgery [25]. The patients undergoing cardiac catheterization should have their projected surgical risks calculated. If any patient then needs CABG, the cardiologists have the data handy to discuss the risk of CABG with the patient, family and surgeon. If the risk is too high, then the patient can be transferred to a larger tertiary center or CABG should be cancelled in favor of medical therapy only [25].

Management with Concrete Solutions

Once the high risk patients are identified, appropriate management requires systematic preoperative, intraoperative, and postoperative approaches. In order to implement effectively these strategies, communication, collaboration and education is required for surgeons, cardiologists, anesthetists, perfusionists, surgical resident-in training, intensive care unit nurses, respiratory therapists, cardiac rehabilitation staff, social workers, and case managers. Weekly meetings address every aspects of problems arising in the cardiac surgical service; separate weekly morbidity and mortality conferences are held. The leadership or coordinating team establishes critical pathways and monitors them. Critical pathways must be constructed internally, not imposed externally. Periodic retreats for staff education on the guidelines, pathways, and to make all practice as consistent and uniform as possible, should be established [26]. The consistency and uniformity of guidelines and pathways will decrease the potential for breakdown of communication between medical and nursing staff. However, in some hospitals, as the staff are focusing on prevention and correction of problems in high risk patients, the management of average- or low-risk patients is put on autopilot and there can be complication. The strategies for improving morbidity and mortality with practical action plans are listed in Table 4.7 [27].

Table 4.7 Strategies to reduce complication and mortality.

Discriminative selection and deselection
1. Reduce the volume of too-high-risk patients
2. Reduce the volume of complications with high fatality
3. Acceptable age-group distribution with preference for younger age; avoid extreme old age

Maximize medical condition
1. Stabilize unstable patients with maximal medical treatment in order to convert urgent cases into elective surgery

Focus care on high-risk patients
1. Identify target patient groups and correct their medical problems before, during and after surgery
2. Take pre- and intra-operative measures to decrease stroke
3. Preferably have off-pump bypass
4. Intra-operative measures to avoid unplanned return to OR
5. Better myoprotection by intra-operative initiatives with anesthesia

Identify windows of opportunity and target patient groups to decrease LOS
1. Off-pump bypass
2. Critical pathways
3. preoperative education of patient and family about the fast tract exercise, rehabilitation and discharge

LOS, length of stay; OR, operating room.

Thorough preoperative evaluation and management

Patient care in cardiac surgery begins with a thorough and precise diagnostic evaluation to define the anatomy and hemodynamic abnormalities of that particular patient. Although an evaluation has usually been performed by the referring cardiologist, it is the surgeon's responsibility to ensure that the evaluation is complete and that all the information needed to plan and perform the proposed surgery is obtained. In addition to developing an operative plan, the surgeon must also identify the patient's coexisting diseases to minimize their risk on surgical outcome. Recently, there has been the shift toward outpatient preoperative management of elective cardiac surgical patients that can complicate the preoperative preparation process. Because the patient is not admitted to the hospital until the day of the operation, it is important to develop a system that ensures that all preoperative issues are addressed prior to the time of surgery. This includes a comprehensive preoperative history and physical examination, risk assessment, abnormal laboratories values (checked and corrected) and patient teaching regarding the planned operation.

Reduce the volume of high risk patients

The outcomes of CABG depend on many modifiable, and many uncontrolled factors. Age, sex, and concomitant valvular replacement cannot be changed.

However, technical skills, experience of surgeons and the surgical teams, severity of co-morbidities can be altered with more training, more resources, more manpower and more focused management before, during and after surgery. In a small CABG program, it is may be wise to avoid the too-severe, moribund patients as their mortality is indeed too high with either medical or surgical management. CABG cannot save every patient with end-stage coronary artery disease (CAD), refractory primary coronary interventions (PCI) with poor LV function, and lack of bypassable run-offs. If the patient is really high risk, then the patient should be transferred to a larger referral center, with more experience, more manpower and higher patient load to dilute the high mortality rate of these extremely sick patients. There are a few surgeons and centers in the US who specialize on difficult cases with third or fourth re-operations. With their experience, and because of their exceptional focus on high risk cases, with the help of a dedicated team, their results are quite impressive. The patients whom a small program should avoid are listed in Table 4.8.

Table 4.8 High risk patients to be avoided in a small coronary artery bypass surgery program.

1. Cardiogenic shock
2. Double valve replacement
3. CABG and aortic root repair
4. LVEF <20%.
5. Redo CABG (possibly second, definitely third or fourth operation)
6. AMI

AMI, acute myocardial infarction; CABG, coronary artery bypass surgery; LVEF, left ventricular ejection fraction.

Medical stabilization before surgery

The medically high risk patient needs excellent stabilization of their medical problems before surgery. As any patient who undergoes surgery, the patient should be on β-blocker. If the patient has LV dysfunction, then angiotensin converting enzyme inhibitors (ACEI) should be given. The patient should be on antiplatelet therapy while waiting for CABG. The patient should be stable and be at a fair New York Heart Association (NYHA) functional level. The medications and exercise schedules would strengthen the patient and speed up the recovery after CABG. If the patient has recent MI, Non-Q MI, or a stroke, then the patient should wait for one month to recover well before undergoing CABG. It is better to convert the urgent case into an elective case.

Intra-operative modifications for high risk patients

During CABG, stress to the myocardium can be caused by the operation itself, ischemia, reperfusion, and cardiopulmonary bypass so there is a need to limit injury to myocardium (so-called myocardial protection). One essential component of myocardial protection is ventricular decompression. The left ventricle may become distended during cardio-pulmonary bypass (CPB), most commonly between ventricular fibrillation; this may impair myocardial perfusion, particularly in the subendocardial region. Prevention of this complication requires venting of the left ventricle using a cannula through the superior pulmonary vein, the left atrium, the mitral valve and then the left ventricle.

A variety of cardioplegia additives have been proposed to enhance myocardial protection, however, none have been proved to be effective. Most often, cardioplegia is administered at a low temperature to reduce myocardial oxygen consumption. It should be administered immediately after induction of aortic cross-clamping to reduce myocardial ischemia.

However, systemic hypothermia might be superior to cold local cardioplegia alone, possibly due to better maintenance of myocardial cooling. Intermittent topical cold hypothermia provides additional and constant myocardial protection to the ventricle.

During surgery, the patient is given heparin so frequent monitoring of anticoagulation should be carried out. Activated clotting time (ACT) is measured before and after administration of heparin, and should be at least 400 seconds. After surgery, heparin is reversed by protamine: this is why during surgery, heparin resistance and heparin induced thrombocytopenia should always be in mind and watched while protamine reaction should also be observed closely during heparin reversal.

Off-pump bypass

The extensive blood device interface intrinsic to the cardiopulmonary bypass equipment results in a profound inflammatory response. The result is activation of clotting factors requiring heparinization, blood loss and red blood cell (RBC) destruction. The Off-Pump Coronary Artery Bypass (OPCAB) involves a sternotomy, but the patient is not placed on cardiopulmonary bypass. The surgeon operates on a beating heart. The published results showed lower incidence of neurologic dysfunction, renal failure, bleeding complications, low cardiac output syndrome and in general lower mortality in high risk patients. However, no matter how much science progresses, the results of surgical or interventional procedures depend on the skill of the surgeon/operator. There were conflicting data about the benefits of OPCAB.

CRITICAL THINKING

OPCAB or CABG, which one is better? A retrospective review revealed that patients who underwent OPCAB had significantly different clinical characteristics compared with those who underwent standard CABG. The patients who underwent OPCAB tended to be older; women; have low EF; had undergone previous CABG; and had a history of prior stroke, peripheral vascular disease, CHF, calcified aortic disease, and renal failure. On the contrary, the patients who underwent standard CABG tended to have had MI, shock, cardiopulmonary resuscitation, left main disease, and more diseased arteries. The propensity-matched retrospective studies suggest that patients who underwent OPCAB tended to have fewer postoperative bleeding complications (including transfusions and re-operations for bleeding), and lower incidence of early neurocognitive dysfunction. The propensity-matched retrospective studies suggest that patients who underwent standard CABG tended to have lower rates of subsequent revascularization procedures, including both percutaneous and repeat open procedures. There are conflicting data regarding mortality, but no strong differences apparent between OPCAB and standard CABG. The meta-analyses also suggest lower rates of postoperative bleeding and stroke associated with OPCAB, but higher rates of subsequent revascularization procedures [28].

In general, patients can expect good outcomes with either procedure, and an individual's outcomes likely depend more on factors other than whether they underwent standard CABG or OPCAB. A large, multicenter, prospective, randomized study that includes patients at higher risk (multivessel or left main disease, impaired LV systolic function) is necessary to better evaluate for differences between the two strategies [28].

Intra-aortic balloon pump
The use of prophylactic IABP as an adjunct to myocardial protection may decrease mortality and overall resource utilization in certain high risk patients. However, the patients who really need IABP are sicker then the stable one who does need any hemodynamic support [4].

Leukocyte depletion
Appreciation of the role of the activated leukocyte in the genesis and exacerbation of myocardial reperfusion injury has led to strategies to remove leukocytes from the coronary blood flow. Clinical studies of leukocyte depletion have shown significant benefit to myocardial performance in the hypertrophied LV and in those with acute or chronic ischemia [29]. Preliminary data seems to support that filtering out leukocytes prior to blood transfusion may reduce the number of postoperative pulmonary infection in high risk patients such as patients with severe COPD and low EF [4].

Internal mammary artery graft
The long-term survival benefit afforded by use of the IMA is well recognized [4]. Less appreciated is the reduction in immediate, operative mortality associated with the use of the mammary artery as opposed to saphenous revascularization. Its use should be encouraged in the elderly [30], the emergent/acutely ischemic patient, and other subgroups that previously were thought not to receive its immediate and long-term benefit. In the large, coronary bypass database available to the STS [31], use of the IMA was associated with reduced operative mortality in all analyzed subgroups.

Graft injury and embolization in re-operative patients

For patients undergoing repeated CABG surgery who previously have had a left IMA-to-LAD (left anterior descending artery) graft, a concern has been the inadvertent transection of the graft during sternotomy [4]. This complication is rare at <3% [32]. The risk of death or serious myocardial dysfunction related to atheroembolism from patent, diseased saphenous vein grafts is high [32]. To avoid these technical catastrophes, the patient should have a CT scan of the chest prior to surgery to visualize the grafts and relationship of the right ventricle, atrium, heart tissues to the sternum. If they are attached to the sternum, alternate surgical strategies (right or left chest thoracotomy), femoral vessel cannulation, etc., could help to prevent injury to these SVGs.

Cardioplegia could be delivered in a retrograde fashion, excluding the atherosclerotic SVGs thus avoiding any chance of distal embolization.

Reducing the risk of perioperative infection

Multiple opportunities exist for infection-risk neutralization in coronary bypass patients [4]. Skin and nasopharyngeal Gram-positive organisms are the leading cause of the most threatening complication: deep sternal wound infection or mediastinitis. Skin preparation with topical antiseptics, clipping rather than shaving the skin, avoidance of hair removal, reduction in OR-traffic, laminar-flow ventilation, shorter operations, minimal electrocautery, avoidance of bone wax [33], use of double-gloving barrier techniques for the operating team, and routine use of an easily constructed pleuropericardial flap [34], have all been shown to be of value in reducing postoperative infection.

Preoperative antibiotic administration reduces the risk of postoperative infection five-fold [35]. Prophylactic antimicrobial efficacy is dependent on adequate drug-tissue levels before microbial exposure [35]. The cephalosporin class of antimicrobials is currently the agent of choice for prophylaxis of infection for coronary operations.

Strict control of blood glucose levels = 200 mg/dL by continuous intravenous (IV) infusion of insulin has been shown to significantly reduce the incidence of sternal infection in diabetic patients [16]. To further avoid mediastinitis: meticulous aseptic technique, minimal perfusion times, use of one IMA, avoidance of unnecessary electrocautery, appropriate use of perioperative antibiotics, and strict control of blood glucose levels during and after operation are suggested. If preventive strategies fail, prompt recognition of deep sternal wound infection or mediastinitis is critical. Aggressive surgical debridement and early vascularized muscle flap coverage are keys to reducing the cost, LOS, and death. Treatment by wound exploration, sternal rewiring, and drainage failed in 88.2% of patients compared with high success in patients treated initially with muscle flap closure [35].

Reducing the need of transfusion

Pre-hospitalization autologous blood donation can be effective [4]. If a patient has no exclusionary criteria (hemoglobin <12, heart failure, unstable angina, left main disease, or symptoms on the proposed day of donation) and can give 1–3 units of blood over 30 days before the operation, the risk of homologous transfusion is significantly lowered (12.6% vs. 46% in a non-preadmission donor control group, $P = 0.001$). An alternative or additional method of pre-CPB blood "donation" is the removal of blood from the patient in the OR immediately before CPB. This blood is then set aside, not exposed to the CPB circuitry, and then reinfused into the patient after the patient is disconnected from CPB. This donation immediately before CPB yielded a significantly higher platelet and hemoglobin count compared with similar postoperative levels in patients who did not undergo harvesting of blood immediately before CPB. This technique translated into a six-fold decrease in the percentage of patients requiring transfusion (10% transfusion rate in pre-CPB donors vs. a 65% transfusion rate in non-pre-CPB donors, $P < 0.01$) [36].

Low hematocrit during CPB was significantly associated with increased risk of in-hospital mortality. Female patients and patients with low surface body area may become more hemodiluted than larger patients. Minimizing intraoperative anemia may result in improved outcomes in these subgroups of patients [37].

Aprotinin: a risk–benefit analysis

During CABG there is a risk of bleeding and subsequent transfusion. However, there are many risks involving transfusion because the blood is combined from many donors. This fact increases the risk of inflammatory reactions during CABG after transfusion. In order to decrease bleeding, there is widespread use of two classes of agents, both proven to mitigate bleeding: the lysine analogues (aminocaproic acid and tranexamic acid) and the serine protease inhibitors (aprotinin).

The effectiveness of aprotinin in reducing the bleeding and transfusion needs in patients undergoing open heart procedures has been documented in a number of reports [3]. There has been speculation, however, that aprotinin might adversely affect the kidneys, causing renal failure. A recent article offered a comprehensive review of the risk associated with aprotinin in cardiac surgery.

CRITICAL THINKING

Benefits and risk of aprotinin. In this observational study that involved 4374 patients undergoing revascularization, three agents (aprotinin [1295 patients], aminocaproic acid [883], and tranexamic acid [822]) as compared with no agent (1374 patients) were prospectively assessed with regard to serious outcomes by propensity and multivariable methods. The results showed that in the propensity-adjusted, multivariable logistic regression (C-index, 0.72), use of aprotinin was associated with a doubling in the risk of renal failure requiring dialysis among patients undergoing complex coronary-artery surgery (OR 2.59; 95% CI 1.36–4.95) or primary surgery (OR 2.34; 95% CI 1.27–4.31). Similarly, use of aprotinin in the latter group was associated with a 55% increase in the risk of MI or heart failure ($P < 0.001$) and a 181% increase in the risk of stroke or encephalopathy ($P = 0.001$). Neither aminocaproic acid nor tranexamic acid was associated with an increased risk of renal, cardiac, or cerebral events. Adjustment according to propensity score for the use of any one of the three agents as compared with no agent yielded nearly identical findings. All the agents reduced blood loss [38].

The conclusion was that the association between aprotinin and serious-end organ damage indicates that continued use is not prudent. In contrast, the less expensive generic medications aminocaproic acid and tranexamic acid are safe alternatives [6].

Reduce volume and/or severity of complications
Although the mortality rates have fallen, the patients presenting for CABG are often older, have more impaired LV systolic function, higher urgency for surgery, fewer single-vessel procedures and multiple co-morbid conditions. Their major postoperative complications were most likely noncardiac: pulmonary (25–40%), renal (15–25%), and neurologic (3–6%). Fewer than 5% had cardiac failure [5].

The lowest possible rate of complications from a premier CABG program are listed in Table 4.9 [5]. They are the benchmarks for any local hospital to achieve.

Table 4.9 Postoperative benchmark for isolated coronary artery bypass surgery.

Bleeding	1.2%
Respiratory failure	3.2%
Sepsis	1%
Transmural MI	2%
Mediastinitis	0.8%
Renal failure – dialysis	0.5%

MI, myocardial infarction.

Prevent stroke
Stroke can be caused by carotid stenosis or LV thrombus, however, proximal aortic atherosclerosis is the strongest predictor of stroke, due to embolization of atheromatous material during manipulation of the aorta [39]. Therefore the detection and the management of the ascending aorta for prevention of atheroembolism is crucial to reduce the stroke rate. Although palpation of the aorta has traditionally been used by surgeons to identify patients with atheromatous disease of the ascending aorta and to find "soft spots" for cannulation or cross clamping, the use of epi-aortic ultrasound has been suggested as a more accurate means of assessing the aorta [16]. Once aortic atherosclerosis is identified, alternative strategies to prevent mobilization of debris from aortic

atheroma include performing CABG without cardio-pulmonary bypass. Off-pump bypass requires technical changes such as axillary artery cannulation, ascending aorta replacement under circulatory arrest, single cross-clamp technique, originating grafts off the left internal mammary artery to avoid ascending aorta proximal anastomosis [40,41]. These approaches are very helpful, especially in elderly patients, peripheral arterial disease, hypertension etc.

In the type 2 deficits, encephalopathic changes may be related to the brain's microcirculation and are more likely to occur after periods of hypotension or inadequate perfusion than by aortic plaque embolization. The preventive measure to avoid stroke are listed in Table 4.10.

Table 4.10 Pre- and intra-operative measures for stroke prevention.

1. Preoperative screening of carotid artery disease by Doppler
2. If patient has recent stroke, wait for 4 weeks after the index event
3. If patient has recent TIA, maximal medical or surgical management as indicated, then wait 4 weeks after the index event
4. If patient has atrial fibrillation, perform TEE looking for atrial thrombus
5. If patient has recent anterior wall MI, be sure patient has no LV thrombus by echocardiography
6. Perform off-pump bypass
7. Perform intraoperatively epi-aortic ultrasound to detect atheromatous plaque on the aortic wall
8. Intraoperative TEE to detect air bubble

LV, left ventricular; MI, myocardial infarction; TEE, transesophageal echocardiography; TIA, transient ischemic attack.

Avoid unplanned return to the OR

The three common causes of unplanned return to the OR are bleeding, valve dysfunction and acute graft occlusion.

In the study of the Northern New England Cardiovascular Disease Study Group [42], the incidence of re-exploration due to bleeding was 3.6%. The mortality of these patients was three times higher at 9.5% and their length of stay was almost doubled at 14 days. The risk factors included prolonged (>150 minutes) of CPB, intraoperative requirement of IABP. The use of thrombolytic therapy within 48 hours of surgery was weakly but not significantly associated with need for re-exploration. To avoid bleeding, meticulous inspections of sites, sutures, prior to closure of the chest. The use of clopidogrel plus aspirin prior to surgery increased significantly the rate of postoperative bleeding compared with acetylsalicyic acid (ASA) alone. Avoidance of clopidogrel prior to surgery is suggested.

To avoid acute reocclusion of the SVG, more delicate handling of the graft during harvesting, implantation, especially when working on a beating heart, is suggested. For the problem of mitral valve dysfunction, the theory is that the structurally normal mitral valve may be regurgitant due to reversible ischemia involving the papillary muscles. Then the dilemma is when it is necessary to inspect the mitral valve for correction. Intraoperative has provided a functional and quantitative assessment before and after CPB. When the mitral regurgitation (MR) is grade 1 to 2, this may decrease during anesthesia induction and/or with complete revascularization, thus eliminating the need to inspect the valve during cross-clamping of the aorta. An added finding by echocardiography or direct inspection at the time of operation is the presence of an enlarged left atrium, which generally signifies chronicity to the MR and adds justification to the consideration of mitral valve repair. This strategy is further assessed by a final post-CPB transesophageal echocardiography (TEE) in the OR. If, under this rare circumstance, the MR is unacceptable, reinstitution of CPB can be performed and the MR corrected. If the MR is grade 3 to 4, it is necessary to inspect the valve and correct the mechanical lesion. It is important to stress that in this situation, it is imperative that an intraoperative TEE be performed to see whether the MR is grade 3 to 4, to assess the reparability of the valve and the success of the repair [4].

Decrease length of stay

The average LOS for a patient undergoing uncomplicated CABG is 6 days post-operatively, including the day of discharge. The data for other types of surgery are listed in Table 4.11 [2]. An increased LOS depends mainly on severe clinical status of patients presenting for surgery: (1) preoperative IABP (OR 3.02); (2) clinical CHF (OR 2.7); (3) acuity status: emergency, salvage surgery (OR 2.4) [21]. The LOS may not be a good indicator of excellent care. The rate of readmission must be added when reducing LOS to ensure patients are not being discharged prematurely. Also, we are treating more elderly patients who are live alone, and it is very difficult to send them home after surgery to care for themselves alone.

Table 4.11 Average length of stay.

Type of surgery	LOS (days)
Uncomplicated CABG	4 days
Mitral valve surgery (minimally invasive) [2]	6 days
Valvular surgery in >80 year-old-patient [21]	9 days (5–56)

CABG, coronary artery bypass surgery; LOS, length of stay.

There are three strategies to decrease the LOS. For the non-complicated patients who were discharged alive without adverse outcome, a risk-adjusted post-procedure average LOS would measure the efficiency of care of a local hospital comparing with a national or regional standard. If almost all the other hospitals in the region can provide the same care, with the same outcome in a shorter LOS, then the LOS of this group of patients needs to be decreased. A further lower LOS would compensate the longer stay of high risk patients, so the average local LOS would be lower. This strategy would permit for the program to accept higher-risk patients rather than turning them away.

The second strategy is to identify the group of patients who had adverse outcomes that were not catastrophic (i.e. not resulting in death or extremely prolonged LOS) and their risk-adjusted excess LOS. The results of LOS in the two above groups of patients would show the magnitude of opportunity to improve the effectiveness of care by reducing the volume and/or severity of patient's adverse outcomes and LOS.

The third strategy is to allocate more manpower and resources to screen high risk patients, correcting their abnormalities before surgery in order to cut morbidity, mortality and LOS. Off-pump bypass showed lower LOS, even in patients with redo-CABG [35].

Early cardiac rehabilitation

Prior to surgery, the patients and families should be instructed to expect early extubation, ambulation, exercise and discharge in day 3 or 4 post-op. Once the patient is transferred to the intensive care unit (ICU) after CABG, the patient should be motivated to follow the active rehabilitation plan. The exercise sessions should be available even on Saturday, Sunday or legal holidays, because the extra cost of staffing would be easily offset by a shorter LOS.

Postoperative Care

Postoperative Atrial Fibrillation

The LOS is increased by postoperative atrial fibrillation (AF), and it is associated with a two- to three-fold increase in postoperative stroke. If AF after CABG persists into a second day, warfarin anticoagulation with a goal international normalized ratio (INR) of 2–3 should be considered [43]. Withdrawal of β-blockers in the perioperative period doubles the incidence of postoperative AF. Propafenone showed no significant benefit over atenolol in the prevention of supraventicular arrhythmias [44]. The former is a less negatively inotropic drug as an alternative to β-blockers in patients in whom underlying LV dysfunction is an important concern, or for patients whose active bronchospasm makes β-blocker use less attractive.

Low-dose sotalol also appears to be effective for reduction of AF after CABG [45]. Amiodarone administered 1 week prior to surgery halves the incidence of postcardiotomy AF (53% placebo to 25% amiodarone, $P = 0.003$) [46]. Digoxin and calcium channel blockers (verapamil has been the most extensively studied) have no consistent benefit for prophylaxis of supraventricular arrhythmias after CABG [47].

In a review of more than 10,000 patients who underwent cardiac surgery, the three risk factors for post-operative atrial fibrillation (AF) are: valvular surgery, increased age, and decreased EF. There was less AF in patients with prior CABG, diabetes, female gender, and smoking [47]. Practically, patients with EF <35% can receive amiodarone 400 mg PO q6H as early post-operatively as tolerated. In patients with EF >35%, patients received orally propafenone 150 mg q8H/metropolol 25 mg q12H [48].

Recently, atrial pacing was randomized in patient right after CABG and continued for 72 hours. The paced rate was adjusted whenever the intrinsic rate equaled or exceeded the paced rate [49]. The patients also received propanolol, a 5 mg test dose orally immediately following extubation and the dose was titrated to a target dose of 20 mg orally four times daily. The results showed a reduction of post-operative AF from 37.5% in patients receiving no post-operative pacing to 17% ($P < 0.005$) in patients with pacing. Two observational studies have explored the value of cardiac denervation at the time of cardiac surgical operation for reducing postoperative AF.

EMERGING TREND

Surgical denervation as prophylaxis for AF The role of ventral cardiac denervation for prevention of AF was examined in 207 patients by removing the nerves around the large vessels at the base of the heart beginning with the right side of the superior vena cava and continuing through the midportion of the anterior pulmonary artery (26). This dissection that removed fat pads surrounding the superior vena cava, aorta, and anterior and right pulmonary arteries required an extra 5 minutes of operative time with no associated operative complications. The 219 subjects considered as nonrandomized controls were similar in baseline and operative characteristics except for fewer grafts per patient in the control group. Postoperative AF occurred in 15 (7%) of 207 patients undergoing ventral cardiac denervation and in 56 (27%) of 219 control subjects ($P < 0.001$). After baseline differences were corrected by multivariable adjustment, ventral cardiac denervation remained the most significant negative predictor of postoperative AF. The 7% reported incidence of AF is remarkably low and, if confirmed in broader experience, would certainly justify adding this minimal modification to cardiac operations [50].

CRITICAL THINKING

Surgical removal of anterior fat pad as a cause of postoperative AF.
The influence of parasympathetic nerves in the anterior fat pad was examined in 55 patients undergoing CABG who were randomly assigned to receive either dissection or no dissection of the anterior fat pad located between the base of the aorta and main pulmonary artery. Evoking sinus cycle length prolongation with stimulation identified the fat pad before cardiopulmonary bypass. Stimulation at the conclusion of surgery documented increased sinus cycle length in patients with the fat pad preserved and failure to increase sinus length documented denervation in patients with the fat pad removed. Removal of the fat pad increased postoperative AF from 37% compared with 7% in patients with the fat pad preserved [51].

Dissection of the anterior fat pad, which often occurs incidental to cardiac surgery, may contribute to postoperative AF. Both of these studies of the influence of operative dissection of cardiac sympathetic and parasympathetic nerves identify a fruitful area for additional work directed toward the important goal of decreasing postoperative AF in cardiac surgical patients [6].

Tight Diabetes Control

The importance of tight diabetic control was assessed in 141 diabetic patients undergoing CABG who were prospectively randomized to glycemic control (serum glucose 1.5–200 mg/dL) with glucose–insulin–potassium or standard therapy using intermittent subcutaneous insulin. Patients treated with glucose–insulin–potassium had lower serum glucose levels, less AF perioperatively, shorter postoperative LOS, and a survival advantage in the initial two years after surgery. Patients with tight diabetic control also had fewer episodes of recurrent ischemia (5% vs. 19%, $P = 0.01$) and fewer sternal or leg wound infections (1% vs. 10%, $P = 0.03$). The results of this study in context of similar benefit found in previous observational studies suggest tight diabetic control should become the standard postoperative management for diabetic patients [7].

Evidence-based Medicine: Diabetic control for CABG

148 diabetic patients undergoing CABG were prospectively randomized to tight glycemic control (serum glucose, 125–200 mg/dL) with a combination of glucose, insulin and potassium (GIK) or standard therapy (serum glucose <250 mg/dL) using intermittent subcutaneous insulin beginning before anesthesia and continuing for 12 hours after surgery. GIK patients had lower serum glucose levels (138 ± 4 vs. 260 ± 6 mg/dL; $P < 0.0001$), a lower incidence of AF (16.6% vs. 42%; $P = 0.0017$), and a shorter postoperative length of stay (6.5 ± 0.1 vs. 9.2 ± 0.3 days; $P = 0.003$). GIK patients also showed a survival advantage over the initial 2 years after surgery ($P = 0.04$) and decreased episodes of recurrent ischemia (5% vs. 19%; $P = 0.01$) and developed fewer recurrent wound infections (1% vs. 10%, $P = 0.03$). So tight glycemic control with GIK in diabetic CABG patients improves perioperative outcomes, enhances survival, and decreases the incidence of ischemic events and wound complications [52].

Management in Specific Subsets of Patients

Elderly Patients

While undergoing CABG, elderly patients have more left main disease, multivessel disease, LV dysfunction, and re-operation, and for many, concomitant valvular surgery [4]. These patients also have more comorbid conditions (diabetes, hypertension, chronic obstructive pulmonary disease (COPD), peripheral vascular disease (PVD), and renal disease). This combination leads to higher rates of intra-operative or postoperative MI, low-output syndrome, stroke, gastrointestinal complications, wound infection, and renal failure.

Their operative mortality has ranged from 5–20% during the past 20 years for isolated CABG, averaging 8.9%. Emergency surgery confers up to a tenfold increase in risk (3.5% to 35%), urgent surgery a three-fold increase (3.5% to 15%), hemodynamic instability a three- to ten-fold increase, and an left ventricular ejection fraction (LVEF) <0.20 up to a ten-fold increase [53].

Predictors of postoperative low cardiac output syndrome are, in descending order of importance, LVEF <0.20, repeated operation, emergency operation, female sex, diabetes mellitus, age >70 years, left main disease, recent MI, and/or three-vessel disease [54]. In general, the patient aged 70 years or older who may be a candidate for CABG surgery has, on average, a higher risk of mortality and morbidity from the operative procedure. Nonetheless, functional recovery and sustained improvement and quality of life may be achieved in the large majority of such patients [54]. In experienced hands, off-pump CABG (OPCABG) is particularly better for this group of patients as it avoids the deleterious effects of heart–lung pump and avoids aortic manipulations. To decrease mortality and morbidity, besides nearly perfect cardiac management, rigorous prevention and correction of non-cardiac problems is strongly suggested.

Octogenarian Patients

Octogenarians have many risk factors when undergoing cardiac surgery. Over 20% of patients had CHF, 21% had prior cardiac procedures, 70% triple-vessel disease and 43% had LM disease. Over 50% of patients had surgery on an urgent or emergent basis. Despite these unfavorable characteristics and circumstances, their in-hospital mortality rate was 8% and stroke was 3.9% [55]. The predictors of in-hospital mortality were similar to the risk factors of other younger patients including urgency, age, prior CABG, vascular disease, history of CHF, renal failure etc. The only difference is that COPD is a risk factor in this age group. Their average LOS was 7 days with 31% experiencing prolonged stay of more than 14 days and 15% were intubated for longer than 48 hours (Table 4.12).

CRITICAL THINKING

Same day percutaneous coronary intervention and aortic valve replacement. In very elderly (>80) patient with symptomatic CAD and aortic stenosis, some surgeons request the patient to have PCI with drug eluting stent (DES) in the morning, while the antiplatelet effect of clopidogrel is still not in full strength (24 hours after the loading dose). Then the surgeon will perform minimally invasive aortic valve replacement (AVR) under the coverage of heparin (as during the PCI). The next day, both procedures are covered by the effect of clopidogrel. Another way to overcome the problem of long term clopidogrel is to stent with a bare metal stent (BMS) and a month later, the patient can undergo AVR with only ASA [56].

Table 4.12 Morbidity and mortality during cardiac surgery.

	CABG		CABG + aortic valve		CABG + mitral valve	
	<80	>80	<80	>80	<80	>80
Mortality (%)	3	8	8	10	12	19
Neurologic events (%)	4.2	10.2	9.1	15.2	11.2	22.5
Stroke only (%)	1.8	3.9	3.2	4.9	4.7	8.8
Renal failure (%)	2.9	6.9	6.8	12.1	11.4	25
Perioperative MI (%)	1.7	2.5	2.0	3.0	2.7	1.5
PLOS days (mean %)	6	7	7	9	9	11

CABG, coronary artery bypass surgery.

Women

Early studies provided evidence that female sex was an independent risk factor for higher in-hospital mortality and morbidity, but that long-term survival and functional recovery were similar in both men and women [4,57]. More recent studies have suggested that on average, women have a disadvantageous preoperative clinical profile such as older age, with poorer LV function, more frequently with unstable angina pectoris, NYHA class IV heart failure, three-vessel and left main disease, and more comorbid conditions including hypothyroidism, renal disease, diabetes mellitus, hypertension, and PVD [58]. Smaller size of the coronary arteries in women, and less use of IMA grafts possibly contribute to a higher mortality [58].

The in-hospital mortality was 2.83% for men, and 4.18% for women, $P < 0.001$ and the 30-day mortality 4.66% and 6.07%; $P = 0.001$, respectively. However, when adjusted for age, peripheral vascular disease, renal failure, preoperative CHF, preoperative EF, preoperative left ventricular end diastolic pressure, re-operation, and surgical priority, no difference in the in-hospital and 30-day mortality rates for women and men was observed. In general, it appears that the in-hospital mortality and morbidity and long-term survival are related more to risk factors and patient characteristics than to gender [59]. However, with more focused care, the in-hospital mortality of women improved [59].

Patients with Carotid Artery Disease

The conventional history and physical examination are neither particularly sensitive nor specific for detecting carotid artery stenosis. The presence of symptoms is alarming, but the absence of symptoms is not particularly protective. The sensitivity of carotid disease detection by auscultation is low at 64% and its specificity is also low at 61% [60]. For the patient with carotid artery stenosis less than 50%, the subsequent risk of stroke was 2%. For stenoses ranging from 50–80%, the risk of stroke increased to 10%. For stenosis greater than 80%, the risk approached 20% [61]. The patients older than 65 years of age, who have LM disease, or central nervous system (CNS) symptoms such as transient ischemic attack (TIA), amaurosis fugax, stroke) should have the carotid artery Doppler screening [61]. Once there is confirmed significant carotid artery disease, the conventional management includes carotid endarterectomy (CEA) then CABG or CEA and CABG in the same setting [61].

In patients with moderate to severe carotid artery disease (50–80% stenosis), the indication of CAE is still controversial. Some surgeons advocate the aggressive management of these patients based on principles of fluid dynamics and rheology. A reduction of diameter of 50% or more leads to a reduction in the cross sectional area of 75% or more, which is associated with a hemodynamically significant flow reduction. The patients undergoing coronary revascularization is at significant risk during the 24- to 72-hour intra-operative and postoperative period for wide ranging variation in blood pressure, cardiac output, rhythm, acid–base balance, temperature, coagulability and in cerebrovascular autoregulation. For a given carotid stenosis, this is likely the highest risk phase the patient will ever see. This background plus the recognized five- to ten-fold increase in stroke risk in patients with 50–80% stenosis justifies consideration of more aggressive approach [61]. Many cardiac surgeons consider CAE as a non-major vascular surgery which does not cause a lot of hemodynamic fluctuations. So they prefer to perform CAE a few days prior to a major CABG.

Patients with Pulmonary Disease

preoperatively, it is important to identify patients with significant obstructive pulmonary disease: pulmonary venous congestion, large pleural effusions, dilated ventricle compressing the lungs, all of which may result in a reduction of lung compliance [4]. Restrictive pulmonary function abnormalities are also found in patients with pulmonary fibrosis, sarcoidosis, pneumoconiosis, and collagen vascular diseases. The most common cause of preoperative pulmonary dysfunction, however, is COPD. Patients with mild COPD and few or mild symptoms generally do well through cardiac surgery. However, patients with moderate to severe COPD, especially elderly patients, are at an increased risk for operative mortality and postoperative complications in a near-direct relation to the severity of the degree of pulmonary dysfunction [62].

Preoperative measures to improve respiratory function may diminish postoperative complications and include the use of antibiotic therapy for lung infections, bronchodilator therapy, cessation of smoking, preoperative incentive spirometry, deep-breathing exercises, and chest physiotherapy [62].

Patients with End-Stage Renal Disease

Many patients with end-stage renal disease (ESRD) who need CABG may have modest decrease in LV function, significant LM disease, three-vessel disease, and unstable angina [4,63]. Although these patients also are at increased risk for operative morbidity and mortality, they are at even higher risk when treated with conservative medical management. Patients with ESRD often have multiple comorbid disorders, including hypertension and diabetes mellitus, each with its own complications and associated impact on both short- and long-term survival [64]. In addition, infection and sepsis, perioperative volume and electrolyte disturbances have been identified as significant causes of morbidity and mortality [64].

The pathophysiology of renal dysfunction is complex, with multiple potential processes contributing; such as hypoperfusion, emboli, toxins, and inflammation. Data on intraoperative strategies to minimize renal injury are limited. The risks for post-operative acute renal dysfunction are showed in Table 4.13.

Table 4.13 Risks for postoperative acute renal dysfunction.

1. Elevated baseline creatinine
2. Congestive heart failure
3. Age >70 years
4. Type 1 diabetes mellitus
5. Re-operation

Patients with Valvular Disease

Many patients with CAD have mitral regurgitation (MR), especially when the mitral valve is structurally normal but functionally regurgitant, most likely caused by ischemia [4]. The quandary this presents is when the MR requires correction at the time of CABG. The question is easily answered if there are structural abnormalities in the mitral apparatus. Mitral repair is indicated in the majority of such circumstances, although occasionally patients require valve replacement.

In patients with low ejection fraction (mean EF: 30%) and mitral valve repair, the 30-day mortality was 9.1% while it was only 2.2% in patients with good EF (mean EF: 57%). The ten-year survival was 33% and 60% respectively [65].

The discussion of combined procedures revolves around overall operative risk, which is dependent on several variables. The most notable of these are age >70 years, female sex, advanced NYHA class, poor LV function, and multiple valve procedures [65]. The simple addition of mitral repair to a coronary bypass without valve correction increases the operative mortality from 3% to 5%.

The results of combined aortic valve and coronary disease have led to the recommendation to graft significantly obstructed vessels (=50%) when an AVR is performed. The operative mortality for patients undergoing AVR who have ungrafted CAD approaches 10%, while those patients having AVR and concomitant CABG for CAD have an operative mortality approaching that of aortic valve replacement alone [66]. It is generally accepted that the risk of adding CABG to a valve replacement or repair will increase the operative mortality over that of an isolated valve procedure. The additional variables of age >70–80 years and poor LVEF will further increase this risk.

Re-operation

The re-operative mortality increases with the urgency or severity of symptoms, age >65 years, <1 year between first and second operations, and low EF [67,68]. The highest risk seems to be associated with a short time interval between the first operation and the subsequent need for re-operation. The re-operative mortality risk was 18% in a group of patients who underwent re-operation <1 year after their first CABG [68]. This figure was compared with an 8% mortality in those patients who had an operation-free time of >1 year. The presence of diabetes was greater in the group undergoing operation in <1 year.

The general higher mortality risk may involve several factors, including older age, presence of more comorbid conditions, LV dysfunction, and more extensive CAD. No randomized trials have compared re-operation and medical therapy in patients with prior CABG. However, retrospective data suggest that patients who undergo medical therapy alone have a lower late survival rate than those who undergo repeat surgical intervention.

Disease of a saphenous venous graft to the LAD is clearly associated with decreased survival, and affected patients indeed have an anatomic indication for surgery. Usually, if patients have an open internal mammary artery to LAD connection, they are less likely to benefit from revascularization in the first five years. Once symptomatic patients are more than 10–15 years post-surgery and have three-vessel disease, surgery may be beneficial even in the presence of an open arterial bypass graft to the LAD. The risk of re-operation is significant. If this surgery is emergent, that risk increases to as high as 12.9% [68].

The potential benefits of re-operation must be measured against the risks and technical difficulties of the surgery. The aspects of re-operation that are challenging to the surgeon include diffuse coronary disease, small or diseased distal coronary arteries, and myocardium that may be scarred rather than ischemic. However, in many clinical scenarios, the best type of treatment is not clear. For example, it is unknown whether documentation of significant ischemia in the absence of severe symptoms is an indication for re-operation [68].

Concomitant Peripheral Vascular Disease

The in-hospital mortality rate with CABG in patients with PVDs was 7.7%, a 2.4-fold higher incidence than in patients without PVD (3.2%) [4,69,70]. The excess risk of in-hospital mortality associated with PVD was particularly notable in patients with lower-extremity occlusive disease (adjusted OR 2.03). The excess mortality rates were due primarily to an increased incidence of heart failure and dysrhythmias rather than cerebrovascular accidents or peripheral arterial complications. Significantly elevated, adjusted hazard ratios occurred in patients with overt cerebrovascular disease, clinical and subclinical lower-extremity occlusive disease, and abdominal aortic aneurysm. The presence of clinical and subclinical PVD is a strong predictor of increased in-hospital and long-term mortality rate in patients undergoing CABG.

Poor Left Ventricular Function

Both low EF and clinical heart failure are predictive of higher operative mortality rates with CABG [4,71]. An operative mortality of 6.6% in patients with an EF <0.35, in comparison with 2.6% in patients with an EF >0.50, was reported. [71] Reports of perioperative mortality rate varied widely, ranging from ~5% in excellent centers in patients of a younger age, with fewer symptoms, and having no comorbid conditions; to >30% in patients who were older, with severe ventricular dysfunction, and having several comorbid conditions [71]. A trend toward lower operative mortality rates in recent years has been reported, due to better myocardial protection techniques and perioperative management.

The success of fibrinolytic and percutaneous coronary interventions has reduced the mortality of acute myocardial infarction. However, the increase in survival has been associated with a larger number of patients with ischemic cardiomyopathy and heart failure. Despite previous teaching to the contrary, it has become apparent that impaired LV dysfunction in patients with coronary heart disease is not an irreversible process. Approximately 40% of segments involved in MI may subsequently recover, either spontaneously or after revascularization, and LV function may improve markedly, and even normalize, in subsets of patients following successful revascularization [72]. The main task is to identify the recoverable, viable or "hibernating" myocardium.

Revascularization may improve symptom status, exercise capacity, and prognosis in selected patients with viable myocardium. As a general rule, the potential for recovery is assumed to be great enough to recommend revascularization when the total of hibernating and ischemic but still functioning myocardium is greater than 60% of the left ventricle. In contrast, when more than 40% of the left ventricle is considered to be scarred or is metabolically inactive, surgical mortality is much higher and the likelihood of the recovery of LV function from revascularization is much lower.

Recently, in order to prevent deterioration of renal function in patients with reduced EF, nesiritide was tried in the NAPA trial.

EMERGING TREND

The NAPA trial In the Nesiritide Administered Peri-Anesthesia in Patients Undergoing Cardiac Surgery trial, 279 patients with heart failure (HF) who underwent CABG with or without mitral valve repair/replacement were randomized with nesiritide or placebo after induction of anesthesia. The maximum mean increase of serum creatinine was 0.15 ± 0.29 mg/dL in nesiritide patients while it was 0.34 ± 0.48 mg/dL in placebo patients. The nesiritide patients also had shorter length of stay [73].

CABG in Acute Coronary Syndromes

To date there is one randomized trial which studied the results of acute coronary syndrome (ACS) patients undergoing CABG [4]. The study has shown a significant mortality reduction accomplished by early revascularization and preceded with antithrombotic treatment in patients with unstable angina [74]. Data from large community hospitals duplicating the above results are needed in order to popularize the concepts and the strategy.

CRITICAL THINKING

CABG in ACS patients: The FRISC-II trial. In the Fragmin during Instability in Coronary Artery Disease study, an early invasive strategy by CABG or PCI reduced the risk of death after 12 months by 44% in patients with unstable angina as compared to a selective approach with invasive procedure only if indicated by symptoms or severe ischemia at exercise testing. The 30-day mortality was quite low at 1.9% for CABG patients, 0.2% for PCI patients and 3.6% for those on medical treatment only. Female sex (OR 5.0) and diabetes (OR 4.2) are independent risk factors for early mortality in patients who underwent CABG [74].

CABG in Acute Myocardial Infarction

CABG has been largely superseded by thrombolysis and primary mechanical interventions [4]. Early coronary bypass for acute infarction may be appropriate in patients with residual ongoing ischemia despite non-surgical therapy, and if other conditions warrant urgent surgery, including left main or three-vessel disease, associated valvular disease, mechanical complications, and anatomy unsuitable for PCI. CABG is reserved for patients with evidence of ongoing ischemia despite maximal medical or percutaneous interventions, or it may be performed with repair of mechanical complications of infarction (i.e., ventricular septal defect or papillary muscle rupture) [75].

Inferior Wall MI with Right Ventricular Involvement

Right ventricular (RV) failure secondary to an ischemic RV (either infarction or stunning) presents a particularly hazardous situation [2,76]. Usually, the patient has an occluded right coronary artery proximal to the major RV branches and presents with an inferior MI with or without recognized RV failure [76,77]. Angiography may demonstrate that the coronary anatomy is best treated surgically, but the opportunity for maximal benefit of an emergency operation (initial 4–6 hours) has often passed. There is substantial risk in operating after this small window of opportunity but before the recovery of RV function, which usually occurs at 4 weeks after injury [78]. During this postinfarct month, the RV is at great risk for severe postoperative dysfunction, which often requires extraordinary levels of perioperative pharmacological and mechanical support and has a very high mortality.

The non-surgical postinfarction patient can most often be supported with pacing, volume loading, and judicious inotropic administration [79]. In the surgical setting, the RV takes on different characteristics. There is loss of the pericardial constraint immediately on exposing the heart, which results in acute dilatation of the dysfunctional RV. The RV often fails to recover in this setting, even when state-of-the-art myocardial protection schemes and revascularization are employed [80]. The parallel effects of RV dilatation and dysfunction on LV diastolic and systolic function are magnified and may be associated with the need for high levels of support, inability to close the chest owing to cardiac dilation, need for ventricular-assist devices, prolonged convalescence, transplantation, or death.

If early angioplasty and/or stenting of the right coronary artery is indicated, this should be performed. It is best to delay surgery for 4 weeks to allow full recovery of RV function prior to CABG.

Take Home Message

CABG is a major modality of treatment of CAD, as medical therapy or PCI. This surgical approach achieves similar or better revascularization benefits as of PCI, even after the availability of drug-coated stent. The results of CABG need to be better, with less mortality, morbidity, LOS, and less costly so it can compete for a niche in the armamentarium of the management of CAD. The goals of any open heart surgery program are to have low mortality, low rate of stroke, mediastinitis, renal failure, postop-AF and short LOS. The strategies are (1) to identify the high risk patients and (2) to correct their problems and (3) to optimize their conditions prior to surgery.

> The patient with CAD and concomitant valve dysfunction needs comprehensive management including valvular repair or replacement for maximal myocardial recovery, and LV function improvement without post-CABG valvular dysfunction. The patients with acute inferior MI should be searched for RV infarction and failure. Any patient with EF <35% should have demonstrable reversible ischemia on non-invasive testing. In order to decrease sequelae from CPB less-invasive coronary bypass surgery is suggested. Avoidance of cardiopulmonary bypass is considered to be an important advantage in order to decrease morbidity, mortality and LOS in general, and particularly in high risk patients: redo-CABG, or patient with renal failure.

References

1 Medicare Program: Changes to the inpatient hospital prospective payment system and fiscal year 2000 rates; Final rule. Federal Register 1999;64:41489–41641.

2 Cohn L, Couper GS, Aranki SF et al. Early and late results of minimally invasive mitral valve surgery. J Am Coll Cardiol 2001;37:475A.

3 Gattuso CF. Negotiating managed care and capitated contracts to minimize risks. Ann Thorac Surg 1997;64:S73–S75.

4 Eagle KA, Guyton RA, Davidoff R et al. ACC/AHA Practice guidelines for Coronary Artery Bypass Graft surgery JACC 1999;34:1262–1347. Recommendations of the ACC/ AHA Task Force in order to decrease morbidity and mortality in patients undergoing CABG. Circulation 1999;100:1464–1480.

5 Department of Thoracic and Cardiovascular surgery, Surgical outcomes 1999. The Cleveland Clinics Foundation, 2000.

6 Jones RH. The Year in Cardiovascular Surgery. J Am Coll Cardiol 2005;45:1517–1528.

7 Roach GW, Kanchuger M, Mangano CM et al. Adverse cerebral outcomes after coronary bypass surgery: Multicenter Study of Perioperative Ischemia Research Group and the Ischemia Research and Education Foundation Investigators. N Engl J Med 1996;335:1857–1863.

8 Mahoney E, Thompson TD, Veledar E et al. Factors associated with the risk of stroke following CABG: Results from the National Cardiovascular network (NCN). J Am Coll Cardiol 2001;37:361A.

9 Newman M, Kirchner JL, Philips-Bute B et al. Longitudinal assessment of neurocognitive function after CABG. J New Engl J Med 2001;344:395–402.

10 Frye RL, Kronmal R, Schaff HV, Myers WO, Gersh BJ. Stroke in coronary artery bypass graft surgery: An analysis of the CASS experience: The participants in the Coronary Artery Surgery Study. Int J Cardiol 1992;36:213–221.

11 Mangano CM, Diamondstone LS, Ramsay JG et al. Renal dysfunction after myocardial revascularization:risk factors, adverse outcomes, and hospital resource utilization: The Multicenter Study of Perioperative Ischemia Research Group. Ann Intern Med 1998; 128:194–203.

12 Chertow GM, Levy EM, Hammermeister KE, Grover F, Daley J. Independent association between acute renal failure and mortality following cardiac surgery. Am J Med 1998; 104:343–348.

13 Cooper WA. O'Brien SM, Thourani VN et al. Impact of Renal Dysfunction on Outcomes of Coronary Artery Bypass Surgery Results From the Society of Thoracic Surgeons National Adult Cardiac Database Circulation 2006;113:1063–1070.

14 Loop FD, Lytle BW, Cosgrove DM *et al*. J. Maxwell Chamberlain memorial paper: Sternal wound complication after isolated CABG: early and late mortality, morbidity, and cost of care. Ann Thorac Surg 1990;49:179–186.

15 Milano CA, Kesler K, Archibald N, Sexton DJ, Jones RH. Mediastinitis after coronary artery bypass graft surgery: risk factors and long-term survival. Circulation 1995;92:2245–2251.

16 Furnary AP, Grunkemeier GL, Floten HS, Swanson JS, Gately HS, Starr A. Continuous intravenous insulin infusion reduces the incidence of deep sternal wound infection in diabetic patients after cardiac surgical procedures. Ann Thorac Surg 1999;67:352–360.

17 Risk factors for deep sternal wound infection after sternotomy: A prospective, multicenter study. J Thorac Cardiovasc Surg 1996;111:1200–1207.

18 Nishida H, Grooters RK, Soltanzadeh H, Thieman KC, Schneider RF, Kim WP Discriminate use of electrocautery on the median sternotomy incision: A 0.16% wound infection rate. J Thorac Cardiovasc Surg 1991;101:488–494.

19 Tu JV, Sykora K, Naylor CD. Assessing the outcomes of coronary artery bypass graft surgery:how many risk factors are enough? Steering Committee of the Cardiac Care Network of Ontario. J Am Coll Cardiol 1997;30:1317–1323.

20 Edwards FH, Grover FL, Shroyer AL, Schwartz M, Bero J. The Society of Thoracic Surgeons National Cardiac Surgery Database:current risk assessment. Ann Thorac Surg 1997;63:903–908.

21 Jones RH, Hannan EL, Hammermeister KE *et al*. Identification of preoperative variables needed for risk adjustment of short-term mortality after coronary artery bypass graft surgery: The Working Group Panel on the Cooperative CABG Database Project. J Am Coll Cardiol 1996;28:1478–1487.

22 Nashef SA, Roques F, Hammill BG *et al*. Validation of European system for cardiac operative risk evaluation (EuroSCORE) in North American cardiac surgery. Eur J Cardiothorac Surg 2002;22:101–105.

23 Dziuban SW Using information from databases to improve clinical practice:Lessons learned under fire. Ann Thorac Surg 1997;64:S64–S67.

24 Malenka DJ, O'Connor GT. The Northern New England Cardiovascular Disease Study Group: A regional collaborative effort for continuous quality improvement in cardiovascular diseases. Jt Comm J Qual Improv 1998;24:594–600.

25 Surgenor SD, O'Connor GT, Lahey SJ *et al*. Predicting the risk of death from heart failure after CABG. Anesth Analg 2001;92:596–601.

26 Cohn L, Rosborough D, Frenandez J. Reducing costs and length of stay and improving efficiency and quality of care in cardiac surgery. Ann Thorac Surg 1997;64:S58–S60.

27 Wechsler AS. CoST-effective management of high-risk patients: A case–map approach. Ann Thorac Surg 1997;64:S76–S79.

28 David S Bach, MD, FACC Sellke FW, DiMaio JM, Caplan LR *et al*. Comparing On–Pump and Off–Pump Coronary Artery Bypass Grafting. Numerous Studies but Few Conclusions: A Scientific Statement From the American Heart Association Council on Cardiovascular Surgery and Anesthesia in Collaboration With the Interdisciplinary Working Group on Quality of Care and Outcomes Research Circulation 2005;111:2858–2864.

29 Lazar HL, Zhang X, Hamasaki T *et al*. Role of leukocyte depletion during cardiopulmonary bypass and cardioplegic arrest. Ann Thorac Surg 1995;60:1745–1748.

30 He GW, Acuff TE, Ryan WH *et al*. Determinants of operative mortality in elderly patients undergoing coronary artery bypass grafting:emphasis on the influence of internal mammary artery grafting on mortality and morbidity. J Thorac Cardiovasc Surg 1994;108:73–81.

31 Edwards FH, Clark RE, Schwartz M. Impact of internal mammary artery conduits on operative mortality in coronary revascularization. Ann Thorac Surg 1994;57:27–32.

32 Lytle BW, McElroy D, McCarthy P et al. Influence of arterial coronary bypass grafts on the mortality in coronary reoperations. J Thorac Cardiovasc Surg 1994;107:675–683.

33 Nelson DR, Buxton TB, Luu QN et al. The promotional effect of bone wax on experimental Staphylococcus aureus osteomyelitis. J Thorac Cardiovasc Surg 1990;99:977–980.

34 Nugent WC, Maislen EL, O'Connor GT, Marrin CA, Plume S.K. Pericardial flap prevents sternal wound complications. Arch Surg 1988;123:636–639.

35 Menges T, Sablotzki A, Welters I et al. Concentration of cefamandole in plasma and tissues of patients undergoing cardiac surgery: The influence of different cefamandole dosage. J Cardiothorac Vasc Anesth 1997;11:565–570.

36 Crosby L, Palarski VA, Cottington E et al. Iron supplementation for acute blood loss anemia after coronary artery bypass surgery: A randomized, placebo-controlled study. Heart Lung 1994;23:493–499.

37 DeFoe GR, Ross CS, Olmstead EM et al. Lowest hematocrit on bypass and adverse outcomes associatedwithCABG. Northern New England Cardiovascular Disease Study Group. Ann Thorac Surg 2001;71:769–776.

38 Mangano, DT, Tudor IC, Dietzel C et al. The risk associated with aprotinin in cardiac surgery N Engl J Med 2006;354:353–365.

39 Duda A.M, Letwin LB, Sutter FP, Goldman SM Does routine use of aortic ultrasonography decrease the stroke rate in coronary artery bypass surgery?. J Vasc Surg 1995;21:98–107.

40 Kouchoukos NT, Wareing TH, Daily BB, Murphy SF Management of the severely atherosclerotic aorta during cardiac operations. J Card Surg 1994;9:490–494.

41 Wareing TH, Davila–Roman VG, Daily BB et al. Strategy for the reduction of stroke incidence in cardiac surgical patients. Ann Thorac Surg 1993;55:1400–1407.

42 Dacey LJ, Munoz JJ, Baribeau YR et al. Reexploration fro hemorrhage following CABG: Incidence and risk factors. Northern New England Cardiovascular Disease Study Group. Arch Surg 1998;133:442–447.

43 Hylek EM, Skates SJ, Sheehan MA, Singer DE An analysis of the lowest effective intensity of prophylactic anticoagulation for patients with nonrheumatic atrial fibrillation. N Engl J Med 1996;335:540–546.

44 Merrick AF, Odom NJ, Keenan DJ, Grotte GJ Comparison of propafenone to atenolol for the prophylaxis of postcardiotomy supraventricular tachyarrhythmias: A prospective trial. Eur J Cardiothorac Surg 1995;9:146–149.

45 Andrews TC, Reimold SC, Berlin JA, Antman EM Prevention of supraventricular arrhythmias after coronary artery bypass surgery: A meta-analysis of randomized control trials. Circulation 1991;84:Suppl III 236–244.

46 Daoud EG, Strickberger SA, Man KC et al. Preoperative amiodarone as prophylaxis against atrial fibrillation after heart surgery. N Engl J Med 1997;337:1785–1791.

47 Veledar E, Thompson T, Mahoney E et al. Predictors of AF following open heart surgery: Implications for coST-effective, targeted, preventive therapy. 493A.

48 Mandrola J, Ruhl S, Brooks–Brun J et al. Prevention of post cardiac surgery atrial fibrillation in a community hospital setting using a post operative to–tiered pharmacologic protocol. J Am Coll Cardiol 2001;37:479A.

49 Greenberg MD, Katz NM, Iuliano S et al. Atrial pacing for the prevention of atrial fibrillation after cardiovascular surgery. J Am Coll Cardiol 2000;35:1416–1422.

50 Melo J, Voight P, Sonmez B, et al. Ventral cardiac denervation reduces the incidence of atrial fibrillation after coronary artery bypass grafting. J Thorac Cardiovasc Surg 2004;127:511–516.

51 Cummings JE, Gill I, Akhrass R, Dery MA, Biblo LA, Quan KJ. Preservation of the anterior fat pad paradoxically decreases the incidence of postoperative atrial fibrillation in humans. J Am Coll Cardiol 2004;43:994–1000.

52 Lazar HL, Chipkin SR, Fitzgerald CA, Bao Y, Cabral H, Apstein CS. Tight glycemic control in diabetic coronary artery bypass graft patients improves perioperative outcomes and decreases recurrent ischemic events. Circulation 2004;109(12):1497–1502.

53 Hannan EL, Burke J. Effect of age on mortality in coronary artery bypass surgery in New York, 1991–1992. Am Heart J 1994;128:1184–1191.

54 Edwards FH, Taylor AJ, Thompson L et al. Current status of coronary artery operation in septuagenarians. Ann Thorac Surg 1991;52:265–269.

55 Alexander KP, Anstrom MS, Muhlbaier Lh et al. Outcomes of cardiac surgery in patients >80 years: Results from the national cardiovascular network. J Am Coll Cardiol 2000;35:731–738.

56 Yacoub MH, Cohn LH. Novel approaches to cardiac valve repair: from structure to function: Part I. Circulation 2004;109:942–950.

57 Czajkowski SM, Terrin M, Lindquist R et al. Comparison of preoperative characteristics of men and women undergoing coronary artery bypass grafting (the Post Coronary Artery Bypass Graft [CABG] Biobehavioral Study). Am J Cardiol 1997;79:1017–1024.

58 O'Connor NJ, Morton JR, Birkmeyer JD et al. Effect of coronary artery diameter in patients undergoing coronary bypass surgery: Northern New England Cardiovascular Disease Study Group. Circulation 1996;93:652–655.

59 O'Rourke DJ, Malenka DJ, Olmstead EM et al. Improved in–hospital mortality in women undergoing CABG. Northern New England Cardiovascular Disease Study Group. Ann Thorac Surg 2001;71:507–511.

60 Sauve JS, Thorpe KE, Scakett DL et al. Can bruits distinguish high grade from moderate symptomatic carotid stenosis? Ann Intern Med 1994;120:633–637.

61 Wennberg DE, Lucas FL, Birkmeyer JD et al. Variation in carotid endarterectomy mortality in the Medicare population: Trial hospitals, volume, and patient characteristics. JAMA 1998;279:1278–1281.

62 Kroenke K, Lawrence VA, Theroux JF, Tuley MR. Operative risk in patients with severe obstructive pulmonary disease. Arch Intern Med 1992;152:967–971.

63 Rutsky EA, Rostand DG. Coronary artery bypass graft surgery in end-stage renal disease:indications, contraindications, and uncertainties. Semin Dial 7 1994:91.

64 Batiuk TD, Kurtz SB, Oh JK, Orszulak TA. The pharmacokinetics of racemic verapamil in patients with impaired renal function:coronary artery bypass operation in dialysis patients. Mayo Clin Proc 1991;66:45–53.

65 Flameng WJ, Herijgers P, Szecsi J et al. Determinants of early and late results of combined valve operations and coronary artery bypass grafting. Ann Thorac Surg 1996;61:621–628.

66 Mullany CJ, Elveback LR, Frye RI et al. Coronary artery disease and its management: Influence on survival inpatients undergoing aortic valve replacement. J Am Coll Cardiol 1987;10:66–72.

67 Pick AW, Mullany CJ, Orszulak TA, Daly RC, Schaff HV. Third and fourth operations for myocardial ischemia:short-term results and long-term survival. Circulation 1997;96 Suppl II:26–31.

68 Christenson JT, Simonet F, Schmuziger M. The impact of a short interval (<:1 year) between primary and reoperative coronary artery bypass grafting procedures. Cardiovasc Surg 1996;4:801–807.

69 Birkmeyer JD, Quinton HB, O'Connor NJ et al. The effect of peripheral vascular disease on long-term mortality after coronary artery bypass surgery: Northern New England Cardiovascular Disease Study Group. Arch Surg 1996;131:316–321.

70 Birkmeyer JD, O'Connor GT, Quinton HB et al. The effect of peripheral vascular disease on in-hospital mortality rates with coronary artery bypass surgery: Northern New England Cardiovascular Disease Study Group. J Vasc Surg 1995;21:445–452.

71 Baker DW, Jones R, Hodges J, Massie BM, Konstam MA, Rose EA. Management of heart failure, III: The role of revascularization in the treatment of patients with moderate or severe left ventricular systolic dysfunction. JAMA 1994;272:1528–1534.

72 Stahle E, Bergstrom R, Edlund B *et al.* Influence of left ventricular function on survival after coronary artery bypass grafting. Ann Thorac Surg 1997;64:437–444.

73 The NAPA investigators Results of the Nesiritide Administered Peri–Anesthesia in Patients Undergoing Cardiac Surgery trial. Circulation May 30th online publication.

74 Fragmin during Instability in Coronary Artery Disease (FRISC) study group. low-molecular-weight heparin during instability in coronary artery disease. Lancet 1996;347:561–568.

75 Gott JP, Han DC. Surgical treatment of acute myocardial infarct:clinical considerations. Semin Thorac Cardiovasc Surg 1995;7:198–207.

76 Serrano CV Jr, Ramires JA, Cesar LA *et al.* Prognostic significance of right ventricular dysfunction in patients with acute inferior myocardial infarction and right ventricular involvement. Clin Cardiol 1995;18:199–205.

77 Berger PB, Ruocco JNA, Ryan TJ *et al.* Frequency and significance of right ventricular dysfunction during inferior wall left ventricular myocardial infarction treated with thrombolytic therapy. Am J Cardiol 1993;71:1148–1152.

78 Bowers TR, O'Neill WW, Grines C, Pica MC, Safian RD, Goldstein JA. Effect of reperfusion on biventricular function and survival after right ventricular infarction. N Engl J Med 1998;338:933–940.

79 Goldstein JA, Barzilai B, Rosamond TL, Eisenberg PR, Jaffe AS. Determinants of hemodynamic compromise with severe right ventricular infarction. Circulation 1990;82:359–368.

80 Calvin JE. Optimal right ventricular filling pressures and the role of pericardial constraint in right ventricular infarction in dogs Circulation 1991;84:852–861.

CHAPTER 5

Care for Patients Undergoing Non-cardiac Surgery

Thach N. Nguyen, Gianluca Rigatelli, Loan T. Pham, Vo Thanh Nhan and Kim Eagle

Introduction

Burdened by disease in the aging process, many middle-aged or elderly cardiac- or possibly-cardiac patients require non-cardiac surgery. The role of the cardiologist is to perform an evaluation of the patient's current medical status, make recommendations concerning the cardiac risk over the entire perioperative and postoperative period, and provide a clinical risk profile that the patient, anesthesiologist, and surgeon can use to make clinical decisions and therapeutic changes [1]. Besides the preoperative evaluation, the cardiologist is expected to provide appropriate pre- and postoperative care in order to lower or neutralize the cardiac risk. Many times, as the most senior consultant handling complex cardiovascular problems, the cardiologist consultant has to orchestrate the non-surgical aspect of care among many other medical consultants (pulmonologist, infectious disease, nephrologist, neurologist, etc.), so there is a coordinating direction and cohesive unity in the care. The ultimate goal is to prevent the occurrence of myocardial infarction (MI), decompensated congestive heart failure (CHF), pulmonary edema, significant arrhythmias or death.

Under best management for elective surgery, the cardiac complications were minimal (<1%) [2]. This is the goal for any surgical program. However, in the litigious climate of the US society and the unrealistically high expectations of some patients and families, any preventable or non-preventable poor outcome may be scrutinized for possible legal recourse. The management strategies during the pre-, peri- and postoperative periods are listed in Table 5.1.

Table 5.1 Management strategies for cardiac patients undergoing non-cardiac surgery.

1. Identify the low risk patients so they can go directly to surgery
2. Identify the high risk patients for invasive work-up prior to surgery
3. Identify the intermediate risk patients for non-invasive testing prior to surgery
4. Optimal medical treatment including β-blockade and control of CHF before surgery

CHF, congestive heart failure.

Initial Consultation

At the first encounter with the patient, the cardiologist reviews the pertinent history and performs a physical examination in the context of the proposed surgical procedure. This preoperative cardiac evaluation must be carefully tailored to the circumstances that have prompted the consultation and nature of the surgical illness. Given an acute surgical emergency, the preoperative evaluation will be limited to a rapid assessment of the cardiovascular vital signs, volume status, and an electrocardiogram (ECG), often performed in the emergency department or the preoperative holding area. Only the most essential tests and interventions are appropriate until the acute surgical emergency is resolved. In some circumstances, surgery is not performed as an emergency procedure, but because good care dictates prompt surgery [1]. Under other less urgent or elective circumstances, a more comprehensive preoperative work-up can be performed.

From the cardiac point of view, the consultant focuses on verifying the presence of four major unstable cardiac conditions which can destabilize the patient or endanger his or her life during the surgical procedure.(Table 5.2). The two most frequent problems are decompensated CHF and unstable coronary artery disease (CAD) which includes previously stable angina now unresponsive to adequate medical therapy, crescendo angina or rest angina. The problems with uncontrolled arrhythmia and significant valvular stenosis or regurgitation are rare. Once identified, these major unstable cardiac conditions mandate intensive management, which may result in delay or cancellation of surgery, unless the condition is emergent. Next the consultant has to unmask conditions, the presence of which triggers the suspicion of occult CAD, often heightens the risk of anesthesia, and thus justifies more in-depth assessment of patient's cardiovascular status [1]. These conditions are classified as intermediate. Other relevant non-cardiac comorbidities which can

Table 5.2 Unstable conditions which increase perioperative cardiac risk.

Major unstable cardiac conditions
1. Unstable coronary syndromes
    (a) Recent MI with ongoing ischemia
    (b) Unstable or severe angina (Canadian Cardiac Society class III or IV)
2. Decompensated CHF
3. Significant arrhythmias
    (a) High grade atrio–ventricular block
    (b) Advanced ventricular arrhythmias
    (c) Supraventricular arrythmias with uncontrolled ventricular rate
4. Severe valvular disease(s)

Intermediate unstable conditions
1. Mild angina (Canadian Cardiac Society class I or II)
2. Prior MI by history or pathological Q waves
3. Compensated or prior heart failure
4. Peripheral arterial diseases
5. Diabetes mellitus
6. Renal insufficiency

Relevant comorbidities
1. Significant chronic pulmonary disease
2. Significant liver disease

CHF, congestive heart failure; MI, mypocardial infarction.

aggravate the surgical process, or prolong the recovery, need also to be identified accurately.

History

Besides a detailed history, accurate recording of current medications including: anticoagulants, aspirin and non-steroidal anti-inflammatory drugs, use of alcohol, over-the-counter herbal medicines and illicit drugs should be documented, owing to the possible detrimental interaction with anesthetic agents [1]. Other important information includes the history of deep vein thrombosis (DVT), history of bleeding complications and prior hospitalization for asthma or intubation. Although an objective measure of exercise tolerance predicts outcome, history alone is frequently sufficient to delineate those persons with good exercise tolerance (Table 5.3) [3]. Poor exercise tolerance is considered when patients cannot walk four blocks or climb two flights of stairs, and manage only activities equivalent to less than four metabolic equivalents (METs) [1,3].

Table 5.3 Assessment of functional status by daily activities [4].

1. 1–4 METS
   a. Can you take care of yourself?
   b. Can you eat, dress, or use the toilet?
   c. Can you walk indoors around the home?
   d. Can you walk one or two blocks on level ground at 2–3 mph?
   e. Can you do light work at home like dusting or washing dishes?

2. 4–9 METS
   a. Can you climb a flight of stairs or walk up a hill?
   b. Can you walk on level ground at 4 mph?
   c. Can you run a short distance?
   d. Can you scrub floors, lifting or moving heavy furniture?
   e. Can you go golfing, bowling, dancing, doubles tennis?

3. 10 METS
   a. Can you participate in strenuous sports like swimming, singles tennis, football, basketball or skiing?

METS, metabolic equivalents.

Physical Examination

A cardiovascular examination should include an assessment of vital signs, blood pressure in both arms, carotid pulse contour and bruits, jugular venous pressure and pulsations, auscultation of the lungs, precordial palpation and auscultation, abdominal palpation, a check for extremities edema and vascular integrity [1]. The goal is to be sure that four possible major cardiac problems are well evaluated and ruled out: unstable angina, decompensated CHF, significant brady-tachy-arrhythmia, and valvular stenosis or regurgitation.

CLINICAL PEARLS
How important is it to evaluate what is not seen or heard in a
preoperative history and physical examination?

- When evaluating the functional level of a patient, lack of activity due to advanced age, deconditioning, chronic arthritis, or pulmonary disease can mask significant problems because these patients may not stress themselves sufficiently in daily life to provoke symptoms of myocardial ischemia or CHF.
- Then peripheral edema is not a reliable indicator of CHF unless the jugular venous pressure is elevated or the hepatojugular reflux is positive [1].
- If a murmur is present, significant mitral or aortic stenosis or regurgitation have to be ruled out because of the increased risk of CHF if a lot of fluid is needed during surgery.
- Detection of significant aortic stenosis (AS) is of particular importance because this lesion with its fixed cardiac output is a traditional high-risk factor for non-cardiac surgery [5].
- Usually, if the second heart sound (S2) is still heard clearly, then there is no severe AS. If the S2 is not heard, then the valve is so calcified it cannot open and close making a click, so AS is quite severe. The systolic murmur also would peak late in severe stenosis.
- The slow rate of rise in the carotid pulse may not be felt in elderly patients owing to generalized stiffness of the whole artery.

In the new revised cardiac risk index [6], AS was not considered as a major risk because judicious management of fluid intake and output could reduce the occurrence of hypotension or fluid overload secondary to AS, and because virtually all symptomatic patients were treated with valve replacement before elective non-cardiac surgery.

The Surgery-specific Risk

The surgery-specific cardiac risk of non-cardiac surgery is related to two important factors. First, the type of surgery itself may identify a patient with a greater likelihood of underlying CAD. Perhaps the best example is vascular surgery, in which underlying CAD is present in a substantial portion of patients. The second aspect is the degree of hemodynamic cardiac stress associated with surgery-specific techniques. Certain operations may be associated with profound alterations in heart rate, blood pressure, vascular volume, pain, bleeding, clotting tendencies, oxygenation, neuro-humoral activation, etc. The intensity of these coronary and myocardial stressors helps determine the likelihood of perioperative cardiac events. This is particularly evident in emergency surgery, where the risk of cardiac complications is substantially elevated. The classification of non-cardiac surgeries and their surgery-specific risk (% rate of cardiovascular complications) are listed in Table 5.4 [1].

Table 5.4 Cardiac risk stratification for non-cardiac surgery.

High (cardiac risk >5%)	Major emergent surgery, particularly in the elderly Aortic surgery and other major vascular surgery Peripheral vascular surgery Anticipated prolonged surgical procedures associated with large fluid shifts and/or blood loss
Intermediate (cardiac risk <5%)	Intra-peritoneal and intra-thoracic surgery Carotid endarterectomy Head and neck surgery Orthopedic surgery Prostatic surgery
Low risk (<1%)	Cataract removal Dermatologic operations Endoscopic procedures Breast surgery

Estimate the Cardiac Risk

At this present time, there are 2 ways to evaluate cardiac patients before non cardiac surgery: the Revised Cardiac Risk Index or the Clinical Algorithm.

The Revised Cardiac Risk Index

In order to identify high risk patients undergoing elective and semi-urgent surgery, a revised cardiac risk index (RCRI) was devised to help clinicians stratify the patient's cardiac risk. Six clinical risk factors were identified and are listed in Table 5.5 [2]. Since these six factors had approximately the same statistical importance, they were each given the same "weight" or one point each. If the patient has two points, he or she is in the intermediate risk group. If there are three or more points, then the patient belongs to the high risk group. The complications mentioned in the study are MI, ventricular fibrillation, primary cardiac arrest, complete heart block, and pulmonary edema [6].

Table 5.5 The revised cardiac risk index.

Assign one point to each of the following variables:
1. High risk surgery (intra-peritoneal, intra-thoracic, supra-inguinal vascular)
2. Ischemic heart disease (history of MI, positive stress test, current ischemic pain, use of nitrate, ECG with Q waves)
3. Congestive Heart Failure (history of HF, pulmonary edema, paroxysmal nocturnal dyspnea, bilateral rales, S3 gallop, CXR with vascular redistribution)
4. Cerebrovascular disease (history of transient ischemic attack or stroke)
5. Diabetes mellitus
6. Pre-operative serum creatinine >2 mg/dl

(Continued)

Table 5.5 (*Continued*)

Total points	Complication rate
Class 1: 0 points	0.4–1%
Class 2: 1 point	2.2%
Class 3: 2 points	6.6%
Class 4: >3 points	9%

CXR, chest X-ray; ECG, electrocardiogram; HF, heart failure; MI, myocardial infarction.

A Clinical Algorithm to Assess the Cardiac Risk

Using the data of the Coronary Artery Surgery Study (CASS) registry, Eagle *et al.* found that patients who underwent major vascular, abdominal, thoracic, or head and neck surgery after previous CABG had fewer perioperative deaths and MI than patients receiving medical therapy [7].

CRITICAL THINKING
The protective effect of coronary artery bypass grafting in the CASS study. 24,959 Coronary Artery Surgery Study registry enrollees were either treated with coronary artery bypass grafting (CABG) or medical therapy. During follow-up, patients who required non-cardiac operations were evaluated for hospital or out-of-hospital death within 30 days of non-cardiac surgery and non-fatal postoperative MI. At a mean follow-up of 4.1 years, 3368 patients underwent non-cardiac surgery. Abdominal, vascular, thoracic, and head and neck surgery each had a combined MI/death rate of >4% among patients with non-revascularized coronary disease. Among 1961 patients undergoing higher-risk surgery, prior CABG was associated with fewer postoperative deaths (1.7% vs. 3.3%, $P = 0.03$) and MIs (0.8% vs. 2.7%, $P = 0.002$) compared with medically managed coronary disease. On the contrary, 1297 patients undergoing urologic, orthopedic, breast, and skin operations had mortality of <1% regardless of prior coronary treatment. Prior CABG was most protective in patients with advanced angina and/or multi-vessel CAD [7].

So, rather using a number to estimate the cardiac risk, these data suggest a clinically oriented pathway to risk-stratify the patients undergoing non-cardiac surgery by going through the steps outlined below [1].

Step 1: What is the urgency of non-cardiac surgery?
Certain emergencies do not allow time for preoperative cardiac evaluation. Postoperative risk stratification may be appropriate for some patients who have not had such an assessment before.

Step 2: Has the patient undergone coronary revascularization in the past 5 years?

If so, and if clinical status has remained stable without recurrent symptoms/ signs of ischemia, further cardiac testing is generally not necessary.

Step 3: Has the patient had a coronary evaluation in the past 2 years?

If coronary risk was adequately assessed and the findings were favorable, it is usually not necessary to repeat testing unless the patient has experienced a change or new symptoms of coronary ischemia since the previous evaluation.

Step 4: Does the patient have an unstable coronary syndrome or a major clinical predictor of risk?

When elective non-cardiac surgery is being considered, the presence of unstable coronary disease, decompensated heart failure (HF), symptomatic arrhythmias, and/or severe valvular heart disease usually leads to cancellation or delay of surgery until the problem has been identified and treated.

Step 5: Does the patient have intermediate clinical predictors of risk?

The presence or absence of prior MI by history or ECG, angina pectoris, compensated or prior HF, preoperative creatinine greater than or equal to 2 mg/dL, and/or diabetes mellitus helps to further stratify clinical risk for perioperative coronary events (Table 5.6). Consideration of functional capacity and level of surgery-specific risk allows a rational approach to identify patients most likely to benefit from further non-invasive testing.

Step 6

Patients without major but with intermediate predictors of clinical risk and moderate or excellent functional capacity can generally undergo intermediate-risk surgery with little likelihood of perioperative death or MI. Conversely, further non-invasive testing is often considered for patients with poor functional capacity or moderate functional capacity but higher-risk surgery, especially for patients with two or more intermediate predictors of risk (Table 5.6).

Step 7

Non-cardiac surgery is generally safe for patients with neither major nor intermediate predictors of clinical risk and moderate or excellent functional capacity (4 METs or greater). Additional testing may be considered on an individual basis for patients without clinical markers but with poor functional capacity who are facing higher-risk operations, particularly those with several minor clinical predictors of risk who are scheduled to undergo vascular surgery.

Step 8

The results of non-invasive testing can be used to determine the need for additional preoperative testing and treatment. In some patients with documented

CAD, the risk of coronary intervention or corrective cardiac surgery may approach or even exceed the risk of the proposed non-cardiac surgery. This approach may be appropriate, however, if it significantly improves the patient's long-term prognosis.

As mentioned above, the patient may need testing if any two of the factors below are present.

Table 5.6 Testing is indicated if any two of the following factors are present.

Intermediate clinical predictors
1. Canadian Cardiac Society class 1 or 2 angina
2. Prior MI by history or presence of pathological Q waves
3. Compensated or prior HF
4. Diabetes

Poor functional capacity (<4 METs)

Procedure with high surgical risk
1. Aortic repair or peripheral vascular surgery
2. Emergency surgery
3. Prolonged surgery with large fluid shift or blood loss

HF, heart failure; METs, metabolic equivalents; MI, myocardial infarction.

CRITICAL THINKING

Which one to use: the cardiac risk index or the clinical algorithm?
After completing a history and physical examination, and reviewing the available laboratories results, for the cardiologist with a mathematic oriented mind, the patient's data can be extrapolated on a simple six-point RCRI formula in order to estimate the patient's operative risk.

- For the cardiologist with practical mind and a lot of clinical experience, there is a friendly clinical-based algorithm to walk through the cardiac evaluation maze.
- Therefore the selection between RCRI or the clinical algorithm is up to the personality or working style of the cardiologist. There is no "one size fits all."
- Any cardiac risk calculation formula or pathway needs to be accurate in predicting peri- or postoperative events. It has to have a favorable benefits–risk trade off too, because auto-pilot preoperative imaging testing, due to high false positive results, may lead to adverse outcome from extra-testing and by delaying necessary surgery [1].

Classification of Patients

With the history, a physical examination and the result of cardiac risk evaluation formula or clinical algorithm, the cardiologist then determines if the patient is in the best (or worst or in-between) medical condition, given the context of the surgical procedure.

The patients who need emergency surgery

In emergency surgical cases, the procedure must be undertaken, regardless of the patient's cardiovascular risk, because without surgery, mortality cannot be avoided [2]. The role of the cardiologist is to support the surgical care by providing recommendations aimed at minimizing the ischemic insult or CHF with vasodilators, careful use of diuretics, and fluid management guided by cardiac filling pressure from a pulmonary artery catheter, if needed. If there are non-specific changes in the ECG, suggesting metabolic and/or electrolyte disturbances, medications, intracranial disease, pulmonary disease, etc, then the role of the cardiologist is to decipher the ECG abnormalities and facilitate resolution of these problems prior to surgery.

The low risk patients

For patients who have no major unstable cardiac problems, nor significant comorbidities, with an excellent functional activity status, (RCRI = 1) there was only 3% incidence of perioperative morbidity. Non-invasive testing adds little to further stratify risk. These patients should undergo the surgical procedure without further testing.

The intermediate risk patients

These patients (RCRI = 1–2) scheduled for intermediate- or high-risk surgery should go for non-invasive testing. If these patients are scheduled for low risk surgery, then β-blockade (BB) is enough [8].

The high risk patients with coronary artery disease

For patients with major clinical risk factors (RCRI > 3) who may have a morbidity rate of 50%, especially in patients with unstable CAD, non-invasive testing for CAD does not further stratify risk [3]. Coronary angiography may be the appropriate next step for possible coronary revascularization. So the indications for coronary revascularization should include patients with poorly controlled ischemic symptoms despite excellent medical therapy, or patients with a large ischemic burden (>25% of the left ventricle) on stress perfusion imaging [9].

The high risk patients who are not eligible for revascularization

In high risk patients for whom myocardial revascularization is not an option, it is often not necessary to perform an exercise stress test. Rather, maximizing best medical therapy is the desired strategy [10]. However, in patients with such extensive ischemia, effective β-blockade may not be sufficient to reduce the rate of perioperative cardiac complications [10].

The forgotten high risk patients

In the cohort of cardiac patients who undergo non-cardiac procedures, patients with HF encountered the highest complications more than the patients with CAD [11]. The HF patients are really forgotten by the cardiology community, as most emphasis in the guidelines is focused on problems with CAD.

 CRITICAL THINKING
Meta-analysis of HF patients undergoing non-cardiac surgery. Using the 1997–1998 standard analytic file 5% sample of Medicare beneficiaries, patients with HF who underwent major non-cardiac surgery were identified. The results showed that of 23,340 HF patients and 28,710 CAD patients, 1,532 (6.56%) HF patients and 1,757 (6.12%) CAD patients underwent major non-cardiac surgery. There were 44,512 patients in the control group with major non-cardiac surgery. After accounting for demographic characteristics, type of surgery, and comorbid conditions, the risk-adjusted operative mortality (death before discharge or within 30 days of surgery) was HF 11.7%, CAD 6.6%, and control 6.2% (HF vs. CAD, $P < 0.001$; CAD vs. control, $P = 0.518$) [12].

So in patients 65 years of age and older, HF patients undergoing major non-cardiac surgery suffer the highest mortality rate despite advances in perioperative care, whereas patients with CAD without HF have similar mortality compared with the general patient population [12]. These results showed the urgent need for BB in the perioperative medical management because BB is first or second essential medication for HF after angiotensin converting enzyme inhibitors (ACEI).

Non-invasive Testing

Exercise Stress Test
Non-invasive testing for ischemia should be considered for patients with high probability of CAD if such risk stratification has not been performed in the last few years, or if there has been some change in the patient's symptomatic status. The test most commonly performed for further risk stratification is the threadmill exercise test. The aim is to provide an objective measure of functional capacity, to identify the presence of important preoperative myocardial ischemia or cardiac arrhythmias, and to estimate perioperative cardiac risk and long-term prognosis. Poor functional capacity in patients with chronic CAD or those convalescing after an acute cardiac event is associated with an increased risk of subsequent cardiac morbidity and mortality [13]. The test is considered abnormal if ischemic changes develop especially when associated with typical chest pain, ischemia occurring at or before 6 METs, or when ischemia is accompanied by a decrease of >10 mmHg from the baseline [13].

CRITICAL THINKING

Why is the nuclear scan falsely negative? The working mechanism of a nuclear scan is its discriminatory capacity between difference of isotope uptake during rest and stress, and between vascular territories. If the difference between two areas is less than 7% then there is no difference noted on the scan.

If the patient has perfusion abnormalities due to severe lesions in all three arteries with a difference of <7% between each, then the uptake on the scan looks homogenous.

If the patient has poor exercise tolerance or the heart is not stressed enough to maximally vasodilate the normal area, then there is no difference between the isotope uptake in a maximally vasodilated area of a significant lesion and a not-yet maximally dilated of a normal area: the scan of isotope uptake would look falsely homogenous.

CLINICAL PEARLS

Why is the stress test in left bundle branch block falsely positive? In patients with pre-existing left bundle branch block (LBBB), pharmacological stress testing with adenosine or dipyridamole is preferable to dobutamine or exercise imaging. The tachycardia induced during exercise, and conceivably also during dobutamine infusion, may result in reversible septal defects even in the absence of left anterior descending artery disease in some patients (a false-positive wall motion finding). This response is unusual with either dipyridamole or adenosine stress testing [1].

Other Imaging Stress Test

The two most common methodologies of imaging exercise- or non-exercise stress testing are dobutamine stress echocardiography and intravenous dipyridamole or adenosine myocardial perfusion imaging [1]. In the stress echocardiography, ischemia is noted when there is development of a new wall motion abnormality in previously normal segment, or akinesis from baseline hypokinesis [3]. As with any diagnostic test, 100% accuracy is not possible. It is important to note that both are extremely operator- and institution-dependent. Nuclear stress testing may be more accurate in one facility and stress echocardiography may be superior in another. It is critical for a physician to recognize the strengths and weaknesses of their individual facilities when selecting a test for their patients.

CRITICAL THINKING

Thallium stress test or stress echocardiography: which is better? In this meta-analysis, thallium imaging (TI) and stress echocardiography (SE) were compared in patients at risk for MI scheduled for elective non-cardiac surgery. Data of 1351 consecutive patients scheduled surgery were analyzed. The results showed that routine screening for myocardial ischemia was used more frequently in SE studies (47.8% vs. 21.2%; $P = 0.008$), and screening dictated treatment more often after TI (72.1%) than after SE (46.3%; $P = 0.027$). The likelihood ratio (LR) for SE was more indicative of a postoperative cardiac event than TI (LR, 4.09; 95% CI, 3.21–6.56 vs. 1.83; 1.59–2.10; $P = 0.001$). This difference was attributable to fewer false-negative SEs. There was no difference in the cumulative Receiver Operating Characteristic curves from qualitative studies (SE, 0.80, 95% CI, 0.76–0.84 vs. TI, 0.75; 95% CI, 0.70–081). Again, the likelihood rate for a negative SE was less (0.23; 95% CI, 0.17–0.32 vs. 0.44; 95% CI, 0.36–0.54). A moderate-to-large defect, seen in 14% of patients by either method, predicts a postoperative cardiac event (LR, 8.35; 95% CI, 5.6–12.45) [14].

This meta-analysis possesses the statistical power to demonstrate that SE has better negative-predicative characteristics than TI. A moderate-to-large perfusion defect by either SE or TI predicts postoperative MI and death. Therefore the SE is superior to TI in predicting postoperative cardiac events [14].

Echocardiogram

The greatest risk of complications after non-cardiac surgery occurs in patients with an "at rest" left ventricular ejection fraction (LVEF) of less than 35%. In the perioperative phase, poor left ventricular (LV) systolic or diastolic function is mainly predictive of postoperative CHF, and in critically ill patients, death. It is noteworthy, however, that resting LV function was not found to be a consistent predictor of perioperative ischemic events [1]. Therefore knowledge of a poor ejection fraction may help the physician to anticipate the risk for CHF and to undertake judicious management of fluids and vasodilator treatment in order to maintain an adequate blood pressure and satisfactory renal function, while effectively avoiding fluid overload.

Management After the Stress test

What should be done once the stress test is performed? A negative nuclear perfusion test result, or a negative dobutamine echocardiography has excellent negative predictive value (100%), and one can generally proceed to surgery without any further work-up. The more problematic patient is the one with an abnormal test result. Their positive predictive value is low (<20%).

CRITICAL THINKING
Why positive stress testing has poor predictive values? In determining the value of preoperative testing, it is important to acknowledge that perioperative cardiac morbidity is multifactorial in origin. Usually MI is caused by plaque rupture, however, during the perioperative period, this pathological mechanism occurs in less than 50% of MI [15,16]; the rest is due to a prolonged

imbalance between myocardial oxygen supply and demand. Myocardial oxygen supply may be diminished by anemia or hypotension, whereas oxygen demand may be increased by tachycardia and hypertension (HTN) resulting from postoperative pain, withdrawal of anesthesia, or shifts in intravascular volume. Perioperative MI usually occurs 1–4 days after surgery [17], when the effects of anesthesia have dissipated and perioperative pain and fluid shifts are occurring [10]. More importantly, the post-operative period is associated with a hypercoagulable state that may promote the formation of postoperative coronary occlusion. Non-invasive testing may identify obstructive lesion distal to which myocardial ischemia may develop, but it cannot predict non-critical stenoses that are susceptible to plaque rupture and development of MI [3].

Another consideration is that several factors limit the predictive value of these clinical indices because more focused preoperative management and risk modifications frequently alter patient's care and outcomes causing lesser predictive values to these indices.

Therefore not all these patients should be referred for cardiac catheterization. The patient with a positive test should first be further risk-stratified. Factors to be considered include the workload at which the test is positive, the number of myocardial segments involved, and whether the LV function is abnormal. A patient with a highly positive test result would likely need a cardiac catheterization prior to surgery, while a mildly positive test may require treatment with medical therapy, such as with β-blockers [2].

CRITICAL THINKING

Can we ever have a perfect postoperative statistical outcome? In patient with low risk, if the pretest probability for cardiac complication is 2.2% (e.g. RCRI = 1), a positive dobutamine stress echo (sensitivity of 85% and specificity of 70%) would yield a post-test probability of 5%. However, in patients with high risk with a pretest probability risk of 20%, a negative stress test (which negates the indication and performance of coronary angiography and revascularization) still yield a 5% probability of cardiac complications. This result is understood to mean that high risk patients may still have 5% perioperative risk despite a negative stress test result [11].

Additional recommendations regarding anesthetic issues, aggressive treatment of hemodynamic disturbances, preoperative medical and coronary interventions, or active monitoring in selective patients are tailored to the individual circumstances [3]. In an era of overpriced health care services, savings from reduced use of postoperative monitoring, treatment or shorter length of stay (LOS) may easily offset the costs of preoperative screening [3].

Preparation of Patients Prior to Surgery

Elective surgery should proceed if: (1) the systolic blood pressure is controlled below 180 mmHg and diastolic pressure below 110 mm Hg; (2) arrhythmia is controlled; (3) no decompensated CHF; (4) no unstable angina; (5) no severe aortic stenosis; and (6) no anemia (ideally hematocrit above 30 g/dl. Furthermore, all patients should be treated with β-blockers when there are no contra-indications and stain in order to improve outcomes.

Maximal Medical Stabilization with β-Blockers

The rationale for β-blocker therapy during the pre-operative period is that it is the only proven intervention (medical or surgical) to reduce the risk of short-term cardiac complications after non-cardiac surgery [18]. The benefits from these medications would presumably be greater if β-blockade titrated to a preoperative heart rate of 60 bpm or less. Therapy should ideally be initiated days or weeks prior to elective surgery. After surgery, β-blockade (BB) is given to avoid the withdrawal symptoms, if the patient was on β-blockers long before surgery. If the patient does not need long term BB therapy, then the patient should receive BB for 7–30 days after surgery.

Evidence-based Medicine: Meta-analysis of β-blockade before surgery

A retrospective study of 782,969 patients, who underwent major non-cardiac surgery. 663,635 (85%) had no recorded contraindications to BB, 122,338 of whom (18%) received such treatment during the first two hospital days, including 14% of patients with a RCRI score of 0 and 44% with a score of 4 or higher. The relationship between perioperative BB treatment and the risk of death varied directly with cardiac risk; among the 580,665 patients with an RCRI score of 0 or 1, treatment was associated with no benefit and possible harm, whereas among the patients with an RCRI score of 2, 3, or 4 or more the adjusted ORs for death in the hospital were 0.88 (95% CI, 0.80–0.98), 0.71 (95% CI, 0.63–0.80), and 0.58 (95% CI, 0.50–0.67), respectively.

Therefore a perioperative BB therapy is associated with a reduced risk of in-hospital death among high-risk-, but not low-risk-, patients undergoing major non-cardiac surgery [19,20] (Table 5.7). One life is saved for every 30–60 high-risk patients treated with BB, but on the contrary, one life could be lost for every 200–500 low-risk patients who received BB.

Table 5.7 Beneficial effect of pre-operative β-blockers [11].

RCRI total points	Complication rate	Complication rate with BB
Class 1: 0 points	0.4–1%	<1%
Class 2–3: 1–2 points	2.2–6.6%	0.8–1.6%
Class 4: >3 points	9%	>3%

BB, β-blockade; RCRI, revised cardiac risk index.

CRITICAL THINKING

How to use β-blockers in patients with contra-indications. In patients with relative contra-indications (reactive airway disease, severe chronic obstructive lung disease, etc), cardio-selective BB may be used and titrated to a resting heart rate of 60–65 [21,22].

- When the patient cannot take medication by mouth, intravenous (IV) β-blocker can be used during the perioperative period. However, all the beneficial effects of BB were proved on randomized trials with oral BB.
- If BB cannot be used, some studies suggested that α-2 agonists might prevent adverse cardiac events when used in the perioperative setting [23].

Congestive Heart Failure

The presence of decompensated CHF before surgery has been associated with the highest incidence of perioperative cardiac morbidity and mortality (double the rate of adverse event in patient with CAD) [12]. Stabilization of ventricular function and treatment of pulmonary congestion is prudent before elective surgery. It is also important to determine the cause of CHF. Congestive symptoms may be caused by non-ischemic cardiomyopathy, CAD, and valvular problems. Because the type of perioperative monitoring and treatments would be different for different conditions, clarifying the cause of CHF is important [3]. However, overzealous use of right heart catheterization (RHC) and monitoring may be detrimental as proved below.

CRITICAL THINKING

Is right heart monitoring detrimental? In an observational cohort study of 4059 patients who underwent major non-cardiac surgery (excluding abdominal aortic aneurysm repair), the value of RHC was underwhelming. Over 200 patients had an RHC, with an overall three-fold increase in the incidence of major postoperative cardiac events and an adjusted OR of 2.0 for postoperative major cardiac events [24].

During surgery, both general and regional anesthesia cause peripheral vasodilation, and venous return is reduced by positive-pressure ventilation, whereas usual perioperative therapy emphasizes fluid replacement. Not surprisingly, the cessation of positive-pressure ventilation and the conclusion of general and regional anesthesia and the third-spaced fluid now mobilized intravascularly can lead to substantial increases in intravascular volume and venous return, causing possible pulmonary congestion and edema. The risk of postoperative edema peaks in the first 36 hours after surgery [25]. Therefore, judicious use of fluid before, during and after surgery is important in preventing hypotension during surgery and HF after surgery. After an exhausting literature search, there are no data documenting an optimal approach or guideline to managing HF before, during, or after non-cardiac surgery [11]. BB did confer benefits to CAD patients and might also help in stabilizing the patients with HF.

Pulmonary Disease

The presence of either obstructive or restrictive pulmonary disease places the patient at increased risk of developing perioperative respiratory complications. Hypoxemia, hypercapnia, acidosis, and increased work of breathing can all lead to further deterioration of an already compromised cardiopulmonary system. If significant pulmonary disease is suspected by history or physical examination, determination of functional capacity, response to bronchodilators, and/or evaluation for the presence of carbon dioxide retention through arterial blood gas analysis may be justified. If there is evidence of infection, appropriate antibiotics are critical. Steroids and bronchodilators may be indicated, although the risk of producing arrhythmia and subsequent or myocardial ischemia by beta-receptor agonists must be considered [1].

Diabetes Mellitus

The presence of diabetes mellitus should heighten suspicion of CAD, since myocardial ischemia is more likely to be silent in the patient with diabetes mellitus. Tight management of blood glucose levels in the perioperative period is needed with frequent adjusted doses or infusions of short-acting insulin based on frequent blood glucose monitoring [1].

Renal Impairment

Azotemia is commonly associated with cardiac disease and often complicates its management. Excessive diuresis in combination with initiation of ACEI may result in an increase in blood urea nitrogen, plasma creatinine concentrations and hypotension from intravascular volume contraction. Maintenance of adequate intravascular volume for renal perfusion during diuresis of a patient with HF is often challenging. Close monitoring of fluid intake and output, daily patient weight measurement helps to maintain a decent blood pressure, and adequate urine output without fluid overload [1].

Coronary Revascularization

Cardiologists must be aware that the cardiac procedures performed in hopes of reducing the perioperative cardiac events have their own inherent risks. Primary coronary interventions (PCI) are still associated with <1% of mortality, <1% emergency CABG, and 2–3% of enzymatic MI. If the expected cardiac morbidity and mortality from the surgical procedures are less than these figures, then PCI is not warranted for the specific intent or the good intention of lowering preoperative risk [26]. Another risk that must be accounted for is the effect of cardiac evaluation in the delaying of the surgical procedure. In some cases, this delay has led to poor surgical outcomes: the patients had required amputation instead of an initially-planned lower extremities revascularization [26]. Until further data are available, the indications for PCI in the perioperative setting are identical to those developed by the joint ACC/AHA Task Force providing guidelines for PCI, regardless of the non-cardiac surgical plan.

When weighing the risk of CABG before non-cardiac surgery, the cumulative complication risk from coronary angiography, followed by CABG, followed by non-cardiac surgery is not likely to be lower than 3.4% seen in the study of patient undergoing non-cardiac surgery treated with BB [18]. No studies have shown that prophylactic CABG decreased the event rate after non-cardiac surgery [19]. Thus, CABG should only be recommended when its performance is likely to relieve symptoms or prolong life, independent of the non-cardiac surgical consideration.

CRITICAL THINKING

How to perform PCI before non-cardiac surgery? Before major elective surgery (e.g. orthopedic or spinal surgery), if a patient needs a stent, a bare metal stent (BMS) rather drug eluting stent (DES), should be used. Then the patient should wait for 4 weeks after PCI while on clopidogrel before the non-cardiac surgery is performed while on acetylsalicyic acid (ASA) to avoid any subacute stent thrombosis [27].

Recently a novel approach was suggested for patients who need CABG and aortic valve replacement. It was applied to >80-year-old patients with significant CAD and AS. The patient could undergo PCI with BMS in the morning with usual anticoagulant therapy during the procedure and bolus dose of clopidogrel before or after the procedure as usual. Then, directly after PCI, the patient could undergo minimally invasive aortic valve replacement with a bioprosthesis while under full dose heparin coverage (ACT >400 seconds). Heparin was reversed by protamine after surgery. The next morning, both the new stent and bioprosthetic valve would benefit from the antiplatelet protection of clopidogrel [28]. One month later, after clopidogrel was discontinued, the patient could undergo the non-cardiac surgery.

Looking at the problem through the same lens, could we perform PCI for a patient who needs any kind of surgery? The patient could undergo PCI with DES and heparin; the therapeutic effect of clopidogrel as usual. Then 4 hours after PCI, when the effect of heparin wears off and the effects of clopidogrel are still subtherapeutic, the patient could undergo surgery as usual. The next day, when the surgery is healing and the patient is recovering well, clopidogrel would kick in and prevent subacute thrombosis of the DES. The main requirements to perform PCI in these patients are that: (1) after PCI, the patients have a strong TIMI (thrombolysis in acute myocardial infarction) 3 flow; (2) there is only minimal residual stenosis (there is never a perfect 100% opening after stenting); and (3) glycoprotein 2b3a inhibition is not used. If the patients meet these three criteria, then this author believes that the patient could undergo the subsequent surgery. If not, surgery should be cancelled, or the BMS could be deployed and the patients go for surgery one month later.

One of the problems with this approach of surgery directly after DES insertion is that there is a concern of heightened coagulable state right after surgery or stenting. We don't have evidence of increased rate of subacute thrombosis (SAT) after freshly implanted DES (<12 hours) in patient undergoing fresh urgent surgery (<12 hours after DES implantation). We need to have a registry of all cases of surgery in <12 hours after DES or BMS implantation to clarify the SAT problem.

Arrhythmia

In the perioperative setting, cardiac arrhythmias or conduction disturbances often reflect the presence of underlying cardiopulmonary disease, drug toxicity, or metabolic derangements [1]. Supraventricular arrhythmias may require either electrical or pharmacological cardioversion if they produce symptoms or hemodynamic compromise. If cardioversion is not possible, satisfactory heart rate control should be accomplished with oral or intravenous digitalis, BB, or calcium channel blockers. Asymptomatic ventricular arrhythmias, whether simple premature ventricular contractions, complex ventricular ectopy, or non-sustained ventricular tachycardia, usually do not require therapy except in the presence of ongoing or threatened myocardial ischemia or moderate to severe LV dysfunction. Sustained or symptomatic ventricular tachycardia should be suppressed preoperatively with IV lidocaine, or amiodarone. The indications for temporary pacemakers are identical to those previously stated for long-term permanent cardiac pacing [29]. Patients with intraventricular conduction delays, bifascicular block (right bundle branch block with left anterior or posterior hemiblock), or LBBB with or without first degree atrioventricular block, do not generally require temporary pacemaker implantation in the absence of a history of syncope or more advanced atrioventricular block.

CLINICAL PEARLS

How to handle pacemakers or defibrillators during surgery In patients who are totally pacemaker-dependent, electrocautery poses a special problem and should be used sparingly, with the indifferent pole placed as far away from the pacemaker and heart as possible.

In pacemaker-dependent patients, use of bipolar pacing will minimize the risk of use of electrocautery. Also, converting the pacemaker to an uninhibited mode such as

AOO, VOO, or DOO with programming or a magnet prevents unwanted inhibition of pacing.

Implanted cardioverter defibrillators (ICD) should be programmed "Off" immediately before surgery and then "On" again postoperatively to prevent unwanted discharge due to spurious signals from the electric surgical equipment that the ICD might interpret as ventricular tachycardia or fibrillation [1].

Patients with Valvular Disease

Experience with managing valvular heart disease during labor and delivery provides insights into the approach to management of the patient for non-cardiac surgery. The vast majority of women with regurgitant valvular heart disease can be managed medically during the course of pregnancy, including labor and delivery, because of the decrease in peripheral vascular resistance [29]. Increased arterial impedance is not well tolerated in patients with aortic and mitral regurgitation. Therefore, increases in blood pressure should be prevented, and LV afterload should be optimized with vasodilators. In contrast, patients with significant aortic (AS) or mitral stenosis (MS) often do not do well with the increased hemodynamic burden of surgery. If the stenosis is severe, percutaneous catheter balloon valvotomy should be considered as definitive therapy (MS) or as a bridge to carry the patient through surgery (AS) [30].

CLINICAL PEARLS

Can the aortic stenosis patient go to emergency hip surgery?

At St Mary Medical Center, Hobart IN, many elderly patients with asymptomatic AS (or where the symptoms are controlled with medication) arrive at the hospital due to fracture of the femur. Often, they are not ideal candidates for cardiac surgery due to age or they have refused valve replacement in the past. Many underwent the orthopedic surgery without problem.

The perioperative medical management requires close monitoring of fluid intake and output in order to avoid quick CHF and pulmonary edema in AS patients who are very sensitive to fluid overload and dehydration, which can cause hypotension because of fixed low cardiac output.

Excessive changes in intravascular volume should be avoided. There were no prospective randomized controlled trial (RCTs) to confirm the above approach.

Patients with Peripheral Arterial Disease

There is an increased risk in performing CABG in patients with peripheral artery disease, and equally, mortality and morbidity following vascular surgery are mostly due to coronary events. If during the history-taking the patient is found to have unstable CAD, coronary angiography for possible revascularization should be undertaken first. In case of dual unstable CAD and carotid artery disease, many patients could safely undergo carotid artery endarterectomy (CEA) first without problem, because many vascular surgeons consider

CAE as a simple vascular procedure without large fluctuating blood pressure and fluid shifting. However, no prospective randomized trials have confirmed this approach. As demonstrated by recent carotid angioplasty trial, in patients with CAD scheduled for carotid surgery, endovascular carotid stenting is the preferable option due to its less invasive approach.

Patients with Congenital Heart Disease

In general, adult patients with undetected and untreated congenital heart disease (CHD) have simple problems such as atrial septal defect, patent foramen ovale, sometimes moderate aortic coarctation or small ventricular septal defect or a congenital coronary anomaly. Usually these patients do not need to specific treatment for heart disease prior to non-cardiac surgery except in two situations. The first one is the patients with congenital coronary anomaly such as ectopic origin of right coronary or left coronary artery from the opposite sinus: this anomaly needs careful preoperative evaluation including stresstest in order to evaluate ischemia-induced by stress during major vascular surgery, which can induce major hemodynamic fluctuation and exacerbate intramural aortic pressure compressing the abnormal coronary artery [31]. The second concern is for patients with patent foramen ovale (PFO) who are scheduled for posterior fossa ovale neurosurgery. In such cases, the clinical significance of their PFO should be assessed with transesophageal echocardiography (TEE) during Valsalva maneuver and transcranial Doppler (TCD) ultrasound should be performed. The results of TEE and TCD are considered abnormal if there is shunt during the Valsalva maneuver on TEE, and shower or curtain pattern of shunt on TCD. Severe hypotension, oxygen desaturation and even major stroke can happen during posterior cranial fossa surgery because of air embolism and hemodynamic instability in patients with right-to-left shunt undergoing neurosurgical procedures in the sitting position. Then transcatheter closure of the PFO should be advised and performed before the elective neurosurgery [32,33]. Patients with pulmonary hypertension, CHF or cyanosis have an increased perioperative risk [34]. The problems of patients with more complex CHD undergoing non-cardiac surgery are discussed in detail in Chapter 14.

Patients with Pulmonary Hypertension

Pulmonary hypertension (PH) is considered to be a significant preoperative risk factor. The predictors of short-term morbidity and mortality (<30 days) after non-cardiac surgery in patients with PH are well documented.

CRITICAL THINKING

Meta-analysis of outcomes of patients with pulmonary hypertension undergoing non-cardiac surgery. Through the PH and surgical databases, 1276 patients in the PH database, 145 patients (73% female) met all study criteria. Right ventricular systolic pressure (RVSP) on the 2D echocardiogram was 68 ± 21 mmHg. There were ten early deaths (7%). A history of pulmonary embolism ($P = 0.04$), right-axis deviation ($P = 0.02$), right ventricular (RV) hypertrophy ($P = 0.04$), RV index of myocardial performance ⩾0.75 ($P = 0.03$), RVSP/systolic blood pressure ⩾0.66 ($P = 0.01$), intraoperative use of vasopressors ($P < 0.01$), and anesthesia when nitrous oxide was not used ($P < 0.01$) were each associated with postoperative mortality. In patients with PH undergoing non-cardiac surgery with general anesthesia, specific clinical, diagnostic, and intraoperative factors may predict worse outcomes [35].

Intraoperative Care

The choice of anesthetic and intraoperative monitors is best left to the discretion of the anesthesia care team. Intraoperative management may be influenced by the perioperative plan, including need for postoperative monitors, ventilation, and postoperative analgesia. Therefore, a discussion of these issues before the planned surgery will allow for a smooth transition through the perioperative period.

In general, most current general anesthetics act as myocardial depressants [36]. They also lower systemic vascular resistance by dilating peripheral vascular beds, thus decreasing the arterial pressure. Autonomic imbalance secondary to catecholamine release during intubation and extubation may cause arrhythmias, arterial pressure changes, or even myocardial ischemia. Spinal and epidural anesthetics also cause sympathetic blockade and decrease arterial pressures [37].

Neuraxial anesthetic techniques include spinal and epidural approaches. Both techniques can result in sympathetic blockade, resulting in decreases in both preload and afterload. The decision to use neuraxial anesthesia for the high-risk cardiac patient may be influenced by the dermatomal level of the surgical procedure. Infrainguinal procedures can be performed under spinal or epidural anesthesia with minimal hemodynamic changes if neuraxial blockade is limited to those dermatomes. Abdominal procedures can also be performed using neuraxial techniques; however, high dermatomal levels of anesthesia may be required and may be associated with detrimental hemodynamic effects. High dermatomal blocks can potentially result in hypotension and reflex tachycardia if preload becomes compromised or blockade of the cardioaccelerators occurs [1].

Postoperative Management

In the preoperative period it is important to avoid the use of medications that may negatively interact with anesthetic agents. Postoperatively, the concern shifts toward avoiding withdrawal symptoms that may develop, and possible progression of the underlying disease if the medications are not restarted in a timely fashion. The potential for decreased gastrointestinal motility in the postoperative patient, which may reduce the efficacy of oral medications, must also be considered. The most favorable option for patients taking cardiovascular agents is to restart taking the agent as soon as they are stable after surgery. For patients who are unable to take oral medications, the medications can be given IV or subcutaneously [38]. If there is a need to confirm or rule out MI, the level of troponin of >2. 6 ng/mL would give the highest diagnostic yield on the postoperative days 1, 2, and 3 [39].

Postoperative Arrhythmias

Postoperative arrhythmias are often due to reversible noncardiac problems such as infection, hypotension, metabolic derangements, and hypoxia. Electrical cardioversion is generally not recommended until correction of the underlying problems has occurred, which frequently leads to a return to normal sinus rhythm. The avoidance of an electrolyte abnormality, especially hypokalemia and hypomagnesemia, may reduce the perioperative incidence and risk of arrhythmias [1].

Take Home Message

Peri-operative cardiac management should aim for both short- and long-term risk assessment and modifications. The approach to cardiac problems in this perioperative arena should mirror that in general cardiovascular practice.

If clinically the patient has low risk for cardiac event, then they should proceed for surgery without further cardiac testing. If the patient has intermediate risk and plans to undergo low-risk surgery, then they should proceed for surgery under protection of BB.

If the patient has intermediate risk and plans to undergo intermediate- or high-risk surgery, then they should have non-invasive testing to stratify the risk. If the patient has a high risk and plans to undergo intermediate or high risk surgery, then the patient either has invasive or non-invasive testing.

The indications for PCI or CABG are followed according to the usual guidelines, independent of the planned non-cardiac surgery.

The patient encounter with the cardiologist for clearance of non-cardiac surgery often represents the first chance for many patients to have their cardiovascular status addressed, and sometimes they have remarkably advanced problems which merit evaluation now simply because they were never properly recognized or treated. Therefore the perioperative cardiac evaluation may increasingly represent an opportunity to initiate or modify cardiac care, including primary and secondary preventive measures that have long-term benefits beyond decreasing surgical morbidity and mortality. The consultant also must seize the moment to identify chronic cardiovascular conditions which merit life-long treatment such as hypertension, diabetes mellitus, smoking, hypercholesterolemia, etc. These interventions should not only improve postoperative prognosis, but also lead to improved long-term cardiovascular outcomes.

References

1 Eagle K, Berger PB, Calkins H *et al*. ACC/AHA guideline update for perioperative cardiovascular evaluation for noncardiac surgery:executive summary: A report of the American College of Cardiology/American Heart Association Task Force on Practice Guidelines (Committee to Update the 1996 Guidelines on Perioperative Cardiovascular Evaluation for Noncardiac Surgery). J Am Coll Cardiol 2002;39:542–553.

2 Lee TH. Assessing and reducing cardiac risk in non cardiac surgery. Cardiology rounds 2000;vol 4 issue 3.

3 Eagle K, Fleisher LA. Screening for cardiac disease in patients having noncardiac surgery. Ann Int Med 1996;124:767–772.

4 Hlatky MA, Boineau RE, Higginbotham MB *et al*. A brief self-administered questionnaire to determine functional capacity (The Duke Activity Status Index). J Am J Cardiol 1989; 89:651–654.

5 Goldman L, Caldera DL, Nussbaum SR *et al*. Multifactorial index of cardiac risk in non cardiac surgical procedures. N Engl J Med 1977;297:845–850.

6 Lee Th, Marcantonio EM, Mangione CM *et al*. Derivation and validation of a simple index for prediction of cardiac risk of major noncardiac surgery. Circulation 1999;100: 1043–1049.

7 Eagle KA, Rihal CS, Mickel MC for the CASS Investigators Influence of Coronary Disease and Type of Surgery in 3368 Operations. Circulation 1997;96:1882–1887.

8 Wesorick DH, Eagle K. The preoperative cardiovascular evaluation of the intermediate-risk patients: New data, changing strategies. The American Journal of Medicine 2005;118:1143–1152.

9 Mukherjee D, Eagle KA. Ischemia, revascularization, and perioperative troponin elevation after vascular surgery. J Am Coll Cardiol 2004;44:576–578.

10 Grayburn PA, Hillis LD. Cardiac Events in Patients Undergoing Noncardiac Surgery:Shifting the Paradigm from Noninvasive Risk Stratification to Therapy. Ann of Intern Med 2003, 138:506–511.

11 Auerbach A, Goldman L. Assessing and reducing the cardiac risk in non cardiac surgery. Circulation 2006;113:1361–1376.

12 Hernandez A, Whellan DJ, Stroud S *et al*. Outcomes in heart failure patients after major noncardiac surgery. J Am Coll Cardiol 2004;44:1446–1453.

13 Morris CK *et al*. The prognostic value of exercise capacity: A review of the literature. Am Heart J 1991;122:1423–1431.

14 Beattie WS, Abdelnaem E, Wijeysundera DM *et al*. A Meta-Analytic Comparison of Preoperative Stress Echocardiography and Nuclear Scintigraphy Imaging. Anesth Analg 2006;102:8–16.

15 Dawood MM, Gutpa DK, Southern J, Walia A, Atkinson JB, Eagle KA. Pathology of fatal perioperative myocardial infarction:Implications regarding pathophysiology and prevention. Int J Cardiol 1996;57:37–44.

16 Cohen MC, Aretz TH. Histological analysis of coronary artery lesions in fatal postoperative myocardial infarction. Cardiovasc Pathol 1999;8:133–139.

17 Grayburn PA, Hillis LD. Cardiac events in patients undergoing noncardiac surgery: Shifting the paradigm from noninvasive risk stratification to therapy. Ann Intern Med 2003;138:506–511.

18 Poldermans D, Boersma E, Bax JJ *et al*. The effect of bisoprolol on perioperative cardiac death and myocardial infarction in high risk patients undergoing vascular surgery. N Engl J Med 1999;341:1789–1794.

19 Lindenauer PK, Pekow P, Wang KW *et al*. Perioperative Beta-Blocker Therapy and Mortality after Major Noncardiac Surgery. NEJM 2005;353:349–361.

20 Boersma E, Poldermans D, Bax JJ *et al*. for the DECREASE Study Group Predictors of Cardiac Events After Major Vascular Surgery: Role of Clinical Characteristics, Dobutamine Echocardiography, and Betablocker Therapy. JAMA 2001;285:1865–1873.

21 Salpeter SR, Ormison TM, Salpeter EE *et al*. Cardioselective β-Blockers in patients with reactive airways disease: A meta-analysis. Ann Intern Med 2002;137:715–725.

22 Salpeter SS, Ormiston ETM, Salpeter EE *et al*. Cardioselective betablockers for chronic obstructive pulmonary disease. Cochrane database Syst rev 2003;3.

23 Wijeysundera DN, NAik JS, Beattie WS. Alpha-2 adrenergic agonists to prevent perioperative cardiovascular complications: A meta-analysis Am J Med 2003;114:742–752.

24 Polanczyk CA, Rohde LE, Goldman L *et al*. Right heart catheterization and cardiac complications in patients undergoing noncardiac surgery: An observational study. JAMA 2001;286:309–314.

25 Arieff Al. Fatal post-operative pulmonary edema: Pathogenesis and literature review. Chest 1999;115:1371–1377.

26 Khot UN, Ellis S. The role of PCI prior to noncardiac surgery. ACC Current Journal Review 2001;10:57–60.

27 Kaluza GL, Joseph J, Lee JR *et al*. Catastrophic outcome of non-cardiac surgery soon after coronary stenting. J Am Coll Cardiol 2000;35:1288–1294.

28 Lawrence Cohn in Expert Opinion. www.cardiosource.com/ExpertOpinions/accel/interviewDetail.asp?interviewID=229 (accessed 4/2/2006).

29 Marcus FI, Ewy GA, O'Rourke RA, Walsh B, Bleich AC. The effect of pregnancy on the murmurs of mitral and aortic regurgitation. Circulation 1970;41:795–805.

30 Reyes VP, Raju BS, Wynne J *et al*. Percutaneous balloon valvuloplasty compared with open surgical commissurotomy for mitral stenosis. N Engl J Med 1994;331:961–967.

31 Warner MA, Lunn RJ, O'Leary PW, Schroeder DR. Outcomes of noncardiac surgical procedures in children and adults with congenital heart disease. Mayo preoperative Outcomes Group. Mayo Clin Proc 1998;73:728–734.

32 Gl Rigatelli, G Rigatelli. Congenital coronary artery anomalies in the adult: A new practical viewpoint. Clin Cardiol 2005 Feb;28(2):61–65.

33 Zanchetta M, Rigatelli G, Ho SY. A mystery featuring right-to-left shunting despite normal intracardiac pressure. Chest 2005;128:998–1002.

34 Zanchetta M, Onorato E, Rigatelli G, Pedon L, Zennaro M, Maiolino P. Can posterior fossa ovale lesions be a place for preventive patent foramen ovale transcathter closure? J Invasive Cardiol 2004;16:346–350.

35 Ramakrishna G, Sprung J, Ravi BS *et al*. Impact of Pulmonary Hypertension on the Outcomes of Noncardiac Surgery Predictors of Perioperative Morbidity and Mortality. J Am Coll Cardiol 2005;45:1691–1699.

36 Vanik PE, Davis HS. Cardiac arrhythmias during halothane anesthesia. Anesth Analg 1968;47:299–307.

37 Goldman L, Caldera DL, Southwick FS, Nussbaum SR, Murray B, O'Malley TA, Goroll AH, Caplan CH, Nolan J, Burke DS, Krogstad D, Carabello B, Slater EE. Cardiac risk factors and complications in non-cardiac surgery. Medicine (Baltimore) 1978;57:357–370.

38 Pass SE, Simpson RW. Discontinuation and Reinstitution of Medications During the Perioperative Period Am J Health-Syst Pharm 2004;61(9):899–912.

39 Martinez EA, Nass CM, Jermyn RM, Rosenbaum SH. Intermittent cardiac troponin-I screening is an effective means of surveillance for a perioperative myocardial infarction. J Cardiothorac Vasc Anesth 2005;19(5):577–582.

CHAPTER 6

Integrated Primary Prevention of Cardiovascular Disease

Huy Van Tran, Olabode Oladeinde, Nguyen Hai Thuy, Huynh Van Minh, Dao Duy An, Dat Nguyen Tran, Thach N. Nguyen, Adolphus Anekwe and Matthew J. Sorrentino

Introduction

Cardiovascular disease (CVD) is a group of major cardiac and vascular diseases, important because of the large number of afflicted patients, and its virulence as the number one killer of men and women in the developed or developing world. Once there is a major cardiovascular event (stroke, acute myocardial infarction (MI), etc.), the survival of these patients is shorter and the lifestyle or level of activity have to be curtailed. There are billion and billions of people in the world who are currently healthy and do not have any single cardiovascular abnormality. These people really need to prevent at earliest any cellular-level injury to the cardiovascular system because this is the best time and way to prevent any occurrence of or progression to CVD. Successful prevention of CVD is the most important and noble mission of the cardiology community toward the patients and society (Table 6.1).

Table 6.1 Management strategies for prevention of cardiovascular disease.

1. Screen and detect subjects at risk
2. Prevent all CVDs (not just coronary artery disease or stroke)
3. Correct and prevent all major risk factors of CVD
4. Initiate diet, exercise and healthy lifestyle change
5. Re-enforce teaching on healthy lifestyle, compliance with medication
6. Schedule for routine follow-up

CVD, cardiovascular disease.

Risk Assessment

An assessment of cardiovascular risk is the key point in the evaluation of apparently healthy subjects or people at risk for of developing CVD. The assessment has three objectives: (1) to classify patients as low-, medium- or high-risk for a cardiovascular event in the next 10 years; (2) to assess the presence or absence of target-organ damage; and (3) to assess lifestyle and identify other cardiovascular risk factors or concomitant disorders in order to form a comprehensive prevention and treatment plan for CVD risk factors.

The traditional major risk factors are hypertension (HTN), dyslipidemia, cigarette smoking, diabetes mellitus (DM), age, and family history of premature coronary artery disease (CAD) [1]. The other confirmed risk factors include obesity, fibrinogen, micro-albuminuria or glomerular filtration rate (GFR) <60 mL/min, impaired glucose tolerance (IGT) and impaired fasting glucose (IFG), alcohol abuse, sedentary lifestyle, etc. [2]. The current understanding and management in the prevention of CVD is incomplete, fractionalized, and piecemeal. Many professional societies: the American College of Cardiology (ACC), the American Heart Association (AHA), the American Hypertension Society (AHS), the American Diabetes Association (ADA), the American Kidney Foundation (AKD), the Heart Failure Society of America (HFSA) and American Stroke Association issued separate lengthy, duplicate guidelines for primary prevention of HTN, diabetes, CAD and heart failure (HF). These preventive strategies have the same message: diet, exercise and treatment of risk factors. A physician cannot say that they prescribe diet, exercise and medication just to prevent CAD and not to prevent stroke. Prevention requires a comprehensive effort because the integrative nature of atherosclerosis as a global disease and the vast numbers of affected patients mandate transcendence of traditional specialty boundaries. This is why instead of having separate chapters on hypertension, hypercholesterolemia, prevention of peripheral, carotid, cerebral or heart disease; we combine all the prevention sections into this one chapter.

Targets of Prevention

The Clinical Diseases

There are many major clinical end-organ problems to be prevented because they all limit functional level and shorten survival. They are: (1) dilated cardiomyopathy from alcohol abuse (EtOH), aortic insufficiency (AI), CAD, etc.; (2) mitral regurgitation (so overwhelmingly common); (3) atrial fibrillation (AF) (very common); (4) hypertrophic cardiomyopathy (non-obstructive) due to long-standing uncontrolled or aortic stenosis (AS), etc.; (5) diastolic dysfunction in old age; thach and (6) many other. A partial list of CVD targets is shown in Table 6.2 and Figure 6.1 [3].

It is understandable to treat risk factors in order to prevent CVD. However, some risk factors are as virulent as CVD itself. Once a patient has diabetes, the

Table 6.2 Cardiovascular disease targets for prevention.

Clinical disease	Causes
CAD	Atherosclerosis, HTN, smoking, DM
Dilated cardiomyopathy	CAD, EtOH, DM, AI, HTN
Hypertrophic cardiomyopathy	HTN, aortic stenosis
Hypertensive CVD	HTN
Stroke	Atherosclerosis, HTN, smoking, DM
Pulmonary HTN	Collagen vascular disease, COPD
Atrial fibrillation	Chronic obstructive pulmonary disease
Mitral or aortic regurgitation	CAD, dilated left ventricle, rheumatic heart disease
Diastolic heart failure	Diastolic dysfunction , aging and HTN
Peripheral arterial disease	Atherosclerosis, HTN, smoking, DM
Retinopathy	Atherosclerosis, HTN, DM

AI, aortic insufficiency; CAD, coronary artery disease; DM, diabetes mellitus; COPD, chronic obstructive pulmonary disease; EtOH, ethanol; HTN, hypertension; LV, left ventricle.

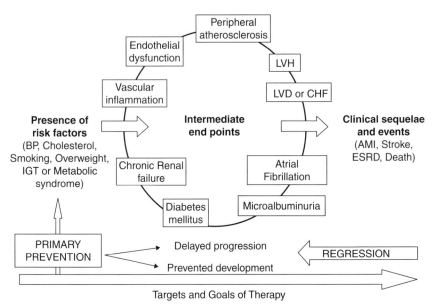

Figure 6.1 Central role of intermediate end points in the cardiovascular and renal continuum and new targets of therapy. From [3] with permission. AMI, acute myocardial infarction; CHF, chronic heart failure; IGT, impaired glucose tolerance; LVH, left ventricular hypertrophy; LVD, left ventricular dysfunction; BP, blood pressure; ESRD, end-stage renal disease.

prognosis is as bad and equivalent as just having an acute MI [4]. So to prevent CVD, besides treating risk factors, it is absolutely essential to prevent risk factors too. There are two major risk factors which need to be prevented: type 2 diabetes and chronic kidney disease (CKD) [5]. It is important to prevent these risk factors as early as possible: at the sub-clinical stage or at the laboratory level.

The Sub-Clinical or Laboratory Precursors

Once there is dilated cardiomyopathy or ventricular hypertrophy, it is difficult to reverse the disease process or its progression. The hemodynamic disturbances are not isolated to the left ventricle (LV) alone. If there is dynamic problem in the LV, we strongly believe there are additional structural changes (remodeling) in the left atrium, right atrium or right ventricle. In the example of atrial fibrillation, besides enlargement of the atria, there should be structural changes (remodeling) in the atria, ventricle and/or pulmonary arteries. The problem is that echocardiography is not sensitive enough to detect these changes. This is why angiotensin converting enzyme inhibitors (ACEI) or angiotensin receptor blockers (ARB) decreased the incidence of AF, most likely due to remodeling in the atria or other parts of the cardiovascular system besides the LV [6]. In patients with congenital heart disease, there would be structural changes in the right ventricle or development of right side failure with or without any obvious involvement of the LV. This is why all patients with congenital heart disease are considered to be at stage B HF. Therefore, there would be many asymptomatic sub-clinical structural or laboratory-detected abnormalities which are the basis of disease. These abnormalities clearly need to be prevented before resulting in minor and major clinical conditions. They are listed in Table 6.3.

Table 6.3 Sub-clinical and laboratory targets for prevention of cardiovascular disease.

Precursor targets	Clinical conditions
HbA1c >6.1	Type 2 diabetes
GFR < 90 mL %	Chronic kidney disease
LVH	Diastolic HF, right HF, dilated LV
Atrial abnormalities and dilation	dilated cardiomyopathy, VT, atrial fibrillation
Left atrium enlargement	Atrial fibrillation
Right ventricular dysfunction	Mitral regurgitation
	Right ventricular failure, RV dilation
	Pulmonary artery hypertension

CKD, chronic kidney disease; HbA1c, hemoglobin A1c; GFR, glomerular filtration rate; HF, heart failure; LV, left ventricle; LVH,. left ventricular hypertrophy; RV, right ventricle; VT, ventricular tachycardia.

Therapeutic Lifestyle Changes

All healthy subjects or patients of all stages of CAD, HF, DM, hypertension, CKD and metabolic syndrome (MS) benefit from a generic lifestyle-behavior change which is the cornerstone of any treatment plan for primary or secondary prevention of CVD. A lifestyle change program includes a well-balanced diet with low sodium, reduced saturated fat and cholesterol, increased aerobic physical activity, no smoking, and weight reduction in obese and overweight individuals. The concrete instructions are highlighted in Table 6.4.

Table 6.4 Concrete instructions about therapeutic lifestyle changes.

Low sodium
Choose and prepare foods with little or no salt
(a) Read label about sodium when buying foods
(b) No salt shaker on table
(c) Use salt substitute for foods seasoning

Low cholesterol diet
Select foods high on polyunsaturated fat
Avoid foods with high level of mono-saturated fat
Cholesterol to <300 mg/day
Avoid use of and exposure to tobacco products

Avoid high glycemic or high protein diet

Daily weight
Weigh every morning on a same scale

Exercise
Exercise at home or exercise in a health club

Fluid restriction
2000–3000 ml/day, if you consume alcohol, do so in moderation

Diet

From a CVD point of view, which diet could best prevent the occurrence of, and progression to, CAD, hypertensive CVD, diabetes, CKD, obesity and diastolic dysfunction? (Table 6.5)

Table 6.5 Diet for prevention of cardiovascular disease.

Type of diet	Clinical entities to be prevented
Low Na diet	Hypertension, heart failure
Fluid restriction	Hypertension, heart failure
Low cholesterol diet	CAD, stroke, PAD, metabolic syndrome
Low protein diet	Chronic kidney disease
Low glucose diet	Diabetes,
Low calorie diet	Diastolic dysfunction due to aging, metabolic syndrome, obesity

CAD, coronary artery disease; PAD, peripheral arterial disease.

Low Sodium Diet

A diet with 1.5 g/day sodium for patients who really need to cut down their sodium intake, such as patients with HF, CKD, or hypertension. However, in view of the available high-sodium food supply and the currently high levels of sodium consumption, a reduction in sodium intake to 1.5 g/day

(65 mmol/day) is not easily achievable at present. In the interim, an achievable recommendation is 2.4 g/day (100 mmol/day) or 6.4 g/day sodium chloride (salt) [7].

Low Carbohydrate Diet

A low-carbohydrate diet, of which the Atkins' Diet is most representative, recommends two weeks of extreme carbohydrate restriction, followed by gradually increasing carbohydrates to 35 g/day. The Atkins' Diet has 68% of total calories from fat, 27% from protein, and 5% from carbohydrates [8]. Low-carbohydrate diets recommend limiting complex and simple sugars, causing the body to oxidize fat to meet energy requirements. During the initial carbohydrate restriction, the body resorts to ketosis for energy needs. Ketones are excreted in the urine with fluid. Rapid initial weight loss may be from this diuretic effect [9,10], which can be encouraging. A drastic reduction in carbohydrates also leads to an overall decrease in caloric intake [11]. Weight loss can be sustained by this reduction in caloric intake. Although palatable for the short term, low-carbohydrate diets raise several nutritional and cardiovascular concerns including high protein diet (with adverse effect on liver and kidneys), atherogenesis because high in saturated fat and cholesterol, lack of fruit, vegetable and whole grain. Low-carbohydrate diets may increase high density lipoprotein (HDL) cholesterol (HDL-C), decrease triglyceride levels, and improve glycemic control, but there appears to be no significant difference in weight loss compared with a low-fat diet at one year [10].

Foods that contain large amounts of fat, sugar, and/or starch, which people have higher tendency to overeat, have low fullness factor (FF). Foods that contain large amounts of water, dietary fiber, and/or protein have the highest FF. These high-FF foods, which include most vegetables, fruits, and lean meats, do a better job of satisfying hunger. Most liquid foods will have above average FF, due to their high water content. By simply selecting foods with high FF, people can improve the chances of consuming fewer calories, while simultaneously minimizing their hunger (Table 6.6). For complete information, please visit the website www.nutritiondata.com/fullness-factor.html (accessed 4/19/2006).

CLINICAL PEARLS

How to eat more but accumulate less calories?   The Fullness Factor (FF) is calculated from the food's nutrient content, using values from those nutrients that have been shown experimentally to have the greatest impact on satiety. The values of the FF range from 0 to 5, with the FF for white bread being 1.8. That means that for servings of equal calories, those foods with FF's above 1.8 are more likely to fill you up than white bread, and foods with FF's below 1.8 are less likely than white bread to fill you up (Table 6.6 and www.nutritiondata.com/fullness-factor.html).

Table 6.6 Fullness factors for common foods.

Food	Fullness factor
Bean sprouts	4.6
Watermelon	4.5
Grapefruit	4.0
Carrots	3.8
Oranges	3.5
Fish, broiled	3.4
Chicken breast, roasted	3.3
Apples	3.3
Sirloin steak, broiled	3.2
Oatmeal	3.0
Popcorn	2.9
Baked potato	2.5
Lowfat yogurt	2.5
Banana	2.5
Macaroni and cheese	2.5
Brown rice	2.3
Spaghetti	2.2
White rice	2.1
Pizza	2.1
Peanuts	2.0
Ice cream	1.8
White bread	1.8
Raisins	1.6
Snickers bar	1.5
Honey	1.4
Sugar (sucrose)	1.3
Glucose	1.3
Potato chips	1.2
Butter	0.5

Very Low Fat Diet

Very-low-fat (VLF) diets allow less than 15% of total calories from fat (with an equal distribution of saturated, monounsaturated, and polyunsaturated fats), 15% from protein, and 70% from carbohydrates [10]. The VLF diet includes variations of vegetarian diets that may include eggs and dairy. The VLF diet and intense life-style changes have significant results in terms of reducing risk factors and cardiac event rates. To check the fat content of each food, please visit the website www.nutritiondata.com/nutrient-search.html (accessed 4/19/2006).

CLINICAL PEARLS
How to select polyunsaturated fat? Saturated fat is a fat or fatty acid in which there are no double bonds between the carbon atoms of the fatty acid chain. Diets high in saturated fat have been shown to cause high both total cholesterol and low density lipoprotein (LDL) cholesterol in the blood. Common

saturated fats include butter, lard, palm oil, coconut oil, cottonseed oil, cream, cheese and meat, etc. Alternative to saturated fats include monosaturated fats such as olive oil and polyunsaturated fats such as canola oil and corn oil. The goal of a low fat diet is to substitute unsaturated fats for saturated fats. To select foods with low saturated and high polyunsaturated fat content, please visit the website www.prevention.com/pdf/ PV-ShoppingList.pdf (accessed 4/19/2006).

However, low fat diet *alone* cannot prevent CVD in high risk patient, because CVD is result of many other risk factors besides high cholesterol level. This concern is confirmed in the study below.

CRITICAL THINKING

Is dieting enough? 48,835 postmenopausal women aged 50–79 years, who participated in the Women's Health Initiative Dietary Modification Trial were randomly assigned to an intervention (19,541) or comparison group (29,294) in a free-living setting. The intervention included intensive behavior modification in group and individual sessions designed to reduce total fat intake to 20% of calories and increase intakes of vegetables/fruits to five servings/day and grains to at least six servings/day. The comparison group received diet-related education materials. By year 6, mean fat intake decreased by 8.2% of energy intake in the intervention vs. the comparison group, with small decreases in saturated (2.9%), monounsaturated (3.3%), and polyunsaturated (1.5%) fat; increases occurred in intakes of vegetables/fruits (1.1 servings/day) and grains (0.5 serving/day). LDL cholesterol levels, diastolic blood pressure, and factor VIIc levels were significantly reduced by 3.55 mg/dL, 0.31 mmHg, and 4.29%, respectively; levels of HDL cholesterol, triglycerides, glucose, and insulin did not significantly differ in the intervention vs. comparison groups. The numbers who developed coronary heart disease (CHD), stroke, and CVD (annualized incidence rates) were 0.63%, 0.28%, and 0.86% in the intervention group, and 0.65%, 0.27%, and 0.88% in the comparison group. The diet had no significant effects on incidence of CHD (hazard ratio [HR], 0.97; 95% CI, 0.90–1.06), stroke (HR, 1.02; 95% CI, 0.90–1.15), or CVD (HR, 0.98; 95% CI, 0.92–1.05). Excluding participants with baseline CVD (3.4%), the HRs (95% CIs) for CHD and stroke were 0.94 (0.86–1.02) and 1.02 (0.90–1.17), respectively. Trends toward greater reductions in CHD risk were observed in those with lower intakes of saturated fat or trans fat or higher intakes of vegetables/fruits [12].

So over a mean of 8.1 years, a dietary intervention that reduced total fat intake and increased intakes of vegetables, fruits, and grains *alone* did not significantly reduce the risk of CHD, stroke, or CVD in postmenopausal women and achieved only modest effects on CVD risk factors, suggesting that more focused diet, lifestyle interventions and drugs may be needed to improve risk factors and reduce further CVD in high risk patients [12].

The Mediterranean Diet

The Mediterranean Diet [10] is characterized by high intake of fruits, vegetables, low-fat dairy products, whole grains, nuts, fish, and poultry, as well as reducing total and saturated fats [13]. Although a Mediterranean-style diet has demonstrated greater weight reduction compared with control diets in randomised controlled trials [14], the most impressive benefits of the diet are related to cardiovascular morbidity and mortality. No isolated aspect of the Mediterranean diet explains these benefits, but much has focused on the omega-3 polyunsaturated fatty acids (N-3 FA). Patients on a Mediterranean diet have been shown to lose more weight, have lower C-reactive protein levels, have less insulin resistance, have lower total cholesterol and triglyceride and higher HDL levels, and have a decreased prevalence of the metabolic syndrome. There are some concerns regarding the Mediterranean diet including a fishy aftertaste, gastrointestinal discomfort, and possibly an increase in LDL cholesterol [14] or mercury exposure. In fact, the Food and Drug Administration currently recommends that children and women who are pregnant and/or lactating should avoid fish consumption due to high mercury level [10].

Diet to Prevent Diabetes

The glycemic index (GI) [10] is a concept that has been used in diets such as the South Beach Diet [15], Sugar Busters [16], and the Zone Diet [17]. These diets allow carbohydrate consumption as long as they have a low GI [18]. The GI is a numerical index that ranks carbohydrates based on their rate of conversion to glucose within the human body. GI uses a scale of 0 to 100, with higher values given to foods that cause the most rapid rise in blood sugar. Pure glucose serves as a reference point, and is given a GI of 100. If the blood glucose rises too fast after ingestion (high GI), the pancreas needs to secrete more insulin which brings the blood glucose down, by converting the excess glucose to stored fat. Then, the greater the rate of increase in blood glucose, the higher will be the level of excess insulin which can cause hypoglycemia. The theory behind the GI is simply to minimize insulin-related problems by identifying and avoiding foods that cause too much swing in blood glucose (and insulin level).

However, it's not the high GI foods that would lead to the increased blood glucose level. The glycemic response depends on both the type *and* the amount of carbohydrate consumed. This concept is known as glycemic load (GL) and calculated as:

$$GL = GI/100 \times Net\ carbs$$

(Net carbs are equal to the total carbohydrates minus dietary fiber)

Therefore, a patient can control the glycemic response by consuming only low GI foods and/or a smaller amount of foods [19]. Table 6.7 shows values of the GI and GL for a few common foods. GI's of 55 or below are considered low, and 70 or above are considered high. GL's of 10 or below are considered low

Table 6.7 Glycemic index and glycemic load for common foods.

Food	GI	Serving size	Net carbs	GL
Peanuts	14	4 oz (113 g)	15	2
Bean sprouts	25	1 cup (104 g)	4	1
Grapefruit	25	½ large (166 g)	11	3
Pizza	30	2 slices (260 g)	42	13
Low fat yogurt	33	1 cup (245 g)	47	16
Apples	38	1 medium (138 g)	16	6
Spaghetti	42	1 cup (140 g)	38	16
Carrots	47	1 large (72 g)	5	2
Oranges	48	1 medium (131 g)	12	6
Bananas	52	1 large (136 g)	27	14
Potato chips	54	4 oz (114 g)	55	30
Snickers bar	55	1 bar (113 g)	64	35
Brown rice	55	1 cup (195 g)	42	23
Honey	55	1 tbsp (21 g)	17	9
Oatmeal	58	1 cup (234 g)	21	12
Ice cream	61	1 cup (72 g)	16	10
Macaroni and cheese	64	1 serving (166 g)	47	30
Raisins	64	1 small box (43 g)	32	20
White rice	64	1 cup (186 g)	52	33
Sugar (sucrose)	68	1 tbsp (12 g)	12	8
White bread	70	1 slice (30 g)	14	10
Watermelon	72	1 cup (154 g)	11	8
Popcorn	72	2 cups (16 g)	10	7
Baked potato	85	1 medium (173 g)	33	28
Glucose	100	50 g	50	50

and 20 or above are considered high. For complete information, please visit the website www.nutritiondata.com/glycemic-index.html (accessed 4/19/2006).

A high-GI diet has been proposed to increase hunger and elevate free fatty acid levels, leading to an increased risk of obesity, diabetes, and CVD [19]. A possible association between a high-GI diet and diabetes has been observed. A meta-analysis of 14 randomized, controlled trials comparing low- and high-GI diets in diabetes management showed that glycated proteins were reduced 7.4% on a low-GI diet [20].

Table 6.8 Best balanced diet and exercise program to prevent diabetes.

1. Total intake of fat to <30% percent of energy consumed
2. Intake of saturated fat to <10% of energy consumed
3. Fiber intake to at least 15 g per 1000 kcal
4. Frequent ingestion of whole-grain products, vegetables, fruits, low-fat milk and meat products, soft margarines, and vegetable oils rich in monounsaturated fatty acids was recommended
4. Moderate exercise (endurance exercise such as walking, jogging, swimming, aerobic ball games, or skiing) for at least 30 minutes per day

Diet to Stop Hypertension

The Dietary Approaches to Stop Hypertension (DASH) Diet is similar to a Mediterranean-type diet, emphasizing high intake of fruits, vegetables, low-fat dairy products, whole grains, nuts, fish, and poultry, as well as reducing total and saturated fats [21]. Reduced intake of red meat, sweets, and sugar-containing beverages is encouraged, which results in a diet high in potassium, calcium, magnesium, and fiber. This dietary approach has been shown to lower blood pressure BP by 10 mmHg.

Diet to Prevent Chronic Kidney Disease

In order to prevent CKD in a patient with normal creatinine level, the diet required is the "renal diet", synonymous with low-protein diet. It is critical to note that by stage 3 CKD and beyond, there is no benefit of a low-protein diet. Such protein restriction will not delay the progression toward end stage renal disease (ESRD) at stage 3 CKD. The target protein intake is approximately 0.8–1.0 g/kg/day and sodium intake is 1500–2000 mg/day [22].

Moderation in Alcohol Consumption

Observational studies consistently show a J-shaped relation between alcohol consumption and total mortality. Moderate alcohol consumption is associated with lower mortality, and higher consumption with higher mortality. The lower mortality appears to be related to CHD death, because CHD accounts for a significant proportion of total deaths. Case-control, cohort, and ecological studies indicate lower risk for CHD at low-to moderate alcohol intake [23]. A moderate amount of alcohol can be defined as no more than one drink per day for women or lighter-weight persons, and no more than two drinks per day for men. A drink is 12 oz of beer, 5 oz of wine, or 1.5 oz of 80-proof liquor [24].

Stop Cigarette Smoking

Epidemiological evidence has unequivocally confirmed that active smoking is a risk factor for CVD and the leading cause of preventable death [25–28]. The risk of death from CVD is elevated at least two-fold among smokers when compared with non-smokers. There is evidence that exposure to, or passive, smoking also increases the risk of CVD, including stroke [26]. Smoking just one or two cigarettes a day is enough to jumpstart the biological processes that lead to atherosclerosis [27].

CLINICAL PEARLS

How to stop smoking? First-line therapies include nicotine replacement and/or bupropion. Second-line treatments include clonidine and nortriptyline.

Additional treatment strategies, with less proven efficacy, include monoamine oxidase inhibitors, selective serotonin reuptake inhibitors, opioid receptor antagonists, bromocriptine, antianxiety drugs, nicotinic receptor antagonists (e.g., mecamylamine), and glucose tablets.

In addition to the above, social support and skills training has been proved to be the most effective approach for quitting [28–30].

Weight Loss Program

Obesity can be defined as an excess of body fat. A surrogate marker for body fat content is the body mass index (BMI), which is determined by weight (kilograms) divided by height squared (square meters). In clinical terms, a BMI of 25–29 kg/m² is called overweight; higher BMIs ($\geqslant 30\,\text{kg/m}^2$) are called obesity. A better way to define obesity would be in terms of percent total body fat [31]. Obesity can be defined as 25% or greater of body fat in men and 35% or greater in women. The exact measurement of percentage body fat is rarely used, because of inconvenience and cost. The best way to estimate obesity in clinical practice is to measure waist circumference. For American patients, abdominal obesity is defined as a waist circumference of 102 cm or more in men, and of 88 cm or more in women [24]. In other countries, the International Diabetes Federation (IDF) defined the waist circumference values according to gender and ethnic group (not country of residence) specific (Table 6.9) [31].

Table 6.9 Ethnic specific values for waist circumference.

Country/ethnic group		Waist circumference	
Europids	Male	$\geqslant$94 cm	In the USA, the ATP III values (102 cm male; 88 cm female are likely to continue to be used for clinical purposes)
	Female	$\geqslant$80 cm	
South Asians and Chinese	Male	$\geqslant$90 cm	Based on a Chinese, Malay and Asian–Indian population
	Female	$\geqslant$80 cm	
Japanese	Male	$\geqslant$90cm	New data support the use of these values
	Female	$\geqslant$80cm	
Ethnic South and Central Americans			Use South Asian recommendations until more special data are available
Sub-Sahara Africans			Use European data until more special data are available
Eastern Mediterranean and Middle East (Arab) populations			Use European data until more special data are available

In clinical and epidemiological studies, obesity is strongly associated with all cardiovascular risk factors (Table 6.10) [32]. The visceral adipose tissue is recognized as a source of several molecules that are potentially pathogenic: excess non-esterified fatty acids, cytokines (tumor necrosis factor), resistin, adiponectin, leptin, and plasminogen activator inhibitor I [33]. However, the mechanisms underlying the association between abdominal obesity (particularly visceral obesity) and the metabolic syndrome are not fully understood. As diet and physical activities exert limited role in weight loss, can medications fill the gap? Can a new drug Rimonabant sustain weight loss and improve the risk profile of obese and overweight patients?

Table 6.10 Relative 10-year risk for diabetes, hypertension, heart disease, and stroke over the next decade among men initially free of disease stratified by baseline body mass index [32].

Body mass index	Diabetes	Hypertension	Heart disease	Stroke
18.5–21.9	1.0	1.0	1.0	1.0
22.0–24.9	1.8	1.5	1.1	1.1
25.0–29.9	5.6	2.4	1.7	1.3
30.0–34.9	18.2	3.8	2.2	2.1
>35.0	41.2	4.2	2.4	2.5

EMERGING TREND

The RIO North American trial 3045 obese (BMI ⩾ 30) or overweight (BMI > 27 and treated or untreated hypertension or dyslipidemia) adult patients were randomized in a double-blind, placebo-controlled trial. Rimonabant-treated patients were re-randomized to receive placebo or continued to receive the same rimonabant dose while the placebo group continued to receive placebo during year 2. The results showed that at year 1, the completion rate was 309 (51%) patients in the placebo group, 620 (51%) patients in the 5 mg of rimonabant group, and 673 (55%) patients in the 20 mg of rimonabant group. Compared with the placebo group, the 20 mg rimonabant group produced greater mean reductions in weight (-6.3 kg vs. -1.6 kg; $P < 0.001$), waist circumference (-6.1 cm vs. -2.5 cm; $P < 0.001$), and level of triglycerides (percentage change, -5.3 vs. 7.9; $P < 0.001$) and a greater increase in level of HDL cholesterol (percentage change, 12.6 vs. 5.4; $P < 0.001$). Patients who were switched from the 20 mg of rimonabant group to the placebo group during year 2 experienced weight regain while those who continued to receive 20 mg of rimonabant maintained their weight loss and favorable changes in cardiometabolic risk factors [34].

In this multi-center trial, treatment with rimonabant plus diet for 2 years promoted modest but sustained reductions in weight and waist circumference and favorable changes in cardiometabolic risk factors. However, the trial was limited by a high drop-out rate and longer-term effects of the drug require further study [34].

Exercise

Substantial evidence exists that physical activity exerts a beneficial effect on multiple cardiovascular risk factors. A plausible explanation is that physical activity tends to lower BP and weight, enhance vasodilatation, improve glucose tolerance, and promote cardiovascular health. Through lifestyle modification, exercise can minimize the need for more intensive medical and pharmacological interventions or enhance treatment end points [28]. While being physically active was found to be associated with a decrease in risk of CHD, a question was raised to see whether the intensity or the amount of exercise accounted for the greatest reduction in risk.

CRITICAL THINKING

Quality of intense exercise or quantity of exercise time? A cohort of 44,452 US men enrolled in the Health Professionals' Follow-up Study, was followed up at 2-year intervals to assess potential CHD risk factors, identify newly diagnosed cases of CHD, and assess levels of leisure-time physical activity. The results showed that total exercise, running, weight training and rowing were all associated with a decreased risk of future CHD. However, running for more than an hour per week was associated with a 42% decreased risk compared with not running; lifting weights for 30 minutes or more per week with a 23% decrease; and rowing for one hour or more per week, with an 18% reduction in risk. Walking briskly for half an hour a day was also associated with an 18% decreased risk of CHD. Overall, the study showed that the intensity of the physical activity was more related to a decreased CHD risk than the amount of time spent exercising [35].

The National Heart, Lung and Blood Institute (NHLBI) recommends that an increase in physical activity is an important part of the weight management program. Most weight loss occurs because of decreased caloric intake. Sustained physical activity is most helpful in the prevention of weight regain. In addition, exercise has a benefit of reducing risks of CVD and diabetes, beyond that produced by weight reduction alone [36]. The exercise can be taken all at one time, or intermittently over the day.

CLINICAL PEARLS

How to exercise? For the beginner, activity level can begin at very light and would include an increase in standing activities, special chores like room painting, pushing a wheelchair, yard work, ironing, cooking, and playing a musical instrument.

The next level would be light activity such as slow walking of 24 min/mile, (walking is particularly attractive because of its safety and accessibility) garage work, carpentry, house cleaning, child care, golf, sailing, and recreational table tennis.

> The next level would be moderate activity such as walking 15 min/mile, weeding and hoeing a garden, carrying a load, cycling, skiing, tennis, and dancing.
> High activity would include walking 10 min/mile or walking with load uphill, heavy manual digging, basketball, climbing, or soccer/kick ball.
> Start exercising slowly and gradually increases the intensity. Trying too hard at first can lead to injury [36].

Intervention for the Modifiable Cardiovascular Risk Factors

The main strategies for correction and prevention of risk factors include control of hypertension, hypercholesterolemia, metabolic syndrome, prevention of diabetes and CKD.

Hypertension

The Seventh Report of The Joint National Committee (JNC) on Prevention, Detection, Evaluation and Treatment of High Blood Pressure provides guidelines for hypertension classification and management (Table 6.11) [37,38]. The new category of prehypertension was proposed because of the observation that patients with high normal BP have twice the risk of developing definite hypertension in their lifetime. These individuals should at the very least be advised about a healthy lifestyle to try to prevent the development of hypertension. Newer evidence has been accumulated to warrant greater attention upon the importance of systolic blood pressure (SBP) as a major risk factor for CVDs. Changing patterns of BP occur with increasing age. The rise in SBP continues throughout life in contrast to diastolic blood pressure (DBP) due to loss of compliance of the arteries. Clinical trials have demonstrated that control of isolated systolic hypertension reduces total mortality, cardiovascular mortality, stroke, and HF events [39].

The Hypertension Writing Group of the American Society of Hypertension proposed an expanded definition and classification of HTN [40]. Cardiovascular risk factors tend to cluster in the same individual. Classification of HTN should

Table 6.11 Classification of blood pressure for adults JNC-7.

BP classification	SBP (mmHg)	DBP (mmHg)
Normal	<120	<80
Prehypertension	120–139	80–89
Stage 1 hypertension	140–159	90–99
Stage 2 hypertension	≥160	≥100

DBP, diastolic blood pressure; SBP, systolic blood pressure.

involve an assessment of global cardiovascular risk that may help determine the aggressiveness of therapy. The Hypertension Writing Group proposed expanding the JNC's definition of HTN by incorporating cardiovascular risk factors and clinical cardiovascular manifestations into the definition (Table 6.12).

Table 6.12 Hypertension Writing Group definition and classification of hypertension.

Classification	Normal	Stage 1 HTN	Stage 2 HTN	Stage 3 HTN
Descriptive category (BP pattern and CVD status)	Normal BP or rare BP elevations and no identifiable CVD	Occasional intermittent BP elevations or risk factors/ markers of early CVD	Sustained BP elevations or evidence of progressive CVD	Marked and sustained BP elevations or advanced CVD
CVD risk factors	None	⩾1 risk factor present	Multiple risk factors	Multiple risk factors
Early disease markers	None	0–1	⩾2	⩾2 with evidence of CVD
Target organ disease	None	None	Early signs present	Overtly present with or without CVD events

BP, blood pressure; CVD, cardiovascular disease; HTN, hypertension.

The cardiovascular risk factors included the classic traditional risk factors such as metabolic syndrome and C-reactive protein, and are listed in Table 6.13. Early markers of hypertensive CVD may become evident in patients at BP

Table 6.13 Cardiovascular risk factors to use for classification of blood pressure [40].

Increasing age (continuous variable)
Elevated BP (⩾140/90 mmHg)
Overweight/obesity (BMI ⩾ 24 kg/m^2)
Abdominal obesity
    Waist circumference >40 inches for men; >35 inches for women
Dyslipidemia
    Elevated LDL cholesterol (⩾130 mg/dL)
    Low HDL cholesterol (<40 mg/dL men; <50 mg/dL women)
    Elevated triglycerides (⩾150 mg/dL)
Elevated fasting blood glucose (⩾100 mg/dL), insulin resistance or diabetes
Smoking
Family history of premature CVD (<50 years in men; <60 years in women)
Sedentary lifestyle
Elevated high-sensitivity C-reactive protein

BMI, body mass index; BP, blood pressure; CVD, cardiovascular disease; HDL, high density lipoprotein; LDL, low density lipoprotein.

levels between 120/80 and 139/89 mmHg (Table 6.14). The presence of these early markers would classify patients as stage 1 HTN. Once target organ damage is present, patients are classified as either stage 2 (early signs) or stage 3 (overt signs) HTN (Tables 6.12 and 6.15).

Table 6.14 Early markers of hypertensive cardiovascular disease [40].

System	Physiologic alterations
Blood pressure	Loss of nocturnal BP dipping Exaggerated BP response to exercise Salt sensitivity Widened pulse pressure
Cardiac	Left ventricular hypertrophy (mild) Increased atrial filling pressure Decreased diastolic relaxation
Vascular	Increased central arterial stiffness or pulse wave velocity Small artery stiffness Increased systemic vascular resistance Increased wave reflection and systolic pressure augmentation Increased carotid intima-media thickness Coronary calcification Endothelial dysfunction
Renal	Microalbuminuria (urinary albumin excretion 30–300 mg/d) Elevated serum creatinine (serum creatinine $>$ 1.6 mmol/L) Reduced estimated GFR (60–90 mL/min)
Retinal	Hypertensive retinal changes

BP, blood pressure; GFR, glomerular filtration rate.

Table 6.15 Hypertensive target organ damage and overt cardiovascular disease [40].

System	Evidence of target organ damage and CVD
Cardiac	LVH (moderate to severe) Systolic or diastolic cardiac dysfunction Symptomatic heart failure Myocardial infarction Angina pectoris Ischemic heart disease or revascularization
Vascular	Peripheral arterial disease Carotid arterial disease Aortic aneurysm Wide pulse pressure ($>$65 mmHg)
Renal	Albuminuria ($>$300 mg/d) CKD (GFR $<$ 60 mL/min) or ESRD
Cerebrovascular	Stroke Transient ischemic attack

CKD, chronic kidney disease; CVD, cardiovascular disease; ESRD, end stage renal disease; GFR, glomerular filtration rate; LVH, left ventricular hypertrophy.

Causes of Hypertension

The most common cause of HTN is still not fully understood and is classified as primary, or essential, HTN. This category accounts for about 90% of all hypertensive patients. Secondary causes of HTN should be considered in HTN that is severe, begins at a young age, or is resistant to standard therapy. Common causes of secondary HTN are listed in Table 6.16.

Table 6.16 Identifiable causes of hypertension [38].

Chronic kidney disease
Coarctation of the aorta
Cushing's syndrome and other glucocorticoid excess states including chronic steroid therapy
Drug induced or drug related (see Table 6.22)
Obstructive uropathy
Pheochromocytoma
Primary aldosteronism and other mineralocorticoid excess states
Renovascular hypertension
Sleep apnea
Thyroid or parathyroid disease

D, chronic kidney disease; HTN, hypertension.

Treatment of Hypertension

The Goal of Therapy

The primary goal of treatment of the hypertensive patient is to achieve the maximum reduction in the long-term total risk of cardiovascular and renal morbidity and mortality. In most patients, the target of the controlled BP is under 140/90 mmHg along with concurrently controlling all of other coexisting modifiable cardiovascular risk factors as the current guidelines. In the special groups of diabetic and CKD patients, the target BP is under 130/80 mmHg. Other groups of patients that are considered for this target BP include the patients with CAD, metabolic syndrome, HF and microalbuminuria.

Lifestyle Modification

A lifestyle modification program including low sodium, low cholesterol diet, fluid restriction, exercise etc. is recommended for all individuals with hypertension or prehypertension and is discussed in detail at the beginning of this chapter.

Pharmacological Treatment

Therapy should be started gradually, and target BP achieved progressively. Choice of drugs monotherapy or combination therapy aim to control BP to reach target which these drugs have been proven by the evidence-based studies decrease the cardiovascular events and death while minimizing side effect or toxicity. These drugs may improve control of HTN by being affordable and available at low cost thus improving compliance to therapy. The single daily dosing provides full 24-hour efficacy should be feasible for virtually all patients (Figure 6.2).

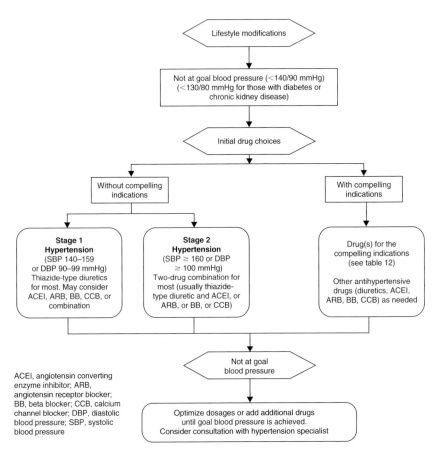

Figure 6.2 Algorithm for treatment of hypertension.
Source: Joint National Committee (JNC)–7, [38].

The JNC-7, World Health Organization (WHO)/International Society of Hypertension (ISH) and Canada guidelines as well as North of England Hypertension Guideline Development Group published by National Institute for Clinical Excellence (NICE), recommend thiazide-type diuretics as the initial therapy for most hypertensive patients, either alone or in combination with one of the other classes [37,38,41–43]. A brief summary of drugs used for essential hypertension is provided in Table 6.17.

Table 6.17 Outline of drugs for hypertension [43].

Class	Common generic names	Mode of action	Usage notes
Thiazide-type diuretic	Bendroflumethiazide, indapamide	Moderate diuresis	Low dose thiazide-type diuretics produce (near) maximum BP lowering; higher dose can cause side effects
Potassium-sparing diuretics	Amiloride	Weakly diuretic, given additionally to, or in combination with, a thiazide to retain potassium	Few side effects. Used to prevent or treat low levels of potassium in the blood. Use with an ACE-inhibitor can cause severely raised levels of potassium in the blood
BB	Atenolol, bisoprolol, metoprolol, propanolol, sotalol	Blocking β-receptors	Contraindicated in asthma, heart-block. Caution applies to patients with diabetes or peripheral vascular diseases
Calcium-channel blockers (CCBs)	'Dihydropyridine' amlodipine, felodipine, lacidipine, nifedipine	Reduced flow of calcium to vascular smooth muscle, reducing contraction efficiency and relaxing vasculature	Reported side-effects include initial headaches, palpitations and facial flushing, ankle swelling
	'Rate limiting' diltiazem, verapamil	Slowing the heart rate	Caution against use in heart failure or in with β-blockers
ACE-inhibitors	Captopril, enalapril, lisinopril, perindopril, ramipril, trandolapril	Prevent conversion of the protein angiotensin I to angiotensin II which raises BP	Dose titration and monitoring is necessary. Contraindicated in pregnancy. Adverse effects include a persistent dry cough, rash, loss of taste
Angiotensin receptor blockers (ARBs)	Candesartan, irbesartan, losartan, valsartan, telmisartan	Blocks the action of angiotensin II by directly blocking the receptor site	Contraindications and side effect profile similar to ACEI but ARBs are not associated with the persistent dry cough sometimes attributed to ACEI
Alpha receptor blockers	Doxazosin, prazosin, terazosin	Blocks receptor sites in blood vessel wall, relaxing vessels	Side-effect: initial dizziness, headache, flushing, nasal congestion, fluid retention, and a rapid heart rate

ACEI, angiotensin converting enzyme inhibitors; ARBs, angiotensin receptor blockers; BP, blood pressure; CCBs, calcium-channel blockers; BB, β-blockers.

Compelling Indications

Compelling indications for specific therapy involve high-risk conditions that can be direct sequelae of HTN (HF, CAD, CKD, recurrent stroke) or commonly associated with HTN (diabetes, high coronary disease risk). The choice of drugs for these compelling indications is on favorable outcome data from the clinical trials [38]. Therapeutic decisions in such individuals should be directed at both the compelling indication and lowering BP (Table 6.18). If a drug is not tolerated or is contraindicated, then one of the other classes proven to reduce cardiovascular events should be used instead.

Table 6.18 Compelling indications for individual drugs classes [38].

Compelling indication	Initial therapy options	Clinical trial basis*
Diabetes	THIAZ, BB, ACEI, ARB, CCB	ADA Guideline [48], UKPDS [49], ALLHAT [50]
Chronic kidney disease	ACEI, ARB	LIFE [56], ESPRIT [52], RENAAL [53], IDNT [54]
Recurrent stroke prevention	THIAZ, ACEI	PROGRESS [57]
Heart failure	THIAZ, BB, ACEI, ARB, ALDO ANT	ACC/AHA Heart Failure Guideline [46], RALES [47]
Post-myocardial infarction	BB, ACEI, ALDO ANT	ACC/AHA post-myocardial infarction Guideline [46]
High coronary disease risk	THIAZ, BB, ACE, CCB	ALLHAT [50], HOPE [57], LIFE [56], EUROPA [45], INVEST [69]

*Conditions for which clinical trials demonstrate the benefit of specific classes of antihypertensive drugs used as part of an antihypertensive regimen to achieve BP goal to test outcomes [38].

ACC/AHA, American College of Cardiology/American Heart Association; ACEI, angiotensin converting enzyme inhibitor; ADA, American Diabetes Association; ALDO ANT , aldosterone antagonist; ALLHAT, Antihypertensive and Lipid-Lowering Treatment to Prevent Heart Attack Trial; ARB, angiotensin receptor blocker; BB, β-blocker; CCB, calcium channel blocker; EUROPA, European Trial on Reduction of Cardiac Events with Perindopril in Stable Coronary Artery Disease; ESPRIT, Efficacy and Safety in Patients with Renal Impairment; treated with Telmisartan; RENAAL, Reduction of Endpoints in Non-Insulin Dependent Diabetes Mellitus with the Angiotensin II Antagonist Losartan Study; IDNT, Irbesartan in Diabetic Nephropathy Trial; HOPE, Heart Outcomes Prevention Evaluation Study; INVEST, The International Verapamil-Trandolapril Study; LIFE, Losartan Intervention for Endpoint Reduction in Hypertension Study; PROGRESS, Perindopril Protection against Recurrent Stroke Study; RALES, Randomized Aldactone Evaluation Study; THIAZ, thiazide; UKPDS, United Kingdom Prospective Diabetes Study.

Treatment of Prehypertension

Prehypertension is considered a precursor of stage 1 HTN and a predictor of excessive cardiovascular risk. The question is whether pharmacologic treatment of prehypertension prevents or postpones stage 1 HTN.

Evidence-based Medicine: The TROPHY trial

In the Trial of Preventing Hypertension, 809 participants with repeated measurements of systolic pressure of 130–139 mmHg and diastolic pressure of 89 mmHg or lower, or systolic pressure of 139 mmHg or lower and diastolic pressure of 85–89 mmHg, were randomly assigned to receive two years of candesartan (Atacand, AstraZeneca) (409) or placebo (400), followed by two years of placebo for all. When a participant reached the study end point of stage 1 hypertension, treatment with antihypertensive agents was initiated. Both the candesartan group and the placebo group were instructed to make changes in lifestyle to reduce blood pressure throughout the trial. During the first two years, hypertension developed in 154 participants in the placebo group and 53 of those in the candesartan group (relative risk reduction, 66.3%; $P < 0.001$). After 4 years, hypertension had developed in 240 participants in the placebo group and 208 of those in the candesartan group (relative risk reduction, 15.6%; $P < 0.007$).

Over a period of 4 years, stage 1 hypertension developed in nearly two thirds of patients with untreated prehypertension (the placebo group). Treatment of prehypertension with candesartan appeared to be well tolerated and reduced the risk of incident hypertension during the study period. Thus, treatment of prehypertension appears to be feasible and effective in preventing the occurrence of stage 1 hypertension [44].

Coronary Artery Disease and Hypertension

Hypertensive patients are at increased risk for MI or other major coronary events and may be at higher risk of death following an acute MI. Lowering both SBP and DBP reduces ischemia and prevents CVD events in patients with CAD, in part by reducing myocardial oxygen demand [45]. One caveat with respect to anti-hypertensive treatment in patients with CAD is the finding in some studies of an apparent increase in coronary risk at low levels of DBP. For example, in the Systolic Hypertension in the Elderly Program (SHEP) study, lowering DBP to <55 or 60 mmHg was associated with an increase in cardiovascular events, including MI [39]. For patients with stable angina and silent ischemia, unless contraindicated, pharmacologic therapy should be initiated with a β-blocker (BB). If angina and BP are not controlled by BB therapy alone, or if BBs are contraindicated (as in the presence of severe reactive airways disease, severe peripheral arterial disease (PAD), high-degree atrio-ventricular block, or sick sinus syndrome), either long-acting dihydropyridine or nondihydropyridine type calcium channel blockers (CCBs) may be used. If angina or BP is still not controlled on this two-drug regimen, nitrates can be added. Short-acting dihydropyridine CCBs should not be used because of their potential to increase mortality, particularly in the setting of acute MI [38].

Heart Failure and Hypertension

For patients with HTN and HF, ACEIs and BBs are indicated [38,46]. In patients intolerant of ACEIs, ARBs may be used. For further BP control, aldosterone antagonists may be of value for both conditions. Aldosterone antagonists may provide additional benefit in patients with severe LV dysfunction, usually late stage C (NYHA class III–IV). In the Randomized Aldactone Evaluation Study (RALES), low dose spironolactone (12.5–25 mg daily), when added to standard therapy, decreased mortality by 34% [47]. However, hyperkalemia is a risk with aldosterone antagonists even at low doses (especially since most patients also are taking ACEIs or ARBs), but its incidence can be reduced by limiting therapy to patients with serum creatinine < 2.5 mg/dL and monitoring carefully serum potassium. BP targets in HF have not been firmly established, but lowering SBP (110–130 mmHg) is almost uniformly beneficial [38,46].

Diabetes and Hypertension

The coexistence of HTN in diabetes is particularly pernicious because of the strong linkage of the two conditions with all CVD, stroke, progression of renal disease, and diabetic retinopathy. Regarding the selection of medications, clinical trials with diuretics, ACEIs, BBs, ARBs, and CCBs have a demonstrated benefit in the treatment of HTN in both type 1 and type 2 diabetics [48–50]. Thiazide-type diuretics are beneficial in diabetics, either alone or as part of a combined regimen [50]. Of potential concern is the tendency for thiazide-type diuretics to worsen hyperglycemia, but this effect tended to be small and did not produce more cardiovascular events compared to the other drug classes [38].

The ADA has recommended ACEIs for diabetic patients older than 55 years of age at high risk for CVD, and BBs for those with known CAD [48]. With respect to microvascular complications, the ADA has recommended both ACEIs and ARBs for use in type 2 diabetic patients with CKD because these agents delay the deterioration in GFR and the worsening of albuminoidal [38,48].

Chronic Kidney Disease and Hypertension

CKD is defined as either: (1) reduced excretory function with an estimated GFR <60 mL/min/1.73 m^2 (approximately corresponding to a creatinine of >1.5 mg/dL in men or >1.3 mg/dL in women); or (2) the presence of albuminuria (>300 mg/day or 200 mg/g creatinine). In a number of laboratories, serum creatinine is being replaced as an index of renal function by estimated GFR, the values of which are derived from newer algorithms that include adjustments for gender, race, and age. The formula to calculate GFR is available on www.hdcn.com/calcf/gfr.htm.

Urinary albumin excretion has diagnostic and prognostic value equivalent to reduced estimated GFR. To avoid inaccuracies associated with 24-hour urine collections, spot urine samples may be used and the albumin/creatinine ratio (ACR) determined. Microalbuminuria is present when the spot urine ACR is between 30–200 mg albumin/g creatinine. ACR values >200 mg albumin/g creatinine signify the presence of CKD [38].

Treatment of HTN in CKD should include specification of target BP levels (<130/80 mmHg), non-pharmacological therapy and specific antihypertensive agents for the prevention of progression of CKD and development of cardiovascular disease [51]. Many drugs can be used safely in chronic renal failure but ACEIs and ARBs were most frequently chosen thanks to their reno-protection effects [52,53,54]. Irbesartan Microalbuminuria Type 2 DM in Hypertensive Patients (IRMA 2) study showed the progression from macroal-buminuria to ESRD can be prevented by inhibition of the renin-angiotensin system with an ARB [55].

Other antihypertensive drugs can be combined with ACEI or ARBs such as diuretics, dihydropyridine CCBs and BBs. When treating HTN in patients with non-diabetic kidney disease, use of combined therapy with ACEI and ARB may offer more renoprotection than with either class of medication alone. Thiazide diuretic may be used if estimated GFR $> 30 \, mL/min/1.73m^2$, but loop diuretics are usually needed for patients with lower kidney function [38]. Potassium-sparing diuretics should be avoided in patients with chronic renal failure. A stable increase of serum creatinine as much as 35% above baseline after ACEI or ARB initiation may be tolerated, as long as hyperkalemia does not occur. ACEI or ARB should be discontinued, or other potentially reversible causes of kidney failure investigated if progressive and rapid rise of serum creatinine continues.

Hypertension and Cerebrovascular Disease

The risk of clinical complications of cerebrovascular disease including ischemic stroke, hemorrhagic stroke, and dementia increases as a function of BP levels. Given the population distribution of BP, most ischemic strokes occur in individuals with prehypertension or stage 1 HTN. The incidence of ischemic or hemorrhagic stroke is reduced substantially by treatment of HTN. No specific agent has been proven to be clearly superior to all others for stroke protection. In the Losartan Intervention for Endpoint Reduction in Hypertension Study (LIFE), there were fewer strokes in the losartan-treated group than in the group treated with atenolol [56]. In the Antihypertensive and Lipid-Lowering Treatment to Prevent Heart Attack Trial (ALLHAT-LLT), the stroke incidence was 15% greater with ACEI than with thiazide-type diuretic or dihydropyridine CCB, but the BP reduction in the lisinopril group was also less than with chlorthalidone or amlodipine [50].

With respect to the prevention of recurrent stroke, the Perindopril Protection Against Recurrent Stroke Study (PROGRESS) demonstrated that addition of the diuretic, indapamide, to the ACEI, perindopril, caused a 43% reduction in stroke occurrence. No significant reduction was present in those on perindopril alone whose BP was only 5/3 mmHg lower than in the control group [57]. The Anglo-Scandinavian Cardiac Outcomes Trial (ASCOT) compared conventional BP lowering based on treatment with a BB (atenolol) with or without a thiazide (bendroflumethiazide-K), with a more contemporary regimen based on a CCB (amlodipine) with or without an ACEI (perindopril). The results show significantly lower rates of coronary and stroke events in individuals allocated an amlodipine-based combination drug regimen than in those allocated an atenolol-based combination drug regimen (HR 0.86 and 0.77, respectively) [58].

CLINICAL PEARLS

How to treat hypertension in acute stroke? The management of BP during an acute stroke remains controversial. BP is often elevated in the immediate post stroke period and is thought by some to be a compensatory physiologic response to improve cerebral perfusion to ischemic brain tissue. The American Stroke Association has provided the following guidelines: in patients with recent ischemic stroke whose SBP is >220 mmHg or DBP 120–140 mmHg, cautious reduction of BP by about 10–15% is suggested, while carefully monitoring the patient for neurologic deterioration related to the lower pressure. If the DBP is >140 mmHg, carefully monitored infusion of sodium nitroprusside should be used to reduce the BP by 10–15%. SBP >185 mmHg or diastolic pressures >110 mmHg are contraindications to the use of tissue plasminogen activator (tPA) within the first 3 hours of an ischemic stroke. Once a thrombolytic agent has been initiated, BP should be monitored closely, especially in the first 24 hours after initiation of treatment. SBP ≥ 180 mmHg or DBP ≥ 105 mmHg usually necessitates therapy with intravenous agents to prevent intracerebral bleeding [38,59]. Avoid large fluctuation of BP.

Left Ventricular Hypertrophy and Hypertension

Left ventricular hypertrophy (LVH) can occur in endurance athletes with normal or supranormal systolic function, large end-diastolic volumes, and elongation of myofibrils (eccentric hypertrophy). LVH due to long standing uncontrolled HTN is usually characterized by "concentric" hypertrophy with circumferential hypertrophy of myofibrils, normal or increased contractility, increased relative wall thickness, normal or low end-diastolic volumes, and at times, impaired relaxation ("diastolic dysfunction"). In population-based samples, 30–50 percent of individuals with stages 1 and 2 hypertension have impaired left ventricular relaxation, and in more severe forms of hypertension, about two-thirds have abnormal left ventricular relaxation. In untreated or poorly treated individuals, LVH becomes a major risk factor for dilated cardiomyopathy and HF [38].

CRITICAL THINKING

Which medications reverse LVH? The LIFE study found that LVH, defined by ECG, was reduced significantly more by a losartan-based than atenolol-based regimen despite equivalent BP lowering [56]. However, in both the Treatment of Mild HTN study and the Veterans Affairs Cooperative Monotherapy trial [60,61] diuretic therapy achieved the greatest benefit in LV mass reduction. So the most consistent reduction in LV mass was achieved with ARBs, the least reduction occurred with BBs, and intermediate benefits occurred for diuretics and CCB [62].

Hypertension in Older People

Elderly patients usually have isolated systolic HTN which is defined as a systolic BP ≥ 140 mmHg in the absence of an elevated diastolic BP (diastolic BP < 90 mmHg). Isolated systolic HTN is a pathologic process due to loss of compliance of the arterial system and is associated with an increased cardiovascular risk. Use of specific drug classes in older people is largely similar to that recommended in the general algorithm and for individual compelling indications. Combination therapy with two or more drugs is generally needed to achieve optimal BP control. In routine practice, if the systolic goal is achieved, the diastolic goal will almost always be reached as well. For elderly with isolated systolic HTN, diuretic and CCBs are the best initial therapy option [50].

Orthostatic Hypotension

Normally, standing is accompanied by a small increase in DBP and a small decrease in SBP when compared to supine values. Orthostatic hypotension (OH) is present when there is a supine-to-standing BP decrease >20 mmHg systolic or >10 mmHg diastolic. There is more OH in diabetic individuals. There is a strong correlation between the severity of OH and premature death, as well as increased incidents of falls and fractures [63]. The causes of OH include severe volume depletion, baroreflex dysfunction, autonomic insufficiency, and certain venodilator antihypertensive drugs, especially alpha blockers and alpha-beta blockers. Diuretics and nitrates may further aggravate OH. In treating older hypertensive patients, clinicians should be alert to potential OH symptoms such as postural unsteadiness, dizziness, or even fainting. Lying and standing BPs should be obtained periodically in all hypertensive individuals over age 50. OH is a common barrier to intensive BP control. Appropriate instruction on sitting up slowly from a lying position or standing up slowly from a sitting position while holding to something firm should be discussed with patients [38].

Hypertension in Women

Oral contraceptives may increase BP and the risk of HTN. Women using oral contraceptives should have their BP checked regularly. HTN in the setting of pregnancy should be followed carefully because of increase risks to mother and fetus. Classification of HTN in pregnancy and treatment is shown in Tables 6.19–21 [38]. Methyldopa, BB, and vasodilators are preferred medications for the safety of fetus. Other antihypertensive have theoretical disadvantage, but none except the ACEI has been proven to increase fetal morbidity and mortality.

Table 6.19 Classification of hypertension in pregnancy [38].

Chronic hypertension	BP >140 mmHg systolic or 90 mmHg diastolic prior to pregnancy pregnancy or before 20 weeks gestation Persists >12 weeks postpartum
Pre-eclampsia	BP >140 mmHg systolic or 90 mmHg diastolic with proteinuria (>300 mg/24 hrs) after 20 weeks gestation Can progress to eclampsia (seizures) More common in nulliparous women, multiple gestation, women with HTN for >4 years, family history of pre-eclampsia, HTN in previous pregnancy, renal disease
Chronic hypertension with superimposed pre-eclampsia	New onset proteinuria after 20 weeks in a woman with HTN In a woman with HTN and proteinuria prior to 20 weeks gestation Sudden two- to threefold increase in proteinuria Sudden increase in BP

(Continued)

Table 6.19 *(Continued)*

	Thrombocytopenia
	Elevated AST or ALT
Gestational hypertension	HTN without proteinuria occurring after 20 weeks gestation
	Temporary diagnosis
	May represent preproteinuric phase of pre-eclampsia or recurrence of chronic HTN abated in midpregnancy
	May evolve to preeclampsia
	If severe, may result in higher rates of premature delivery and growth retardation than mild pre-eclampsia
Transient hypertension	Retrospective diagnosis
	BP normal by 12 weeks postpartum
	May recur in subsequent pregnancies
	Predictive of future primary HTN

ALT, aspartate aminotransaminase; AST, alanine aminotransferase; BP, blood pressure; HTN, hypertension.

Table 6.20 Treatment of chronic hypertension in pregnancy [38].

Agent	Comments
Methyldopa	Preferred based on long-term follow-up studies supporting safety
Betablockers	Reports of intrauterine growth retardation (atenolol)
	Generally safe
Labetalol	Increasingly preferred to methyldopa due to reduced side effects
Clonidine	Limited data
Calcium antagonists	Limited data
	No increase in major teratogenicity with exposure
Diuretics	Not first-line agents
	Probably safe
ACEIs, ARB	Contraindicated
	Reported fetal toxicity and death

ACEI, angiotensin converting enzyme inhibitors; ARB, angiotensin receptor blockers; BB, β-blocker.

Table 6.21 Treatment of acute severe hypertension in pre-eclampsia [38].

Hydralazine	5 mg IV bolus, then 10 mg every 20–30 minutes to a maximum of 25 mg, repeat in several hours as necessary
Labetalol	20 mg IV bolus, then 40 mg 10 minutes later, 80 mg every 10 minutes for two additional doses to a maximum of 220 mg
Nifedipine (controversial)	10 mg PO, repeat every 20 minutes to a maximum of 30 mg
	Caution when using nifedipine with magnesium sulfate, can see precipitous BP drop
	Short-acting nifedipine is not approved by the Food and Drug Administration for managing HTN
Sodium nitroprusside (rarely, when others fail)	0.25 μg/kg/min to a maximum of 5 μg/kg/min
	Fetal cyanide poisoning may occur if used for more than 4 hours

BP, blood pressure; HTN, hypertension; IV, intravenous; PO, by mouth.

Resistant Hypertension

The term "resistant HTN" is used for the persistence of a BP that is usually above 140/90 mmHg despite a combination of three or more antihypertensive drugs at full doses including a diuretic. After excluding potential identifiable HTN (see Table 6.16), physicians should carefully explore reasons why the patient is not at target BP. Specific causes of resistant HTN are listed in Table 6.22. They can usually be identified by appropriate evaluation, and once identified can almost always be treated effectively. The prevalence of truly resistant HTN is small [38,64].

Table 6.22 Causes of resistant hypertension [38].

Improper BP measurement
Volume overload and pseudo tolerance
Excess sodium intake
Volume retention from kidney disease
Inadequate diuretic therapy

Drug-induced or other causes
Non-compliance
Inadequate doses
Inappropriate combinations
NSAIDs; cyclooxygenase 2 inhibitors
Cocaine, amphetamines, other illicit drugs
Sympathomimetics (decongestants, anorectics)
Oral contraceptives
Adrenal steroids
Cyclosporine and tacrolimus
Erythropoietin licorice (including some chewing tobacco)
Selected over-the-counter dietary supplements and medicines
  (e.g., ephedra, ma huang, bitter orange)

Associated conditions
Obesity
Excess alcohol intake

BP, blood pressure; NSAID, non-steroidal anti-inflammatory drug.

Hypertensive Crises

These include hypertensive emergencies and urgencies.

Hypertensive emergencies are characterized by severe elevations in BP (>180/120 mmHg) complicated by evidence of impending or progressive target organ dysfunction. They require immediate BP reduction (not necessarily to normal level) to prevent or limit target organ damage [38]. Patients may require hospitalization and parenteral drug therapy (Table 6.23). The initial goal of therapy in hypertensive emergencies is to reduce mean arterial BP by no more than 25% (within minutes to 1 hour), then if stable, to 160/100–110 mmHg within the next 2–6 hours [38].

Hypertensive urgencies are those situations associated with severe elevations in BP without progressive target organ dysfunction. Examples include upper levels of stage 2 hypertension associated with severe headache, shortness of

Table 6.23 Parenteral drugs for treatment of hypertensive emergency* [38].

Drug	Dose	Onset of action	Duration of action	Adverse effects[†]	Special indications
Vasodilators					
Sodium nitroprusside	0.25–10 µg/kg/min as IV infusion[#]	Immediate	1–2 min	Nausea, vomiting, muscle twitching, sweating, thiocynate; and cyanide toxicity	Most hypertensive emergencies caution with high intracranial pressure or azotemia
Nicardipine hydrochloride	5–15 mg/h IV	5–10 min	15–30 min may exceed 4 h	Tachycardia, headache flushing, local phlebitis	Most hypertensive emergencies except acute heart failure; caution with coronary ischemia
Fenoldopam mesylate	0.1–0.3 µg/kg per min IV infusion[#]	<5 min	30 min	Tachycardia, headache nausea, flushing	Most hypertensive emergencies; caution with glaucoma
Nitroglycerin	5–100 µg/min as IV infusion	2–5 min	5–10 min	Headache, vomiting methemoglobinemia, tolerance with prolonged use	Coronary ischemia
Enalaprilat	1.25–5 mg every 6 hrs IV	15–30 min	6–12 h	Precipitous fall in pressure in high-renin states; variable response	Acute LV failure; avoid in acute myocardial infarction
Hydralazine hydrochloride	10–20 mg IV 10–40 mg IM	10–20 min IV 20–30 min IM	1–4 h IV 4–6 h IM	Tachycardia, flushing, headache, vomiting, aggravation of angina	Eclampsia
Adrenergic inhibitors					
Labetalol hydrochloride	20–80 mg IV bolus every 10 min 0.5–2.0 mg/min IV infusion	5–10 min	3–6 h	Vomiting, bronchoconstriction, dizziness, nausea, heart block, orthostatic hypotension	Most hypertensive emergencies except acute heart failure
Esmolol hydrochloride	250–500 µg/kg/min IV bolus, then 50–100 µg/kg/min by infusion; may repeat bolus after 5 min or increase infusion to 300 µg/min	1–2 min	10–30 min	Hypotension, nausea, asthma – first degree heart block, heart failure	Aortic dissection, perioperative
Phentolamine	5–15 mg IV bolus	1–2 min	10–30 min	Tachycardia, flushing, headache	Catecholamine excess

IV, intravenous; LV, left ventricle; IM, intramuscular; [†]Hypotension may occur with all agents; *These doses may vary from those in the Physicians' Desk Reference (51st ed.).
[#]Require special delivery system.

breath, epistaxis, or severe anxiety. The majority of these patients present as non-compliant or inadequately treated hypertensive individuals, often with little or no evidence of target organ damage [38]. The BP control can be lowered by the oral agents. The initial goal of therapy should be archived a diastolic BP of 100–110 mmHg in the several hours following admission. Normal BP can be attained gradually over several days as tolerated by the individual patient. Excessive or rapid decrease in BP should be avoided to minimize the risk of cerebral hypoperfusion or coronary insufficiency.

Patients Undergoing Surgery

Uncontrolled HTN is associated with wider fluctuations of BP during induction of anesthesia and intubations, and may increase the risk for perioperative ischemic events. BP levels of >180/110 mmHg should be controlled prior to surgery. For elective surgery, effective BP control can be achieved over several days to weeks of outpatient treatment. In urgent situations, rapidly acting parenteral agents, such as sodium nitroprusside, nicardipine, and labetalol, can be utilized to attain effective control very rapidly. Surgical candidates with controlled HTN should maintain their medications until the time of surgery, and therapy should be reinstated as soon as possible postoperatively [38].

Hypertension in African-Americans

Hypertension is more prevalent and severe in African descendent populations living outside of Africa than in any other populations. The racial difference is even more remarkable for its most severe forms and complications. Excess morbidity and mortality among African-Americans are more related to a multitude of factors including late diagnosis, genetic, racial and biologic factors which all work in concert with environmental factors (including smoking and "western" lifestyle, diets and habits) and co-existing conditions including diabetes, obesity, insulin resistance, sedentary lifestyles and metabolic syndrome. The prevalence of HTN in African-Americans is 37.5%. African-Americans with HTN predominantly have a low serum/plasma renin and consequently a low serum/plasma angiotensin II, conversely this is associated with a robust tissue renin and angiotensin II levels, hence large doses of ACEI and ARBs required to block these vasoactive substances [65,66]. The target BP for African-Americans is 130/80 mmHg. For patients with diabetes and renal disease, it is <130/80 mmHg; for patient with proteinuria (1 g/dL), it is <125/75 mmHg.

CLINICAL PEARLS

Treatment of hypertension in African-Americans Emphasis on the importance of therapeutic lifestyle modification such as diet, weight loss and exercise. Carefully controlled diet rich in fruits, vegetables, low fat dairy products, low saturated fats, low in total fat, cholesterol, and low dietary sodium < 2.4 g/day (100 mM/day), well supplemented in potassium = 90 mmol/day produce reduction in BP. Aerobic exercise of moderate intensity is associated with significant decrease in BP, decreased LV mass.

Response to ACEI and BB is blunted in African-Americans when used as monotherapy, combination regimen including a diuretic narrows the response in this racial divide. African-Americans exhibit the most profound response of lower BP to diuretics, followed by CCB. Adequate BP control is common denominator in good outcomes regardless of agents used [50,66,67].

Use of ACEI or ARBs in adequate doses with other classes of anti-hypertension translates into improved renal and cardiac indices [66–68], and prevent or stem progression of new onset diabetes [69]. CCB are not deleterious to cardiovascular outcomes [50].

Follow-up

The JNC-7 guidelines recommend that most patients should return for follow-up and adjustment of medications at approximately monthly intervals until the BP goal is reached. More frequent visits will be necessary for patients with stage 2 HTN or with complicating co-morbid conditions. Serum potassium and creatinine should be monitored at least 1–2 times per year. After BP is at goal and stable, follow-up visits can usually be at 3- to 6-month intervals [38].

Hypercholesterolemia

The Adult Treatment Panel III (ATP III) of the National Cholesterol Education Program (NCEP) recommends that LDL cholesterol be the primary target of therapy with LDL goals based on risk levels (Table 6.24) [24,70]. Risk calculators for these goals are available at www.nhlbi.nih.gov/guidelines/cholesterol. The very high risk category includes patient with established CHD plus (1) multiple major risk factors (especially diabetes), (2) severe and poorly controlled risk factors (especially continued cigarette smoking), (3) multiple risk factors of the metabolic syndrome (especially high triglycerides 200 mg/dL plus non-HDL cholesterol 130 mg/dL with low-HDL cholesterol [40 mg/dL]) and (4) with acute coronary syndromes (ACS) [70]. The clinical trials add further support for the NCEP priority on high serum LDL cholesterol. Four trials; including Heart Protection Study (HPS) [71], PROspective Study of Pravastatin in the Elderly at Risk (PROSPER) [72], Angio-Scandinavian Cardiac Outcomes Trial–Lipid Lowering Arm (ASCOT–LLA) [73], and Pravastatin or Atorvastatin Evaluation and Infection Therapy–Thrombolysis in Myocardial Infarction 22 Investigators (PROVE-IT-TIMI-22) [74] demonstrate that effective LDL cholesterol reduction substantially reduces risk for CHD, whereas one trial, ALLHAT-LLT, [74b] failed to produce a sizable differential in LDL cholesterol levels between treatment and control groups and did not yield a significant risk reduction.

Although LDL cholesterol is the primary target of therapy, other lipid risk factors besides elevated LDL affect CHD risk. Among these are low HDL cholesterol, elevated triglyceride (especially very low-density lipoprotein (VLDL) remnants), and possibly small LDL particles. This "lipid triad" has been called *atherogenic dyslipidemia*. Therefore, the ATP III introduced a secondary target of therapy namely non-HDL cholesterol, in patients with elevated triglyc-erides ($\geqslant 200\,\text{mg}/\text{dL}$). VLDL + LDL cholesterol, termed non-HDL cholesterol, equals total cholesterol minus HDL cholesterol, which represents *atherogenic cholesterol*. Relations among the different lipoprotein fractions are as follows:

1) Total cholesterol = LDL + VLDL + HDL
2) Total cholesterol − HDL = LDL + VLDL = non-HDL

The non-HDL cholesterol goal is $30\,\text{mg}/\text{dL}$ higher than the LDL cholesterol goal. Non-HDL cholesterol was added as a secondary target of therapy to take into account the atherogenic potential associated with remnant lipoproteins in patients with hypertriglyceridemia [24,70]. The CHD risk equivalents men-tioned in Table 6.24 are clinical manifestations of noncoronary forms of athero-sclerotic disease (transient ischemic attacks or stroke of carotid origin, $>50\%$ obstruction of a carotid artery), diabetes, and 2 + risk factors with 10-year risk $>20\%$ for hard CHD [24,70].

Table 6.24 Categories of risk that modify low density lipoprotein cholesterol goals [70].

Risk category	LDL goal (mg/dL)
Very high risk: high risk features (e.g. CHD + DM)	Optional goal < 70
High risk: CHD and CHD risk equivalents; 10 year risk > 20%	<100
Moderately high risk: 10 year risk 10–20%	<130, optional goal < 100
Moderate risk: 2+ risk factors; 10-year risk < 10%	<130
Lower risk: 0–1 risk factors (<10% ten-year risk)	<160

CHD, coronary heart disease; LDL, low density lipoprotein; DM, diabetes mellitus.

Lipid Lowering with Statin

The statin drugs are considered the agents of first choice for lowering LDL cholesterol based on their efficacy and multiple studies across the risk spectrum showing a reduction in cardiovascular morbidity and mortality with these agents. Statin works by inhibiting the enzyme HMG-CoA reductase, thus reducing the cholesterol content in the hepatocytes, and enhancing removal cholesterol from the ciruculation. There are currently six statins on the US mar-ket (Table 4.25). They differ in terms of efficacy, half-life and metabolism. The statins work by inhibiting the enzyme that catalyzes the rate-limiting step in cholesterol synthesis. This leads to clearance of LDL cholesterol particles from the circulation by the liver. In addition, statins minimally raise HDL choles-terol and lower triglyceride-containing particles. They all reduce levels of high-sensitivity C-reactive protein and other inflammatory markers.

Primary Prevention

Two important primary prevention trials have shown that treatment with statins can reduce cardiovascular events between 19–37%. Individuals with multiple risk factors have a greater potential for benefit. The West of Scotland

Table 6.25 Available statins.

Statin (generic)	Brands available	Available doses (mg)	LDL lowering efficacy (%)
Lovastatin	Lovastatin Mevacor (Merck) Altocor (Andrix)	10, 20, 40, 60 SR (Altocor)	21–42
Pravastatin	Pravachol (Bristol-Myers Squibb)	10, 20, 40, 80	22–37
Fluvastatin	Lescol (Novartis) Lescol XL	20, 40, 80 SR	22–36
Simvastatin	Zocor (Merck)	10, 20, 40, 80	26–47
Atorvastatin	Lipitor (Pfizer)	10, 20, 40, 80	39–60
Rosuvastatin	Crestor (AstraZeneca)	5, 10, 20, 40	40–60

Coronary Prevention (WOSCOP) study used pravastatin in a high-risk cohort of middle-aged men with high cholesterol levels and showed that a 26% reduction in LDL cholesterol resulted in a 31% relative reduction in risk of non-fatal MI and death from CAD [75]. The Air Force/Texas Coronary Atherosclerosis Prevention Study (AFCAPS/TexCAPS) evaluated whether cholesterol lowering with statin therapy can benefit individuals with average cholesterol levels but low HDL cholesterol levels. In this study, lovastatin reduced the risk of a first major cardiac event by 37% [76]. However, should the LDL cholesterol level be lowered further? Will there be further benefits?

Evidence-based Medicine: The ASTEROID trial

In A Study to Evaluate the Effect of Rosuvastatin on Intravascular Ultrasound (IVUS)-Derived Coronary Atheroma Burden trial, 349 patients received intensive statin therapy with rosuvastatin, 40 mg/day and had evaluable serial IVUS examinations. Two primary efficacy parameters were prespecified: the change in plaque atheroma volume (PAV) and the change in nominal atheroma volume in the 10-mm sub-segment with the greatest disease severity at baseline. A secondary efficacy variable, change in normalized total atheroma volume for the entire artery, was also prespecified. The results showed that the mean baseline LDL cholesterol level of 130.4 mg/dL declined to 60.8 mg/dL, a mean reduction of 53.2% ($P < 0.001$). Mean HDL cholesterol level at baseline was 43.1 mg/dL, increasing to 49.0 mg/dL, an increase of 14.7% ($P < 0.001$). The mean change in PAV for the entire vessel was −0.98% (3.15%), with a median of −0.79% (97.5% CI, −1.21% to −0.53%) ($P < 0.001$ vs. baseline). The mean (SD) change in atheroma volume in the most diseased 10-mm subsegment was −6.1(10.1)mm^3, with a median of −5.6 mm^3 (97.5% CI, −6.8 to −4.0 mm^3) ($P < 0.001$ vs. baseline). Change in total atheroma volume showed a 6.8% median reduction; with a mean (SD) reduction of −14.7 (25.7) mm^3, with a median of −12.5 mm^3 (95% CI, −15.1 to −10.5 mm^3) ($P < 0.001$ vs. baseline).

Adverse events were infrequent and similar to other statin trials. Very high-intensity statin therapy using rosuvastatin 40 mg/day achieved an average LDL cholesterol of 60.8 mg/dL and increased HDL cholesterol by 14.7%, resulting in significant regression of atherosclerosis for all three prespecified IVUS measures of disease burden [77].

Secondary Prevention

The use of statins in patients already diagnosed with CAD was studied in secondary prevention trials to determine if these agents would reduce subsequent cardiac events. The Scandinavian Simvastatin Survival Study (4S) evaluated the effect of cholesterol lowering with simvastatin in 4444 patients with angina or a previous MI, and reported a 30% reduction in risk of death compared with the placebo group [78]. This was the first major study to show that long-term treatment with simvastatin is safe and improves survival in CHD patients. Additional studies such as the Cholesterol and Recurrent Events (CARE) trial using pravastatin demonstrated similar results in individuals with lower average cholesterol levels than the 4S study [79].

The Medical Research Council Heart Protection Study extended these findings to CHD risk equivalent patients. This large collaborative study of over 20,000 individuals treated patients with CAD, other atherosclerotic disease including carotid artery disease and PAD, or diabetes [71]. Patients were randomized to simvastatin 40 mg/day or placebo. The treatmentgroup had a 24% reduction in major vascular events regardless of their disease category.

Evidence-based Medicine: Intensive vs standard therapy

A recent meta-analysis cardiovascular outcomes with high-dose statin therapy vs standard dosing; from four randomized trials, including TNT (Treating to New Targets), IDEAL (Incremental Decrease in End Points Through Aggressive Lipid Lowering), PROVE-IT-TMI-22 and A–Z (Aggrastat-to-Zocor) yielded a population of 27,548 patients with either stable CHD or ACSs showed a significant 16% odds reduction in coronary death or myocardial infarction ($p < 0.00001$), as well as a significant 16% odds reduction of coronary death or any cardiovascular event ($p < 0.00001$) [79a]. These trials achieved final mean LDL cholesterol levels of 62–81 mg/dL (1.6–2.1 mmol/L), which are well below the current 100 mg/dL (2.6 mmol/L) guideline target for patients at elevated cardiovascular risk [24]. No difference was observed in total or non-cardiovascular mortality, but a trend toward decreased cardiovascular mortality (odds reduction 12%, $p = 0.054$) [79a]. Thus, it appears that intensive therapy for LDL lowering does indeed provide additional clinical cardiovascular benefit to 'standard' intervention with these statins. However, these benefits are modest, and the potential for further benefits may be limited. A prospective meta-analysis of data from 90,056 individuals in 14 randomised trials of statins has shown that the relative risk of CHD or of any adverse vascular event during statin treatment declined by about 20% for each 1 mmol/L (39 mg/dL) reduction in LDL cholesterol [80a]. In addition, for some patients, increased cost or emergence of side-effects may limit the practicability of intensive statin therapy.

CLINICAL PEARLS

How to treat high cholesterolemia? The general strategy for initiation and progression of drug therapy is outlined in Figure 6.3. Consideration of drug therapy often occurs simultaneously with the decision to initiate lifestyle change. Thus weight reduction and exercise may begin at the same time as drug treatment.

After 6 weeks, the response to therapy should be assessed. If the LDL cholesterol goal is still not achieved, further intensification of therapy should be considered, with re-evaluation in another 6 weeks. Once the LDL cholesterol goal has been attained, attention turns to other lipid risk factors when present.

If triglycerides are high (≥200 mg/dL), the secondary target of treatment becomes non-HDL cholesterol. If the LDL cholesterol goal has been attained but not the non-HDL cholesterol goal, there are two alternative approaches: (1) the dose of the LDL-lowering drug can be increased to reduce both LDL and VLDL; or (2) consideration can be given to adding a triglyceride-lowering drug (fibrate or nicotinic acid) to LDL-lowering therapy, which will mainly lower VLDL.

Once the patient has achieved the treatment goal(s), follow-up intervals may be reduced to every 4–6 months (Figure 6.3). The primary focus of these visits is encouragement of long-term compliance with therapy and side effects. Monitoring parameters and follow-up schedule listed in the Table 6.26 [24].

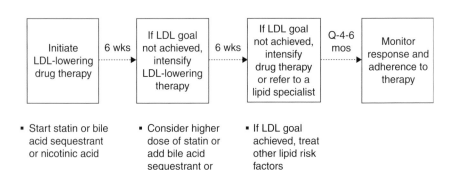

Figure 6.3 Progression of drug therapy [24].

Table 6.26 Monitoring parameters and follow-up schedule [24].

Drug	*Monitoring parameters*	*Follow-up schedule*
Bile acid sequestrants	Indigestion, bloating, constipation, abdominal pain, flatulence, nausea	Evaluate symptoms initially, and at each follow-up visit. Also check time of administration of other drugs

(Continued)

Table 6.26 (*Continued*)

Drug	Monitoring parameters	Follow-up schedule
Nicotinic acid	Flushing, itching, tingling, headache, nausea, gas, heartburn, fatigue, rash	Evaluate symptoms initially, and at each follow-up visit
	Peptic ulcer	Evaluate symptoms initially, then as needed
	Fasting blood sugar; uric acid	Obtain an FBS and uric acid initially, 6–8 weeks after starting therapy, then annually or more frequently if indicated to monitor for hyperglycemia and hyperuricemia
	ALT and AST	Obtain an ALT/AST initially, 6–8 weeks after reaching a daily dose of 1500 mg, 6–8 weeks after reaching the maximum daily dose, then annually or more frequently if indicated
Statins	Muscle soreness, tenderness or pain	Evaluate muscle symptoms and CK initially. Evaluate muscle symptoms at each follow-up visit. Obtain a CK when persons have muscle soreness, tenderness, or pain
	ALT, AST	Evaluate ALT/AST initially, approximately 12 weeks after starting, then annually or more frequently if indicated
Fibrates	Abdominal pain, dyspepsia, headache, drowsiness	Evaluate symptoms initially, and at each follow-up visit
	Cholelithiasis	Evaluate history and symptoms initially, and then as needed

ALT, aspartate aminotransaminase; AST, alanine aminotransferase; CK, creatine kinase; FBS, fasting blood sugar.

Combination Therapy

Statins are currently the most prescribed lipid-altering drugs because of their efficacy in favorably altering blood lipid levels, safety and tolerability, and proven benefits on reducing atherosclerotic CHD events. However, some patients require combination lipid-altering treatment to achieve their LDL cholesterol and non-HDL cholesterol goals. How to choose between the higher dose statin monotherapy or combination of two different classes of drugs? The lipid-altering agents most commonly used in combination with statins include ezetimibe, bile acid sequestrants, peroxisome proliferator–activated receptor (PPAR) agonists, fish oils, and niacin.

CLINICAL PEARLS

When to combine drugs for hypercholesterolemia? Combination lipid-altering drug therapy with statins is often indicated for the following patients.

1 Patients who are unable to achieve recommended treatment LDL cholesterol and non-HDL cholesterol goals with statin monotherapy.
2 Patients who may be at risk for intolerance, toxicity, or adverse drug interactions with higher-dose statin monotherapy. *Or*
3 Patients who may benefit from the use of one or more lipid-altering drugs in combination with statins resulting in complementary benefits towards further reduction in CHD risk.

Statin and Ezetimibe

Ezetimibe blocks the synthesis of a key protein in the intestinal villi, thus preventing the absorption of dietary cholesterol. By itself, the drug has been shown to modestly reduce the serum levels of LDL cholesterol, but it works synergistically when combined with a statin. In the Ezetimibe Study with 628 patients diagnosed of primary hypercholesterolemia, ezetimibe plus 10 mg of atorvastatin was more effective than atorvastatin 10 mg, 20 mg, or 40 mg in lowering LDL cholesterol levels. In fact, the LDL cholesterol-lowering efficacy of 10 mg of ezetimibe plus 10 mg of atorvastatin was similar to 80 mg of atorvastatin (the "formula" of "10 + 10 = 80") [80]. Two other studies with a total of 1555 participants, demonstrated ezetimibe/simvastatin to be more effective in lowering LDL cholesterol levels than simvastatin monotherapy, with a mean reduction of 51–53% compared with 37–39% with simvastatin alone [81,82].

Evidence-based Medicine: The VYVA trial

In the Vytorin vs. Atorvastatin trial, 1902 patients with LDL cholesterol above ATP III goal were randomized to atorvastatin (10 mg, 20 mg, 40 mg, or 80 mg) or to ezetimibe/simvastatin (10/10 mg, 10/20 mg, 10/40 mg, or 10/80 mg). The results showed that at each milligram-equivalent statin dose comparison, and averaged across doses, ezetimibe/simvastatin provided greater LDL cholesterol reductions (47–59%) than atorvastatin (36–53%). Ezetimibe/simvastatin 10/40 mg and 10/80 mg also provided significantly greater HDL cholesterol increases than atorvastatin 40 mg and 80 mg. Triglyceride reductions were similar for all comparisons. More ezetimibe/simvastatin than atorvastatin patients with CHD or CHD risk equivalents attained the ATP III LDL cholesterol goal of <100 mg/dL and the optional LDL cholesterol target of <70 mg/dL. C-reactive protein reductions were similar between treatment groups [83].

No studies of ezetimibe alone or the combination of ezetimibe and simvastatin have examined cardiovascular morbidity or mortality or all-cause mortality.

Statin and Niacin

Several clinical trials supported the efficacy of nicotinic acid for reduction of CHD risk, both when used alone [84] and in combination with statins [85]. The combination of a statin with nicotinic acid produces a marked reduction of LDL cholesterol and a striking rise in HDL cholesterol (the ADvicor vs. Other Cholesterol-Modulating Agents Trial Evaluation [ADVOCATE) [85]. Although the majority of patients can tolerate nicotinic acid therapy, a sizable minority are intolerant because of a variety of side effects.

Statin and Fibrate

For the combination of fibrate and statin, although the evidence base to support fibrate therapy is not as strong as that for statins, fibrates may have an adjunctive role in the treatment of patients with high triglycerides/low HDL, especially in combination with statins. Concern about development of myopathy with this combination has been lessened somewhat by the recent finding that one fibrate, fenofibrate, does not interfere with catabolism of statins and thus likely does not substantially increase the risk for clinical myopathy in patients treated with moderate doses of statins [86]. A statin plus fibrate can reduce both LDL cholesterol and VLDL cholesterol (i.e., non-HDL cholesterol) in patients with elevated triglycerides. Since the primary aim of cholesterol management is LDL reduction, statin therapy usually will be introduced before fibrates. In some patients with high triglycerides, both LDL and non-HDL goals can be attained with higher doses of statins or by an alternative approach with statin and fibrate [24].

Management of Specific Dyslipidemias

Familial Hypercholesterolemia, Very High LDL cholesterol

Severe forms of elevated LDL cholesterol are defined as those in which LDL concentrations are persistently $\geq 190\,mg/dL$ after therapeutic lifestyle changes. Most elevations of this degree have a strong genetic component. It is caused by a mutation of the gene for the LDL receptor which is located on chromosome 19. In heterozygous familial hypercholesterolaemia (FH), one of the LDL-receptor genes has a mutation; in homozygous FH both LDL-receptor genes are affected. This mutation prevents the receptor from participating efficiently in LDL uptake. In patients with FH, LDL remains in the circulation for longer, from the average of 2.5 days to about 4.5 days in heterozygous FH, to even longer in homozygous FH. By adulthood the serum cholesterol level in heterozygous FH can be double what it would have been in the absence of the mutation, and typically can be 9.0–14.0 mmol/L (360–560 mg/dL). In homozygous FH, serum total cholesterol levels are almost always greater than 15 mmol/L (600 mg/dL) and can be as high as 30 mmol/L (1200 mg/dL). The symptoms of FH are tendon xanthomata, corneal arcus and xanthelamata. All of these symptoms tend to occur earlier in patients with homozygous FH than in patients with heterozygous FH, and can even occur in childhood. Patients with FH have increased risk of early-onset CVD. MI has been recorded in patients with homozygous FH at 2 years of age, and life expectancy does not usually extend beyond the early twenties. The use of statin therapy in patients with FH represents a major advancement in the treatment of these patients [87]. Clinical features, clinical outcomes, and therapeutic considerations are listed in Table 6.27 [24].

Table 6.27 Familial disorders that cause very high low density lipoprotein cholesterol levels (≥190 mg/dL) [24].

Clinical condition	Clinical features and clinical outcomes	Therapeutic considerations
Heterozygous FH	Due to mutated LDL receptor (half normal-expression) Prevalence: 1/500 in US LDL cholesterol levels: twice normal (e.g., 190–350 mg/dL) Tendon xanthomas common Premature CHD common	Begin LDL-lowering drugs in young adulthood TLC indicated for all persons Statins: first line of therapy (start dietary therapy simultaneously) BAS (if necessary in combination with statins) If needed, consider triple-drug therapy (statins + BAS + nicotinic acid)
Homozygous FH	Due to two mutated LDL receptors Prevalence: 1/1,000,000 in US LDL cholesterol levels: 4-fold increase (e.g., 400–1000 mg/dL) Xanthomas: tendinous, tuberous, dermal Widespread, atherosclerosis (multiple arterial beds affected) Very severe clinical atherosclerotic disease Aortic valve disease	Dietary therapy not effective BAS not effective Nicotinic acid mildly effective Statins may be moderately effective in some persons Ileal exclusion operation not effective Liver transplant effective, but impractical LDL-pheresis currently employed therapy (in some persons, statin therapy may slow down rebound hypercholesterolemia)
FDB	Due to mutated apo B-100 (position 3500 A-G) Prevalence 1/700–1000 LDL cholesterol levels: 1.5–2-fold increase (e.g., 160–300 mg/dL) Xanthomas: tendon Premature CHD CHD 40–65 year common in men Uncertain in women	TLC indicated All LDL-lowering drugs are effective Combined drug therapy required less often than in heterozygous FH
Polygenic hypercholesterolemia	Due to multiple gene polymorphisms (often combined with dietary excesses) Prevalence: 1/10–20 (depending on age) LDL cholesterol: ≥ 190 mg/dL Prevalence of CHD: 3–4-fold increase (above average)	TLC indicated for all persons Consider for drug therapy (if LDL cholesterol ≥ 190 mg/dL after dietary therapy [all persons]) All LDL-lowering drugs are effective; if necessary to reach LDL cholesterol goals, consider combined drug therapy

BAS, bile acid sequestrants; CHD, coronary heart disease; FDB, familial defective apolipoprotein B-100; FH, familial hypercholesterolemia; LDL, low density lipoprotein; TLC, therapeutic lifestyle changes.

Elevated Triglycerides

Triglycerides are major lipids in chylomicrons and VLDL particles. Increased triglyceride levels, especially in individuals with additional lipoprotein abnormalities (mixed hyperlipidemia), predict higher cardiovascular risk. Elevated triglyceride level is marker for the metabolic syndrome and predicts the presence of small dense LDL particles. Small dense LDL particles are more susceptible to oxidation which may increase their atherogenicity. Classification and causes of elevated serum triglycerides are listed in Table 6.28 [24].

Table 6.28 Classification and causes of elevated serum triglycerides [24].

Classification of serum triglycerides	Causes of elevated serum triglycerides
Normal triglycerides (<150 mg/dL)	
Borderline high triglycerides (150–199 mg/dL)	Acquired causes – Overweight and obesity – Physical inactivity – Cigarette smoking – Excess alcohol intake – High carbohydrate intake (>60% of total energy) Secondary causes* Genetic causes – Various genetic polymorphism
High triglycerides (200–499 mg/dL)	Acquired causes – Same as for borderline high triglycerides (usually combined with foregoing causes) Secondary causes* Genetic patterns – Familial combined hyperlipidemia – Familial hypertriglyceridemia – Polygenic hypertriglyceridemia – Familial dysbetalipoproteinemia
Very high triglycerides (≥500 mg/dL)	Usually combined causes – Same as for high triglycerides Familial lipoprotein lipase deficiency Familial apolipoprotein C-II deficiency

*Secondary causes of elevated triglycerides: diabetes mellitus (see Diabetic dyslipidemia), chronic renal failure, nephrotic syndrome, Cushing's disease, lipodystrophy, pregnancy, and various drugs (corticosteroids, β-blockers, retinoids, oral estrogens [not transcutaneous estrogen], tomoxifen, protease inhibitors for AIDS).

Treatment of hypertriglyceridemia consists of both a lifestyle modification program and pharmacological therapy. Table 6.29 gives a summary of a lifestyle modification and drug therapy to reduce elevated triglyceride levels [24,88].

For many patients with mild increases in triglycerides a lifestyle program alone will normalize the triglyceride levels. The limitation of the intake of complex carbohydrates can be very beneficial in lowering triglyceride levels [88]. When lifestyle modification cannot achieve the desired triglyceride goal,

Table 6.29 Treatment considerations for elevated serum triglycerides.

Serum triglyceride category	Special treatment considerations
Borderline high triglycerides (150–199 mg/dL)	Primary goal: achieve LDL cholesterol goal Life-habit changes: first-line therapy for borderline high triglycerides – Body weight control – Regular physical activity – Smoking cessation – Restriction of alcohol use (when consumed in excess) – Avoid high carbohydrate intakes (>60% of calories) Drug therapy: – Triglycerides in this range not a direct target of drug therapy
High triglycerides (200–499 mg/dL)	Primary goal: achieve LDL cholesterol goal Secondary goal: achieve non-HDL cholesterol goal: 30 mg/dL higher than LDL cholesterol goal First-line therapy for high triglycerides: TLC-emphasize weight reduction and increased physical activity Second-line therapy: drugs to achieve non-HDL cholesterol goal – Statins: lowers both LDL cholesterol and VLDL cholesterol – Fibrates: lowers VLDL-triglycerides and VLDL cholesterol – Nicotinic acid: lowers VLDL-triglycerides and VLDL cholesterol Alternate approaches to drug therapy for lowering non-HDL cholesterol – High doses of statins (lower both LDL cholesterol and VLDL cholesterol) – Moderate doses of statins and triglyceride-lowering drug (fibrate or nicotinic acid): **Caution:** increased frequency of myopathy with statins + fibrates
Very high triglycerides (≥500 mg/dL)	Goals of therapy: – Triglyceride lowering to prevent acute pancreatitis (first priority) – Prevention of CHD (second priority) Triglyceride lowering to prevent pancreatitis: – Very low-fat diet when TG >1000 mg/dL (<15% of total calories as fat) – Medium-chain triglycerides when TG >1000 mg/dL (can replace long-chain triglycerides in diet) – Institude weight reduction/physical activity – Fish oils (replace some long-chain triglycerides in diet) – Triglyceride-lowering drugs (fibrate or nicotinic acid): most effective – Statins: not first-line agent for very high triglycerides (statins not powerful triglyceride-lowering drugs) – Bile acid sequestrants: contraindicated—tend to raise triglycerides Triglyceride lowering to prevent CHD: – Efficacy of drug therapy to prevent CHD in persons with very high triglycerides not demonstrated by clinical trials

CHD, coronary heart disease; HDL, high density lipoprotein; LDL, low density lipoprotein; TG, triglyceride; TLC, therapeutic lifestyle changes; VLDL, very low-density lipoprotein.

pharmacological therapy will need to be considered. Triglyceride values greater than 500 mg/dL usually require drug therapy. The fibric acid derivatives are most commonly used for isolated hypertriglyceridemia although these agents typically lower triglyceride levels only about 30%. Omega-3 fatty acids in the form of dietary fish or fish oil supplements can help to lower triglyceride levels. Prospective data and clinical trial evidence in secondary CHD prevention suggest that higher intakes of n-3 fatty acids reduce risk for coronary events or coronary mortality. ATP III supports the AHA recommendation that fish be included as part of a CHD risk-reduction diet [24]. Doses of 4 g of omega-3 fish oils a day may be needed to achieve about a 30% reduction in triglyceride levels [89].

Strategies for Raising HDL cholesterol

HDL cholesterol levels are inversely correlated with CHD risk. The AFCAPS/ TexCAPS trial suggested that a treatment strategy using statins to primarily lower LDL cholesterol could achieve risk reduction in individuals with lower than average HDL cholesterol values [76]. Strategies to raise HDL cholesterol have also been studied. The fibrates are a class of medications that lower triglyceride levels and mildly raise HDL cholesterol. They may lower LDL cholesterol although if there is a substantial decrease in triglyceride levels, LDL cholesterol may increase slightly in some patients. This increase in LDL cholesterol may be due to an increase in size and thus cholesterol content of the LDL particles and not an increase in absolute number of LDL particles. These less dense LDL particles may be less atherogenic than small dense LDL. There are currently four available fibrates (three in the US), although clofibrate is rarely used because of potential gastrointestinal toxicity (Table 6.30).

Table 6.30 Fibrates.

Fibrate (generic)	Brands available	Doses available (mg)
Gemfibrozil	Lopid (Parke–Davis, NY)	600
Fenofibrate	Tricor (Abbott, Abbott Park IL)	45, 160
	Fenofibrate micronized	67, 134, 200
Bezafibrate (not in US)	Bezalip (Roche, Manati PR),	200, 400
	Bezalip SR and generic	
Clofibrate (not widely	Atromid-S (Wyeth,	
available)	Philadelphia PA) and generic	500

The Veterans Affairs High-Density Lipoprotein Cholesterol Intervention Trial (VA-HIT) compared 1200 mg of gemfibrozil with placebo in over 2500 men with CHD and low HDL cholesterol levels (40 mg/dL or less) [68,90]. HDL cholesterol levels were increased by 6%, triglycerides lowered 31% and no change was observed in LDL cholesterol levels with gemfibrozil therapy. There was a 24% reduction in the combined endpoint of death from CAD, non-fatal MI and stroke. This risk reduction is comparable to findings in many of the statin trials.

Niacin therapy has the greatest potential to raise HDL cholesterol levels. Niacin is available as a short-acting supplement or as a prolonged release preparation to attempt to avoid cutaneous side effects such as flushing. Brands available in the US include Niaspan (Kos Pharmaceutical Inc, Miami FL) and Slo-Niacin (Upsher-Smith, Minneapolis MN). High doses of niacin can raise HDL cholesterol greater than any other currently available therapy. There have been few outcome studies, however, that document cardiovascular risk reduction with niacin. The Coronary Drug Project conducted between 1966 and 1975 evaluated the long-term efficacy of 3 g of niacin daily in a group of men who had previous MI [91]. Mortality in the niacin group was 11% lower than in the placebo group (52.0 versus 58.2%; $p = 0.0004$). No further studies with niacin have been performed that clearly show risk reduction. Niacin is difficult to take and nearly 50% of individuals cannot tolerate the drug because of side effects. Niacin is used in lower doses in combination with statins with the hope that a combined effect of lowering LDL cholesterol with the statin and raising HDL cholesterol with niacin will translate into further risk reduction. The product Advicor (Kos Pharmaceutical Inc, Miami FL) combining lovastatin with extended-release niacin can lower LDL cholesterol from 30–42% and raise HDL cholesterol up to 30% with currently available doses. Studies will need to be performed to determine if these favorable lipid changes bring about further event reduction.

Emerging therapies are being developed to increase HDL cholesterol since HDL is an independent cardiovascular risk factor and high HDL cholesterol levels appear to protect against the development of CAD. Investigators have targeted cholesteryl ester transfer protein (CETP) for raising HDL. Individuals with CETP deficiency have a marked increase in HDL levels. A number of CETP inhibitors are in development. Torcetrapib has been studied in phase two multidose trials and has resulted in HDL cholesterol increases from 16–91% from baseline, LDL cholesterol decreased 21–42% [92]. Further studies will be carried out to determine if these impressive changes in lipid values will lead to significant cardiovascular risk reduction [93]. So, these effects of CETP inhibition resemble those observed in partial CETP deficiency. This work serves as a prelude to further studies in subjects with low HDL, or combinations of dyslipidemia, in assessing the role of CETP in atherosclerosis.

Diabetic Dyslipidemia

The term *diabetic dyslipidemia* essentially refers to *atherogenic dyslipidemia* occurring in persons with type 2 diabetes. It is characterized by elevated triglyceride-rich lipoproteins, small LDL particles, and low HDL cholesterol concentrations. Diabetic dyslipidemia must be considered as one component of the metabolic syndrome, which is exceedingly common in persons with type 2 diabetes. Since diabetes falls into the category of CHD risk equivalent, the goal for LDL cholesterol in persons with diabetes, particularly type 2 diabetes, is <100 mg/dL and optimally <70 mg/dL.

If the patient also has high triglycerides (≥200 mg/dL), non-HDL cholesterol will be a secondary target [24]. Simultaneous control of other risk factors is essential. For treatment, statins are first-line therapy for reducing LDL choles-terol levels in persons with diabetes and they are generally well tolerated [94–96]. They have the advantage of lowering VLDL cholesterol as well as LDL cholesterol; thus they can assist in attaining the non-HDL cholesterol goal when triglyceride levels are ≥200 mg/dL. Fibrates favorably modify diabetic dyslipi-demia. They are well tolerated, and do not worsen hyperglycemia. The Fenofibrate Intervention and Event Lowering in Diabetes (FIELD) trial, has shown that patients with type 2 diabetes, use of fenofibrate should be consid-ered in the context of well-established statin therapy, where its main use is likely to be in combination. It was demonstrated to be well tolerated, alone and in com-bination with statin therapy [97]. However, we need to note that more answers to questions about the safety and efficacy of combined use of fenofibrate and a statin in diabetes patients should come from the ongoing Action to Control Cardiovascular Risk in Diabetes (ACCORD) trial. Nicotinic acid also has a favor-able effect on diabetic dyslipidemia. Unfortunately, nicotinic acid therapy can increase insulin resistance and clinical experience has shown that in rare instances, diabetic dyslipidemia is worsened with nicotinic acid therapy [98].

Dyslipidemia in Patients with Liver Disease
Biliary obstruction can lead to severe hypercholesterolemia that is resistant to conventional cholesterol-lowering drugs. The only effective therapy is treatment of the underlying liver or biliary tract disease [24]. In patients with borderline elevation of liver enzyme, if the patient needs to be on medication, the patient should be on statin with more frequent checks of liver enzyme. If there is per-sistent and substantial elevation of liver enzyme, then statin should be dis-continued [99].

CLINICAL PEARLS
Use of statin in patients with baseline elevation of liver enzyme
Measure baseline electrolyte, liver function, renal function and thyroid stimulating hormone.

Look for non-drug causes of elevation of aminotransferase (ALT or AST) such as alcohol use, non-immune hepatitis, infectious hepatitis, or non-alcoholic fatty liver disease.

Statin can be started if the ALT and AST level is not >3 times the upper limit of normal.

After starting statin, monitor ALT and AST every 6 and 12 weeks and after dose increase.

If the level of AST and ALT is elevated >3 times of normal during monitoring: repeat measurement in 1 week.

If level still high, decrease the dose or stop the medication if the patient has chronic liver disease or chronic alcohol abuse.

If decrease the dose, repeat measurement in 2–4 weeks.

If level return to baseline, continue lower dose and monitor.

If statin is discontinued, consider rechallenge the same statin at lower dose or another statin [99].

Dyslipidemia in HIV Patients Taking Protease Inhibitor

Dyslipidaemia associated with the treatment of HIV infection, particularly with the use of protease inhibitors, can raise cholesterol and triglyceride levels to the thresholds indicated for intervention. Diet and exercise should be tried first. If there is no satisfactory result, the other options are to switch antiretroviral agents and to start lipid-lowering drugs. Selection of drug therapy for lipid lowering depends on the type of predominating dyslipidemia and the potential for drug interactions. The use of the statins is recommended for the treatment of patients with elevated LDL cholesterol levels and gemfibrozil or fenofibrate for patients with elevated triglycerides concentrations. Because atorvastatin and some antiretroviral drugs are metabolized by the same cytochrome C-450 isoenzyme CYP3A4, inhibition of the isoenzyme may result in excessive high level of statin (raising the risk of rhabdomyolysis). So simvastatin, lovastatin should be avoided, while atorvastatin should be used at lower dose. Pravastatin can be used, however, its efficacy is questioned. Rosuvastatin is a better choice for the patients receiving antiretroviral drugs, because it may have slightly more CYP3A4 activity [100,101].

Metabolic Syndrome

The metabolic syndrome is a constellation of interrelated risk factors of metabolic origin – *metabolic risk factors* – that appear to directly promote the development of atherosclerotic CVD as well as increase the risk for developing type 2 diabetes. In patients with the metabolic syndrome, relative risk for CVD ranges from 1.5–3.0 depending on the stage of progression [102]. When diabetes is not yet present, risk for progression to type 2 diabetes averages about five-fold increase compared with those without the syndrome [103]. The ATP III criteria required no single factor for diagnosis, but instead made the presence of three of five factors the basis for establishing the diagnosis. The AHA and NHLBI recently reaffirmed the utility of ATP III criteria, with minor modification (Table 6.31) [104,105]. According to the new IDF definition for a person to be defined as having the metabolic syndrome they must have central obesity (defined by waist circumference in Table 6.9) plus any two of four other factors of updated ATP III cut-points in Table 6.3 [31].

The pathogenesis of the metabolic syndrome is multifactorial. The major *underlying risk factors* are obesity and insulin resistance. Risk associated with obesity is best identified by increased waist circumference (abdominal obesity). Insulin resistance can be secondary to obesity but can have genetic components as well. Several factors further exacerbate the syndrome: physical inactivity, advancing age, endocrine dysfunction, and genetic aberrations affecting individual risk factors [106]. The increasing prevalence of metabolic syndrome in the US and worldwide [107,108], however, seems to be driven largely by more obesity exacerbated by sedentary lifestyles [109].

The primary goal of clinical management in individuals with the metabolic syndrome is to reduce risk for clinical atherosclerotic disease. Even in people

Table 6.31 Criteria for clinical diagnosis of metabolic syndrome.

Any three of five constitute diagnosis of metabolic syndrome
Elevated waist circumference
102 cm (40 inches) in men
88 cm (35 inches) in women

Elevated triglycerides
150 mg/dL (1.7 mmol/L) or on drug treatment for elevated triglycerides

Reduced HDL cholesterol
<40 mg/dL (1.03 mmol/L) in men
<50 mg/dL (1.3 mmol/L) in women
or on drug treatment for reduced HDL cholesterol

Elevated blood pressure
130 mmHg systolic BP
or 85 mmHg diastolic BP
Or on antihypertensive drug treatment in a patient with a history of HTN

Elevated fasting glucose
100 mg/dL (5.6 mMol/L), or on drug treatment for elevated glucose

BP, blood pressure; HDL, high density lipoprotein; HTN, hypertension.

CLINICAL PEARLS

How to measure waist circumference? Locate top of right iliac crest.
Place a measuring tape in a horizontal plane around abdomen at level of
iliac crest. Before reading tape measure, ensure that tape is snug but does
not compress the skin and is parallel to floor. Measurement is made at the end of a
normal expiration.

Some US adults of non-Asian origin (e.g., White, Black, Hispanic) with marginally
increased waist circumference (e.g., 94–101 cm [37–39 inches] in men and 80–87 cm
[31–34 inches] in women) may have strong genetic contribution to insulin resistance
and should benefit from changes in lifestyle habits, similar to men with categorical
increases in waist circumference. Lower waist circumference cutpoint (e.g., 90 cm [35
inches] in men and 80 cm [31 inches] in women) appears to be appropriate for Asian
Americans. In other countries, IDF defined the waist circumference values according to
gender and ethnic group (see Table 6.9) [31,104].

with the metabolic syndrome, first-line therapy is directed toward the major
risk factors: LDL cholesterol above goal, hypertension, and diabetes.
Prevention of type 2 diabetes is another important goal when it is not present
in a person with the metabolic syndrome. For individuals with established
diabetes, risk factor management must be intensified to diminish their higher
risk for atherosclerotic CVD [104–106].

The metabolic syndrome itself is not a robust risk assessment tool for estimating absolute 10-year risk; but its presence calls for more extensive short-
term risk assessment, either by risk-factor scoring or imaging for sub-clinical

atherosclerosis. The primary intervention is lifestyle therapy, particularly weight reduction and increased exercise. Many studies have shown the clinical benefits of lifestyle change [110]. In people for whom lifestyle intervention is not enough and who are considered to be a high risk for atherosclerotic CVD, more aggressive drug therapy may be required to treat the metabolic syndrome. Drug therapies should be based on global risk assessment and should follow current treatment guidelines for each of the risk factors [31,105]. Both the results of the Rimonabant in Obesity-Lipids (RIO-Lipids) Study with the investigational cannabinoid receptor 1 (CB1) antagonist rimonabant, along with another trial, have shown that a combined drug/counseling approach to obesity is better than either alone [111]. Rimonabant suppresses endogenous activation of the endocannabinoid system. The drug causes a 5–10% weight loss up to 2 years and might have systemic actions that independently reduce risk factors for the metabolic syndrome [112]. Dual PPAR agonists combine PPAR-alpha and PPAR-gamma agonism in a single agent and thus have favorable effects on several metabolic risk factors [113]. In spite of promise, all of these drugs have outcome hurdles to mount before they can be approved for routine use in patients with the metabolic syndrome. Until now, there are no effective new drugs specifically for metabolic syndrome available yet. Bariatric surgery may lead to improvement in patient with class II/III obesity: significant weight loss (>44 kg), decreased SBP and DBP, total cholesterol decreased by 45 mg/dL, LDL decreased by 40 mg/dL [114].

Primary Prevention of Diabetes

Normal fasting glucose is defined as glucose <100 mg/dL (5.6 mmol/L), and IFG has been defined at levels between 100–126 mg/dL (5.6–6.9 mmol/L). A fasting plasma glucose level >126 mg/dL (7.0 mmol/L) or a random plasma glucose >200 mg/dL (11.1 mmol/L) meets the threshold for the diagnosis of diabetes [48]. Hemoglobin A_{1c} level >7% is defined as inadequate control of hyperglycemia. The evolution of type 2 diabetes can be seen as a continuum, from normal glucose tolerance, to IGT, to early and late stage type 2 diabetes. A range of interventions, involving lifestyle modification and/or pharmacologic therapy has been shown to positively influence the risk of developing type 2 diabetes. Table 6.32 summarizes the results of key intervention studies in patients with IGT or other cardiovascular risk factors. These studies suggest that the development of strategies to prevent or delay the onset of type 2 diabetes is a realistic goal [115].

Multifactorial approaches with intensive treatments to control hyperglycemia, HTN, dyslipidemia, and microalbuminuria have demonstrated reductions in the risk of cardiovascular events [119]. These intensive approaches included behavioral measures and the use of a statin, ACEI, ARB, and antiplatelet drug as appropriate. Intensive treatment of HTN in diabetics also significantly reduced the risk of the combined end point of MI, sudden death, stroke, and peripheral vascular disease by 34% ($P = 0.019$) [67]. Although

Table 6.32 Diabetes prevention strategies and outcomes.

Intervention therapy	Study	Risk reduction (%)
Intensive lifestyle	DPP [114b], FDP [115]	58*
Metformin	DPP [114b]	31*
Acarbose	STOP-NIDDM [116]	25*
Pravastatin	WOSCOPS [75]	30*
Ramipril	HOPE [67]	34*
Oestrogen/progesterone	HERS [117]	35*
Intensive lifestyle + Orlistat	XENDOS [118]	37†

*Versus standard lifestyle advice.
†Versus intensive lifestyle advice.
DPP, Diabetes Prevention Program; FDP, Finish Diabetes Prevention Study: STOP-NIDDM, Study to Prevent: Non-Insulin Dependent Diabetes Mellitus Trial; WOSCOP, West of Scotland Coronary Prevention; HOPE, Heart Outcomes Prevention Evaluation Study; HERS, The Heart and Estrogen/Progestin Replacement Study; XENDOS, XENical in the prevention of Diabetes in Obese Subjects.

most of these studies did not reach the goal BP of 130/80 mmHg, epidemiological analyses suggest a continual reduction in cardiovascular events to a BP of 120/80 mmHg [49]. Thiazide diuretics, BBs, ACEIs, and ARBs are beneficial in reducing cardiovascular events and stroke incidence in patients with diabetes [49,50,90,120] and are therefore preferred for the initial treatment of HTN. ACEI- and ARB-based treatments have been shown to favorably affect the progression of diabetic nephropathy and to reduce albuminuria, and ARBs have been shown to reduce the progression to macroalbuminuria [53,54,121].

Evidence-based Medicine: Which β-blocker decreases microalbuminuria? The GEMINI trial

A pre-specified secondary end point of the Glycemic Effects in Diabetes Mellitus Carvedilol-Metoprolol Comparison in Hypertensives trial was to examine the effects of different β-blockers on changes in albuminuria in the presence of renin-angiotensin system blockade. Participants with HTN and type 2 diabetes were randomized to either metoprolol tartrate ($n = 737$) or carvedilol ($n = 498$) in blinded fashion after a washout period of all antihypertensive agents except for ACEI or ARB. Blinded medication was titrated to achieve target BP, with a 5-month follow-up period. The results showed that a greater reduction in microalbuminuria was observed for those randomized to carvedilol (−16.2% δ; 95% CI, −25.3, −5.9; $P = 0.003$). Of those with normoalbuminuria at baseline, fewer progressed to microalbuminuria on carvedilol vs. metoprolol (20 of 302 [6.6%] vs. 48 of 431 [11.1%], respectively; $P = 0.03$). Microalbuminuria development was not related to differences in BP or achievement of BP goal (68% carvedilol vs. 67%, metoprolol). Presence of metabolic syndrome at baseline was the only independent predictor of worsening albuminuria throughout the study ($P = 0.004$). β-blockers have differential effects on microalbuminuria in the presence of renin-angiotensin system blockade. These differences cannot be explained by effects on BP or α 1-antagonism but may relate to antioxidant properties of carvedilol [122].

The ADA now recommends that all patients with diabetes and hypertension should be treated with a regimen that includes either an ACEI or an ARB [48]. Some studies have shown an excess of selected cardiac events in patients treated with CCBs compared with ACEIs [123]. Glycemic control, shown to reduce the occurrence of microvascular complications (nephropathy, retinopathy, and peripheral neuropathy) in several clinical trials [124] is recommended in multiple guidelines of both primary and secondary prevention of stroke and cardiovascular disease [48].

Evidence-based Medicine: ACEI or ARB for prevention of type 2 diabetes

A meta-analysis of 12 randomized controlled clinical trials of ACEIs or ARBs to study the efficacy of these medications in diabetes prevention. The results showed that ACEIs and ARBs were associated with reductions in the incidence of newly diagnosed diabetes by 27% and 23%, respectively, and by 25% in the pooled analysis. So ACE inhibitor or ARB should be given to patients with pre-diabetic conditions such as metabolic syndrome, hypertension, IFG, family history of diabetes, obesity, HF, or CAD [125].

In summary, the effectiveness of lifestyle intervention in delaying the onset of diabetes indicates strongly that subjects with IGT or IFG should receive lifestyle advice (Table 6.8). Pharmacological treatment can also be considered when lifestyle intervention fails.

Primary Prevention for Chronic Kidney Disease

CKD is a worldwide public health problem. In the US there is an increasing incidence and prevalence of renal failure with poor outcome and high costs and an even higher prevalence of earlier stages of CKD (approximately 80 times greater than ESRD prevalence). Moreover, CKD is associated with elevated cardiovascular morbidity and mortality. Therefore, strategies that are aimed at identifying, preventing, and treating CKD and its related risk factors are needed. The patients at risk for CKD include persons with diabetes, hypertension, or close relatives with ESRD. The risks in these categories are markedly amplified in African-American, Native American, and Hispanic groups. The tools for screening are cost-effective and include spot urine samples for protein-creatinine ratio (obviating the need for 24-hour urine collections) and a urine-free calculation of GFR requiring a serum creatinine measurement and anthropometric measures of the patient [126]. The main plan for prevention of CKD is to control hypertension, prevent diabetes, low protein diet, exercise, lower cholesterol level.

Evidence-based Medicine: ACEI for prevention of the onset of microalbuminuria: The BENEDICT Trial

The Bergamo Nephrologic Diabetes Complication Trial was a prospective, randomized, double-blind, parallel-group study that was organized in two phases. Phase A included 1204 patients and was aimed at assessing the efficacy of the ACEI (trandolapril), the non-dihydropyridine CCB (verapamil), and the trandolapril plus verapamil combination as compared with placebo in prevention of microalbuminuria in hypertensive patients with type 2 diabetes and normal urinary albumin excretion rate. Phase B was aimed at assessing the efficacy of the combination as compared with trandolapril alone in prevention of macroalbuminuria in patients with microalbuminuria. The BENEDICT Phase A study showed microalbuminuria developed in 17 (5.7%) of 300 patients in the group that received verapamil SR plus trandolapril and in 30 (10%) of 300 patients in the placebo group. The onset of microalbuminuria was significantly delayed by a factor of 2.6 ($P = 0.02$). Microalbuminuria developed in 18 (6.0%) of 301 patients who were taking trandolapril alone and in 36 (11.9%) of 303 patients who were taking verapamil $P < 0.001$. Verapamil SR alone (11.9%) was compared with placebo (10.0%) $P = 0.54$. These findings suggest that in hypertensive patients with type 2 diabetes and normal renal function, an ACEI may be the medication of choice for controlling BP [127].

The apparent advantage of ACEI over other agents includes a protective effect on the kidney against the development of microalbuminuria, which is a major risk factor for cardiovascular events and death in this population. Not only cardiologists but nephrologists and diabetologists now have a new goal: to prevent patients with diabetes from progressing to nephropathy, the final aim being to limit cardiovascular events and death [127].

Influenza Vaccination and Prevention for CVD

Influenza-related death is more common among individuals with CVD than among patients with any other chronic condition. Influenza can exacerbate underlying medical conditions, including CVD and diabetes, and can also lead to viral pneumonia, secondary bacterial pneumonia, or a coinfection with other viruses or bacteria [128,129]. Clinical trials and observational studies have demonstrated that vaccination against influenza is associated with significantly reduced risk of cardiovascular death and nonfatal events, or

Evidence-based Medicine: FLUVACS trial

The strongest evidence for a protective effect comes from a randomized, controlled trial of influenza vaccination (FLU Vaccination in Acute Coronary Syndromes [FLUVACS]) in which 301 patients hospitalized for either myocardial infarction (MI) or planned angioplasty/stenting were randomly assigned to receive influenza vaccination or remain unvaccinated [130–131]. At 1 year, the relative risk of cardiovascular mortality in the vaccinated group was 0.25 (95% CI 0.07 to 0.86) compared with the unvaccinated group (overall rates 2% versus 8%), and the relative risk of a composite end point (cardiovascular death, nonfatal MI, or severe ischemia) was 0.59 (95% CI 0.30 to 0.86; 11% versus 23%) [130]. At 2 years, although risk reductions of similar magnitude were measured, the remaining sample size after loss to follow-up was too small to find statistical significance [131]. Of note, the FLUVACS trial was conducted without financial support from the influenza vaccine industry [131]. No study has indicated higher rates of cardiovascular events for individuals who receive influenza vaccination [128].

According to the US Centers for Disease Control and Prevention, and the AHA and ACC, vaccination with inactivated influenza vaccine is recommended for individuals who have chronic disorders of the cardiovascular system [128].

Take Home Message

Medical therapy designed to lower BP, HbA1c, cholesterol levels and reduce proteinuria is the main strategy in prevention of CVD. All we need are to achieve the goals set as:

Fasting plasma glucose <100 mg/dL
Hemglobin A1c <7%
Blood pressure <140/90 mmHg (optimal <130/80 mmHg)
LDL-**cholesterol** <100 mg/dL (optimal <70 mg/dL)
HDL-cholesterol >40 mg/dL
Total cholesterol <200 mg/dL
Triglycerides <150 mg/dL
Ideal BMI, waist circumference

unplanned angioplasty and stenting (presented at the American Heart Association 2006 Scientific Sessions in Chicago).

However, despite accumulating evidence of the benefits of LDL and BP lowering over the past two decades, initiation of treatment and long-term compliance to therapy remain far from optimal. Lack of compliance is causing individuals to miss the risk-reducing benefit of treatment, and is creating enormous costs in the health system to treat cardiovascular events that could have been prevented [24]. Therefore, effective strategies for compliance are needed for the success in prevention of CVD.

CLINICAL PEARLS
How to improve compliance? [24]
Keep the medication regimen as simple as possible
Give the patient clear instructions
Discuss compliance for at least a minute at each visit
Concentrate on those who don't reach treatment goals
Always call patients who miss visit appointments
Use two or more strategies for those who miss treatment goals
Use systems to reinforce compliance and maintain contact with the patient
Encourage the support of family and friends
Involve patients in their own care through self-monitoring
Develop a standardized treatment plan to structure care
Use feedback from past performance to foster change in future care

If a person has normal BP at rest and with exercise, no DM, no metabolic syndrome, exercises well and has good diet, then this is an excellent gift for him-or herself, his/her family and a great contribution to society: that person would use less health care resources. To achieve these goals is a noble contribution of the cardiology community to the society. It is do-able and achievable. What are we waiting for?

References

1 Anderson KM, Castelli WP, Levy D. Cholesterol and mortality: 30 years of follow – up from the Framingham study. JAMA 1987;257:2176–2180.
2 Neaton JD, Wentworth D. Serum cholesterol, blood pressure, cigarette smoking, and death from coronary heart disease: Overall findings and differences by age for 316,099 white men. Multiple Risk Factor Intervention Trial Research Group. Arch Intern Med 1992;152:56–64.
3 Volpe, M., Tocci, G., Pagannone, E. Fewer Mega–Trials and More Clinically Oriented Studies in Hypertension Research? The Case of Blocking the Renin–Angiotensin– Aldosterone System. J Am Soc Nephrol 2006.17: S36–S43 [Abstract] [Full Text].
4 Mehta JL, Rasouli N, Sinha AK, Molavi B. Oxidative stress in diabetes: a mechanistic overview of its effects on atherogenesis and myocardial dysfunction. Int J Biochem Cell Biol. 2006;38(5–6):794–803.
5 Meisinger C, Doring A, Lowel H. Chronic kidney disease and risk of incident myocardial infarction and all–cause and cardiovascular disease mortality in middle-aged men and women from the general population. Eur Heart J. May;27(10):1245–1250.
6 Healey JS, Baranchuk A, Crystal E et al. Prevention of atrial fibrillation with angiotensin-converting enzyme inhibitors and angiotensin receptor blockers: a meta-analysis. J Am Coll Cardiol. 2005 Jun 7;45(11):1832–1839.
7 Lichtenstein AH et al. Diet and lifestyle recommendations revision 2006: a scientific statement from the American Heart Association Nutrition Committee. Circulation. 2006 Jul 4;114(1):e27.

8 St. Jeor ST, Howard BV, Prewitt TE *et al.* Dietary protein and weight reduction: a statement for healthcare professionals from the Nutrition Committee of the Council on Nutrition, Physical Activity, and Metabolism of the American Heart Association. Circulation 2001;104:1869–1874.

9 Bonow RO, Eckel RH. Diet, obesity, and cardiovascular risk N Engl J Med 2003;348: 2057–2058.

10 Parin P, Michael CM, Dominique A *et al.* Diets and Cardiovascular Disease J Am Coll Cardiol, 2005; 45:1379–1387.

11 Bravata DM, Sander L, Huang J *et al.* Efficacy and safety of low-carbohydrate diets: a systematic review. JAMA 2003;289:1837–1850.

12 Howard BV, Horn LV, Hsia J *et al.* Low-Fat Dietary Pattern and Risk of Cardiovascular Disease The Women's Health Initiative Randomized Controlled Dietary Modification Trial *JAMA*2006;295:655–666.

13 Hu FB. The Mediterranean Diet and mortality – olive oil and beyond N Engl J Med 2003;348:2595–2596.

14 Kris-Etherton PM, Harris WS, Appel LJ *et al.* Fish consumption, fish oil, omega-3 fatty acids, and cardiovascular disease Circulation 2002;106:2747–2757.

15 Agatston A. The South Beach Diet, The Delicious, Doctor–Designed, Foolproof Plan for Fast and Healthy Weight Loss. New York, NY: Rodale; 2003.

16 Sugar Busters! Concept 2004 http://www.sugarbusters.com/filessb/concept.html. Accessed May 11.

17 ZonePerfect Nutrition Program 2004 http://www.zoneperfect.com/site/content/guide_02_ZoneDiet.asp. Accessed May 11.

18 Jenkins DJA, Thomas DM, Wolever S *et al.* Glycemic index of food: a physiological basis for carbohydrate exchange. Am J Clin Nutr 1981;34:362–366.

19 Foster–Powell K, Holt SHA, Brand-Miller JC. International table of glycemic index and glycemic load values 2002. Am J Clin Nutr 2002;76:5–56.

20 Brand–Miller J, Hayne S, Petocz P, Colagiuri S. Low-glycemic index diets in the management of diabetes: a meta–analysis of randomized controlled trials. Diabetes Care 2003;26: 2261–2267.

21 Champagne CM. Dietary interventions on blood pressure: the Dietary Approaches to Stop Hypertension (DASH) trials. Nutr Rev 2006 Feb;64(2 Pt 2):S53–56.

22 Teta D, Phan O, Halabi G *et al.* Chronic renal failure: what diet?Rev Med Suisse. 2006 Mar 1;2(55):566–569.

23 Criqui MH. Alcohol and coronary heart disease: consistent relationship and public health implications. Clinica Chimica Acta 1996;246:51–57.

24 Third Report of the National Cholesterol Education Program (NCEP) Expert Panel on Detection, Evaluation, and Treatment of High Blood Cholesterol in Adults (Adult Treatment Panel III) final report. Circulation 2002;106:3143–3421.

25 Ockene IS, Miller NH. Cigarette smoking, cardiovascular disease, and stroke: a statement for healthcare professionals from the American Heart Association. American Heart Association Task Force on Risk Reduction. Circulation 1997;96:3243–3247.

26 Tobias Raupach, Katrin Schäfer, Stavros Konstantinides, Stefan Andreas. Secondhand smoke as an acute threat for the cardiovascular system: a change in paradigm. EHJ 2006 27: 386–392.

27 Barua RS, Ambrose JA, Eales-Reynolds LJ, DeVoe MC, Zervas JG, Saha DC. Heavy and light cigarette smokers have similar dysfunction of endothelial vasoregulatory activity: an *in vivo* and *in vitro* correlation. J Am Coll Cardiol. 2002 Jun 5; 39(11):1758–1763.

28 Sacco RL, Adams R, Albers G *et al.* Guidelines for Prevention of Stroke in Patients With Ischemic Stroke or Transient Ischemic Attack A Statement for Healthcare Professionals From

the American Heart Association/American Stroke Association Council on Stroke: Co–Sponsored by the Council on Cardiovascular Radiology and Intervention: The American Academy of Neurology affirms the value of this guideline. Stroke 2006;37: 577–617.

29 Frishman WH, Mitta W, Kupersmith A, Ky T. Nicotine and non-nicotine smoking cessation pharmacotherapies. Cardiol Rev 2006 Mar–Apr;14(2):57–73.).

30 The Health Consequences of Smoking: a Report of the Surgeon General.

31 International Diabetes Federation: The IDF consensus worldwide definition of the metabolic syndrome [article online], 2006. Available from www.idf.org/webdata/docs/IDF_Meta_def_final.pdf.

32 Field AE et al. Impact of overweight on the risk of developing common chronic diseases during a 10–year period. Arch Intern Med 2001;161:1581–1586.

33 Turkoglu C, Duman BS, Gunay D et al. Effect of abdominal obesity on insulin resistance and the components of the metabolic syndrome: evidence supporting obesity as the central feature. Obes Surg 2003;13(5):699–705.

34 Pi–Sunyer FX, Aronne L J, Heshmati HM et al. for the RIO-North America Study Group Effect of Rimonabant, a Cannabinoid-1 Receptor Blocker, on Weight and Cardiometabolic Risk Factors in Overweight or Obese Patients RIO-North America: A Randomized Controlled Trial J AMA2006;295:761–775.

35 Tanasescu M, Leitzmann MF, Rimm EB, Willett WC, Stampfer MJ, Hu FB. Exercise type and intensity in relation to coronary heart disease in men. JAMA 2002 Oct 23–30;288(16): 1994–2000.

36 National Heat, Lung, and Blood Institute. Guide to Physical Activity. http://www.nhlbi.nih.gov/health/public/heart/obesity/lose_wt/phy_act.htm).

37 Chobanian AV, Bakris GL, Black HR et al.; National Heart, Lung, and Blood Institute Joint National Committee on Prevention, Detection, Evaluation, and Treatment of High Blood Pressure; National High Blood Pressure Education Program Coordinating Committee. The Seventh Report of the Joint National Committee on Prevention, Detection, Evaluation, and Treatment of High Blood Pressure: the JNC 7 report. JAMA 2003;289:2560–2572.

38 Chobanian AV et al. Complete Report. The Seventh Report of the Joint National Committee on Prevention, Detection, Evaluation, and Treatment of High Blood Pressure. NIH Publication No. 04–5230. August 2004.

39 SHEP Cooperative Research Group. Prevention of stroke by antihypertensive drug treatment in older persons with isolated systolic hypertension. Final results of the Systolic Hypertension in the Elderly Program (SHEP). JAMA 1991;265:3255–3264.

40 Giles TD, Berk BC, Black HR et al. Expanding the definition and classification of hypertension. J Clin Hypertens 2005;7:505–512.

41 World Health Organization, International Society of Hypertension Writing.Group. 2003 World Health Organization (WHO)/International Society of Hypertension (ISH) statement on management of hypertension. J Hypertens 21:1983–1992 & 2003.

42 Khan NA et al. 2004 Canadian Recommendations for the Management of Hypertension. Can J Cardiol 2004;20:41–54.

43 National Institute of Clinical Excellence (NICE) Clinical Guideline 18 – management of hypertension in adults in primary care, 2004. Available at: www.nice.org.uk/CG018NICEguideline.

44 Julius S, Nesbitt SD, Egan BM et al. for the Trial of Preventing Hypertension (TROPHY) Study Investigators Feasibility of Treating Prehypertension with an Angiotensin-Receptor Blocker NEJM 534;1685–1697.

45 The European Trial on Reduction of Cardiac Events with Perindopril in Stable Coronary Artery Disease Investigators. Efficacy of perindopril in reduction of cardiovascular

events among patients with stable coronary artery disease: Randomised, double-blind, placebo-controlled, multicentre trial (the EUROPA study). Lancet 2003;362: 782–788.

46 Hunt SA, Baker DW, Chin MH, Cinquegrani MP,Feldman AM, Francis GS *et al.* ACC/AHA 2005 Guideline Update for the Diagnosis and Management of Chronic Heart Failure in the Adult A Report of the American College of Cardiology/American Heart Association Task Force on Practice Guidelines. American College of Cardiology Web Site. Available at: http://www.acc.org/clinical/guidelines/failure//index.pdf.

47 Pitt B, Zannad F, Remme WJ *et al.* The effect of spironolactone on morbidity and mortality in patients with severe heart failure. Randomized Aldactone Evaluation Study Investigators. N Engl J Med 1999;341:709–717.

48 American Diabetes Association. ADA clinical practice recommendations. Diabetes Care 2004;27:S1–S143.

49 Adler AI, Stratton IM, Neil HA *et al.* Association of systolic blood pressure with macrovascular and microvascular complications of type 2 diabetes (UKPDS 36): prospective observational study. BMJ. 2000;321:412–419.

50 The ALLHAT Officers and Coordinators for the ALLHAT Collaborative Research Group. Major outcomes in high–risk hypertensive patients randomized to angiotensin-converting enzyme inhibitor or calcium channel blocker vs diuretic: The Antihypertensive and Lipid-Lowering Treatment to Prevent Heart Attack Trial (ALLHAT–LLT).). JAMA 2002; 288:2981–2997.

51 Wenzel RR. Renal protection in hypertensive patients: selection of antihypertensive therapy. Drugs 2005;65(Suppl 2):29–39.

52 Sharma AM, Hollander A, Koster J. Efficacy and Safety in Patients with Renal Impairment; treated with Telmisartan (ESPRIT) Study Group. Telmisartan in patients with mild/moderate hypertension and chronic kidney disease. Clin Nephrol 2005;63(4): 250–257.

53 Brenner BM, Cooper ME, de Zeeuw D *et al.* Effects of losartan on renal and cardiovascular outcomes in patients with type 2 diabetes and nephropathy. N Engl J Med 2001;345:861–869.

54 Lewis EJ, Hunsicker LG, Clarke WR *et al.* Renoprotective effect of the angiotensin-receptor antagonist irbesartan in patients with nephropathy due to type 2 diabetes. N Engl J Med 2001;345:851–860.

55 Sasso FC, Carbonara O, Persico M *et al.* Irbesartan reduces the albumin excretion rate in microalbuminuric type 2 diabetic patients independently of hypertension: a randomized double–blind placebo–controlled crossover study. Diabetes Care 2002 Nov;25(11):1909–1913.

56 Dahlof B, Devereux RB, Kjeldsen SE *et al.* Cardiovascular morbidity and mortality in the Losartan Intervention For Endpoint Reduction in Hypertension Sudy (LIFE): A randomised trial against atenolol. Lancet 2002;359:995–1003.

57 PROGRESS Collaborative Group. Randomised trial of a perindopril–based blood–pressure–lowering regimen among 6,105 individuals with previous stroke or transient ischaemic attack. Lancet 2001;358:1033–1041.

58 Dahlof B, Sever PS, Poulter NR *et al.* ASCOT Investigators. Prevention of cardiovascular events with an antihypertensive regimen of amlodipine adding perindopril as required vs. atenolol adding bendroflumethiazide as required, in the Anglo– Scandinavian Cardiac Outcomes Trial–Blood Pressure Lowering Arm (ASCOT–BPLA): a multicentre randomised controlled trial. Lancet 2005 Sep 10–16;366(9489):895–906.

59 Adams HP, Jr., Adams RJ, Brott T *et al.* Guidelines for the early management of patients with ischemic stroke: A scientific statement from the Stroke Council of the American Stroke Association. Stroke 2003;34:1056–1083.

60 Liebson PR, Grandits GA, Dianzumba S *et al.* Comparison of five antihypertensive monotherapies and placebo for change in left ventricular mass in patients receiving nutritional–hygienic therapy in the Treatment of Mild Hypertension Study (TOMHS). Circulation 1995;91:698–706.

61 Gottdiener JS, Reda DJ, Massie BM, Materson BJ, Williams DW, Anderson RJ. Effect of single–drug therapy on reduction of left ventricular mass in mild to moderate hypertension: Comparison of six antihypertensive agents. The Department of Veterans Affairs Cooperative Study Group on Antihypertensive Agents. Circulation 1997;95: 2007–2014 .

62 Schmieder RE, Schlaich MP, Klingbeil AU, Martus P. Update on reversal of left ventricular hypertrophy in essential hypertension (a meta-analysis of all randomized double-blind studies until December 1996). Nephrol Dial Transplant 1998;13:564–569.

63 Masaki KH, Schatz IJ, Burchfiel CM *et al.* Orthostatic hypotension predicts mortality in elderly men: The Honolulu Heart Program. *Circulation* 1998;98:2290–2295.

64 Norman M. Kaplan. Resistant hypertension J Hypertens 2005; 23:1441–1444.

65 Douglas JG. Clinical guidelines for the treatment of hypertension in African Americans. Am J Cardiovasc Drugs 2005;5(1):1–6.

66 Wright JT Jr, Bakris G, Greene T *et al.* Effect of blood pressure lowering and antihypertensive drug class on progression of hypertensive kidney disease: Results from the AASK trial. JAMA 2002;288:2421–2431.

67 Holman R, Turner R, Stratton I *et al.* Effects of ramipril on cardiovascular and microvascular outcomes in people with diabetes mellitus: results of the HOPE study and MICRO–HOPE substudy: Heart Outcomes Prevention Evaluation Study Investigators. Lancet 2000;355:253–259.

68 Weber MA, Julius S, Kjeldsen S *et al.* Blood pressure dependent and independent effects of antihypertensive treatment on clinical events in the VALUE Trial. Lancet 2004;363: 2049–2051.

69 Pepine C, Handberg E, Cooper-DeHoff R *et al.* for the INVEST Investigators. A calcium antagonist vs a noncalcium antagonist hypertension treatment strategy for patients with coronary artery disease. The International Verapamil–Trandolapril Study (INVEST): A Randomized Controlled Trial. JAMA 2003;290:2805–2816.

70 Grundy SM, Cleeman JI, Merz CNB *et al.* Implications of recent clinical trials for the National Cholesterol Education Program Adult Treatment Panel III guidelines. Circ 2004;110:227–239.

71 Heart Protection Study Collaborative Group. MRC/BHF Heart Protection Study of cholesterol lowering with simvastatin in 20,536 high–risk individuals: a randomised placebo-controlled trial. Lancet 2002;360(9326):7–22.

72 Shepherd J, Blauw GJ, Murphy MB *et al.* PROSPER study group. Pravastatin in elderly individuals at risk of vascular disease (PROSPER): a randomised controlled trial. PROspective Study of Pravastatin in the Elderly at Risk. Lancet 2002;360:1623–1630.

73 Sever PS, Dahlof B, Poulter NR, Wedel H, Beevers G, Caulfield M, Collins R, Kjeldsen SE, Kristinsson A, McInnes GT, et al; ASCOT investigators. Prevention of coronary and stroke events with atorvastatin in hypertensive patients who have average or lower-than-average cholesterol concentrations, in the Anglo-Scandinavian Cardiac Outcomes Trial–Lipid Lowering Arm (ASCOT–LLA): a multicentre randomised controlled trial. Lancet 2003;361:1149–1158.

74 Cannon CP, Braunwald E, McCabe CH *et al.* Pravastatin or Atorvastatin Evaluation and Infection Therapy–Thrombolysis in Myocardial Infarction 22 Investigators. Intensive vs. moderate lipid lowering with statins after acute coronary syndromes. N Engl J Med 2004;350:1495–1504.

74b ALLHAT Officers and Coordinators for the ALLHAT Collaborative Research Group. Major outcomes in moderately hypercholesterolemic, hypertensive patients randomized to pravastatin vs. usual care: the Antihypertensive and Lipid-Lowering Treatment to Prevent Heart Attack Trial (ALLHATLLT). JAMA 2002;288:2998–3007.

75 Shepherd J, Cobbe SM, Ford I *et al.* Prevention of coronary heart disease with pravastatin in men with hypercholesterolemia. N Engl J Med 1995;333:1302–1307.

76 Downs JR, Clearfield M, Weis S *et al.* Primary prevention of acute coronary events with lovastatin in men and women with average cholesterol levels: results of AFCAPS/TexCAPS. JAMA 1998;279:1615–1622.

77 Nissen SE; Nicholls SJ; Sipahi I *et al.*; for the ASTEROID Investigators. Effect of Very High-Intensity Statin Therapy on Regression of Coronary Atherosclerosis: The ASTEROID Trial. JAMA 2006 Apr 5;295(13):1583–1584.

78 Scandinavian Simvastatin Survival Study Group. Randomised trial of cholesterol lowering in 4444 patients with coronary heart disease: the Scandinavian Simvastatin Survival Study (4S). Lancet 1994;344:1383–1389.

79 Sacks FM, Pfeffer MA, Moye LA *et al.* The effect of paravastatin on coronary events after myocardial infarction in patients with average cholesterol levels. N Engl J Med 1996;335:1001–1009.

79a Christopher P Cannon, Benjamin A *et al.* Meta-Analysis of Cardiovascular Outcomes Trials Comparing Intensive Versus Moderate Statin Therapy. J. Am. Coll. Cardiol. 2006;48:438–445.

80 Ballantyne CM, Houri J, Notarbartolo A *et al.*, for the Ezetimibe Study Group. Effect of ezetimibe coadministered with atorvastatin in 628 patients with primary hypercholesterolemia: a prospective, randomized, double–blind trial. Circulation 2003;107; 2409–2415.

80a Baigent C, Keech A, Kearney PM, Blackwell L, Buck G *et al.* Efficacy and safety of cholesterol-lowering treatment: prospective meta-analysis of data from 90,056 participants in 14 randomised trials of statins. Lancet 2005;366:1267–1278.

81 Davidson MH, McGarry T, Bettis R *et al.* Ezetimibe coadministered with simvastatin in patients with primary hypercholesterolemia. J Am Coll Cardiol 2002;40:2125–2134.

82 Feldman T, Koren M, Insull W Jr *et al.* Treatment of high–risk patients with ezetimibe plus simvastatin co–administration vs. simvastatin alone to attain National Cholesterol Education Program Adult Treatment Panel III low–density lipoprotein cholesterol goals. Am J Cardiol 2004;93:1481–1486.

83 Ballantyne CM, Abate N, Yuan Z *et al.* Dose-Comparison Study of the Combination of Ezetimibe and Simvastatin (Vytorin) vs. Atorvastatin in Patients With hypercholesterolemia: The Vytorin vs. Atorvastatin (VYVA) Study. Am Heart J 2005;149(3):464–473.

84 Brown BG, Zhao XQ, Chait A *et al.* Simvastatin and niacin, antioxidant vitamins, or the combination for the prevention of coronary disease. N Engl J Med 2001;345: 1583–1592.

85 Bays HE, Dujovne CA, McGovern ME *et al.*; ADvicor vs. Other Cholesterol-Modulating Agents Trial Evaluation. Comparison of once-daily, niacin extended-release/lovastatin with standard doses of atorvastatin and simvastatin (the ADvicor vs. Other Cholesterol-Modulating Agents Trial Evaluation [ADVOCATE]). Am J Cardiol. 2003;91:667–672.

86 Prueksaritanont T, Tang C, Qiu Y, Mu L, Subramanian R, Lin JH. Effects of fibrates on metabolism of statins in human hepatocytes. Drug Metab Dispos 2002;30:1280–1287.

87 Fast Facts – Hyperlipidaemia. Eds Durrington P, Sniderman A. Health Press Ltd, Oxford, Second Edition, 2002. 34–47.

88 Coughlan BJ, Sorrentino MJ. Does hypertriglyceridemia increase risk for CAD? PostGraduate Medicine 2000;108:77–84.

89 U.S. Department of Agriculture and U.S. Department of Health and Human Services. Nutrition and your health: dietary guidelines for Americans, 5th edition. Home and arden Bulletin no. 232. Washington, D.C.: U.S. Department of Agriculture, 2000.

90 Rubins HB, Robins SJ, Collins D *et al.* Gemfibrozil for the secondary prevention of coronary heart disease in men with low levels of high–density lipoprotein cholesterol. Veterans Affairs High–Density Lipoprotein Cholesterol Intervention Trial Study Group. N Engl J Med 1999;341:410–418.

91 Canner PL, Berge KG, Wenger NK *et al.* Fifteen year mortality in Coronary Drug Project patients: Long–term benefit with niacin. J Am Coll Cardiol 1986;8:1245–1255.

92 Clark RW, Sutfin TA, Ruggeri RB *et al.* Raising high-density lipoprotein in humans through inhibition of cholesteryl ester transfer protein: An initial multidose study of Torcetrapib. Arterioscler Thromb Vasc Biol 2004;24:1–9.

93 Barter PJ, Kastelein .J JP Targeting Cholesteryl Ester Transfer Protein for the Prevention and Management of Cardiovascular Disease J Am Coll Cardiol, 2006; 47:492–499.

94 Goldberg RB, Mellies MJ, Sacks FM et al., for the CARE Investigators. Cardiovascular events and their eduction with pravastatin in diabetic and glucose-intolerant myocardial infarction survivors with average cholesterol levels: subgroup analyses in the Cholesterol and RecurrentEvents (CARE) trial. Circulation 1998;98:2513–2519.

95 Keech A, Colquhoun D, Best J *et al.* LIPID Study Group. Secondary prevention of cardiovascular events with long–term pravastatin in patients with diabetes or impaired fasting glucose: results from the LIPID trial. Diabetes Care 2003; 26:2713–2721.

96 LaRosa JC, Grundy SM, Waters DD *et al.* Treating to New Targets (TNT) Investigators. Intensive lipid lowering with atorvastatin in patients with stable coronary disease. *N Engl J Med* 2005;352:1425–1435.

97 Keech A, Simes RJ, Barter P *et al.* FIELD study investigators.The FIELD study investigators. Effects of long–term fenofibrate therapy on cardiovascular events in 9795 people with type 2 diabetes mellitus (the FIELD study): randomised controlled trial. Lancet 2005;366(9500):1849–1861.

98 Kelly JJ, Lawson JA, Campbell LV, Storlien LH, Jenkins AB, Whitworth JA, O'Sullivan AJ. Effects of nicotinic acid on insulin sensitivity and blood pressure in healthy subjects. *J Hum Hypertens* 2000;14:567–572.

99 Vasudevan A, Hamirani Y, Jones P. Safety of statin: Effects on the Muscle and liver. CCJM 2005;72:990–1000.

100 Martinez E, Tuset M, Milinkovic A, Miro JM, Gatell JM. Management of dyslipidaemia in HIV–infected patients receiving antiretroviral therapy. Antivir Ther 2004 Oct;9(5): 649–663. Review.

101 Calza L, Colangeli V, Manfredi R, Legnani G, Tampellini L, Pocaterra D, Chiodo F. Rosuvastatin for the treatment of hyperlipidaemia in HIV-infected patients receiving protease inhibitors: a pilot study. AIDS. 2005 Jul 1;19(10):1103–1105.

102 Dekker JM, Girman C, Rhodes T *et al.* Metabolic syndrome and 10-year cardiovascular disease risk in the Hoorn Study Circulation 2005;112:666–673.

103 Schmidt MI, Duncan BB, Bang H *et al.* The Atherosclerosis Risk in Communities Investigators Identifying individuals at high risk for diabetes The Atherosclerosis Risk in Communities study. Diabetes Care 2005;28:2013–2018.

104 Grundy SM, Cleeman JI, Daniels SR *et al.* Diagnosis and management of the metabolic syndrome. An American Heart Association/National Heart, Lung, and Blood Institute Scientific Statement. Circulation 2005;112:2735–2752.

105   Grundy SM. Metabolic Syndrome Scientific Statement by the American Heart Association and the National Heart, Lung, and Blood Institute. Arterioscler Thromb Vasc Biol 2005;25:2243–2244.

106   Scott M. Grundy. Metabolic Syndrome: Connecting and Reconciling Cardiovascular and Diabetes Worlds. J Am Coll Cardiol, 2006; 47:1093–1100.

107   Ford ES, Giles WH, Dietz WH. Prevalence of the metabolic syndrome among US adults: findings from the third National Health and Nutrition Examination Survey. JAMA 2002;287(3):356–359.

108   Huy V Tran, M.T. Truong, Thach Nguyen. Prevalence of metabolic syndrome in adults in Khanh Hoa, Viet Nam. J Geriatr Cardiol 2004;1(2):9–100.

109   Park YW, Zhu S, Palaniappan L, Heshka S, Carnethon MR, Heymsfield SB. The metabolic syndrome prevalence and associated risk factor findings in the US population from the Third National Health and Nutrition Examination Survey, 1988–1994. Arch Intern Med 2003;163:427–436.

110   Tuomilehto J, Lindstrom J, Eriksson JG, et al. Finnish Diabetes Prevention Study Group. Prevention of Type 2 Diabetes Mellitus by Changes in Lifestyle among Subjects with Impaired Glucose Tolerance. N Engl J Med 2001;344:1343–1350.

111   Després JP, Golay A, Sjostrom L et al. Effects of rimonabant on metabolic risk factors in overweight patients with dyslipidemia. N Engl J Med 2005;353:2121–2134.

112   Wadden TA, Berkowitz RI, Womble LG et al. Randomized trial of lifestyle modification and pharmacotherapy for obesity. N Engl J Med 2005;353:2111–2120.

113   Fagerberg B, Edwards S, Halmos T et al. Tesaglitazar, a novel dual peroxisome proliferator-activated receptor alpha/gamma agonist, dose-dependently improves the metabolic abnormalities associated with insulin resistance in a non-diabetic population Diabetologia 2005;48:1716–1725.

114   Batsis JA. Effects of bariatric surgery on cardiovascular risk factors and predicted effect on CV events and mortality of class II/III obesity. Abstract #842–848. Presented at the American College of Cardiology Scientific Session 2006. March 11–14 Atlanta.

114b Kriska AM, Edelstein SL, Hamman RF, Otto A et al. Physical activity in individuals at risk for diabetes: Diabetes Prevention Program. Med Sci Sports Exerc. 2006 May;38(5): 826–32.

115   Tuomilehto J, Lindstrom J, Eriksson JG et al. Prevention of type 2 diabetes mellitus by changes in lifestyle among subjects with impaired glucose tolerance. N Engl J Med 2001;344:1343–1350.

116   Chiasson JL, Josse RG, Gomis R et al. Acarbose for prevention of type 2 diabetes mellitus: the STOP–NIDDM randomised trial. Lancet 2002;359:2072–2077).

117   Chiasson JL, Brindisi MC, Rabasa-Lhoret R. The prevention of type 2 diabetes: what is the evidence? Minerva Endocrinol 2005 Sep;30(3):179–91. Review.

118   Torgerson JS, Hauptman J, Boldrin MN, Sjostrom L. XENical in the prevention of diabetes in obese subjects (XENDOS) study: a randomized study of orlistat as an adjunct to lifestyle changes for the prevention of type 2 diabetes in obese patients. Diabetes Care. 2004 Jan;27(1):155–61. Erratum in: Diabetes Care 2004 Mar;27(3):856.

119   Gaede P, Vedel P, Larsen N, Jensen GV, Parving HH, Pedersen O. Multifactorial intervention and cardiovascular disease in patients with type 2 diabetes. N Engl J Med. 2003;348:383–393.

120   Hansson L, Hedner T, Lund-Johansen P et al. Randomised trial of effects of calcium antagonists compared with diuretics and beta–blockers on cardiovascular morbidity and mortality in hypertension: the Nordic Diltiazem (NORDIL) study. Lancet 2000;356:359–365.

121 Parving HH, Lehnert H, Brochner–Mortensen J, Gomis R, Andersen S, Arner P, for the Irbesartan in Patients with Type 2 Diabetes and Microalbuminuria Study Group. The effect of irbesartan on the development of diabetic nephropathy in patients with type 2 diabetes. N Engl J Med 2001;345:870–878.

122 Bakris GL, Fonseca V, Katholi RE et al. for the GEMINI Investigators Differential Effects of β–Blockers on Albuminuria in Patients With Type 2 Diabetes. Hypertension 2005;46: 1309–1315.

123 Tatti P, Pahor M, Byington RP, Di Mauro P, Guarisco R, Strollo G, Strollo F. Outcome results of the Fosinopril vs. Amlodipine Cardiovascular Events Randomized Trial (FACET) in patients with hypertension and NIDDM. Diabetes Care 1998;21:597–603.

124 Ohkubo Y, Kishikawa H, Araki E, Miyata T, Isami S, Motoyoshi S, Kojima Y, Furuyoshi N, Shichiri M. Intensive insulin therapy prevents the progression of diabetic microvascular complications in Japanese patients with non-insulin–dependent diabetes mellitus: a randomized prospective 6-year study. Diabetes Res Clin Pract 1995;28:103–117.

125 Abuissa H, Jones PG,. Marso SP, et al. Angiotensin-Converting Enzyme Inhibitors or Angiotensin Receptor Blockers for Prevention of Type 2 Diabetes A Meta-Analysis of Randomized Clinical Trials J Am Coll Cardiol 2005; 46:821–826.

126 Eddy AA. Interstitial nephritis induced by protein-overload proteinuria. Am J Pathol 135:719–733,1998.

127 Remuzzi G, Macia M, Ruggenenti P. Prevention and Treatment of Diabetic Renal Disease in Type 2 Diabetes: The BENEDICT Study. J Am Soc Nephrol 2006;17:S90–S97.

128 AHA/ACC Science Advisory. Matthew MD: Kathryn Taubert et al. influenza Vaccination as Secondary Prevention for Cardiovascular Disease. Circulation. 2006;114: 1549–1553.)

129 Smith JC Jr, Allen J, Blair SN et al; AHA/ACC; NHLBI. AHA/ACC guidelines for secondary prevention for patients with coronary and other atherosclerotic vascular disease: 2006 update. Circulation 2006;113:2363–2372.

130 Gurfinkel EP, Leon de la Fuente R, Mendiz O, Mautner B. Flu vaccination in acute coronary syndromes and planned percutaneous coronary interventions (FLUVACS) Study, Eur Heart J. 2004;25:25–31.

131 Gurfinkel EP, de la Fuente RL. Two-year follow-up of the FLU Vaccination Acute Coronary Syndromes (FLUVACS) Registry. Tex Heart Inst J. 2004;31:28–32.

CHAPTER 7

Pulmonary Hypertension

Michael D. McGoon

Introduction

Pulmonary hypertension (PH) is a hemodynamic term which refers to pulmonary arterial pressure exceeding the normal range. Among otherwise normal individuals, the average mean pulmonary artery pressure (mPAP) is 15 mmHg. However, clinically significant PH is generally accepted as an mPAP greater than 25 mmHg at rest, with a pulmonary vascular resistance greater than 3 Wood units [1]. Pulmonary arterial hypertension (PAH) is a clinical term referring to a constellation of disorders which exhibit PH, and which, though different in many ways, have certain characteristics in common including key pulmonary vascular pathologic features, pathobiologic mechanisms, and responses to pharmacologic intervention.

Definition of Pulmonary Arterial Hypertension

The definition of PAH was refined at the Third World Symposium on Pulmonary Arterial Hypertension in 2003. PAH is synonymous with the Group 1 category shown in Table 7.1. This chapter will focus specifically on the diagnosis, treatment and management problems of patients with PAH.

Table 7.1 Third World Symposium classification of Pulmonary Hypertension [1].

1. **Pulmonary arterial hypertension**
   1.1 Idiopathic (IPAH)
   1.2 Familial (FPAH)
   1.3 Associated with (APAH)
      1.3.1 Collagen vascular disease
      1.3.2 Congenital systemic-to-pulmonary shunts
      1.3.3 Portal hypertension
      1.3.4 HIV infection
      1.3.5 Drugs and toxins
      1.3.6 Other (thyroid disorders, glycogen storage disease, Gaucher's disease, hereditary hemorrhagic telangiectasia, hemoglobinopathies, chronic myeloproliferative disorders, splenectomy)
   1.4 Associated with significant venous or capillary involvement
      1.4.1 Pulmonary veno-occlusive disease (PVOD)
      1.4.2 Pulmonary capillary hemangiomatosis (PCH)
   1.5 Persistent pulmonary hypertension of the newborn
2. **Pulmonary hypertension with left heart disease**
   2.1 Left-sided atrial or ventricular heart disease
   2.2 Left-sided valvular heart disease
3. **Pulmonary hypertension associated with lung diseases and/or hypoxemia**
   3.1 Chronic obstructive pulmonary disease
   3.2 Interstitial lung disease
   3.3 Sleep-disordered breathing
   3.4 Alveolar hypoventilation disorders
   3.5 Chronic exposure to high altitude
   3.6 Developmental abnormalities
4. **Pulmonary hypertension due to chronic thrombotic and/or embolic disease (CTEPH)**
   4.1 Thromboembolic obstruction of proximal pulmonary arteries
   4.2 Thromboembolic obstruction of distal pulmonary arteries
   4.3 Non-thrombotic pulmonary embolism (tumor, parasites, foreign material)
5. **Miscellaneous**
   Sarcoidosis, histiocytosis X, lymphangiomatosis, compression of pulmonary vessels (adenopathy, tumor, fibrosing mediastinitis)

Pathophysiology of Pulmonary Arterial Hypertension

The occurrence of PAH can often be traced to one predominant predisposing factor, such as a left-to-right intracardiac shunt caused by a congenital cardiac defect. In most cases, "risk" factors do not inevitably lead to clinical PAH; the presence of a second triggering factor is thought to be required [1]. The presence of two (or more) initiating components, such as a genetic substrate and an environmental condition, may precipitate vascular constriction, cellular proliferation and a prothrombotic state which set the stage for the development of PAH. Recognition of underlying permissive and provocative factors, and the cellular and molecular mechanisms of disease that ensue, has permitted insights into preventive, early detection and aggressive treatment strategies.

Genetics of Pulmonary Arterial Hypertension

Although PAH has been recognized to be a heritable condition based on family studies and the observation that 6% of patients in a national registry had first degree relatives with PAH [1], the genetic basis for at least some familial transmission was first recognized in 2000, when mutations of the gene on chromosome 2 encoding for bone morphogenetic protein receptor type-2 (BMPR2) were found to be associated with familial PAH (FPAH) [1]. BMPR2 is part of the receptor on the vascular smooth muscle cell membrane which is one of the superfamily of transforming growth factor-β (TGFβ) receptors. A mutation in the BMPR2 receptor protein results in interrupted signal transduction in the pulmonary vascular smooth muscle cell which appears to reduce the process of apoptosis and consequently promotes cellular proliferation. Up to 65% of families with FPAH have exonic or intronic mutations in BMPR2 which are transmitted in an autosomal dominant fashion, and approximately 10% of apparently sporadic cases of idiopathic PAH (IPAH) have isolated exonic mutations [2]. Whether these latter cases represent a spontaneous new mutation or occur in families without a phenotypic presentation of PAH remains unclear. The penetrance of the mutation is low (only 20%, but variable between families) [2], meaning that only one in five people with BMPR2 mutation exhibit features of PAH.

Activin-like kinase type-1 (ALK-1) is another TGFβ receptor, encoded by a gene on chromosome 12, which is located on endothelial cells. Mutations in this receptor have been identified in some families with hereditary hemorrhagic telangiectasia (HHT) and PAH [2]. Although ALK-1 mutations are most commonly associated with HHT and PAH, mutations in another TGF receptor gene (on chromosome 9), endoglin, have also been identified in some patients [2].

5-hydroxytryptamine (serotonin) transporter (5-HTT) activity is associated with pulmonary artery smooth muscle cell proliferation. The L-allelic variant of the 5-HTT gene promoter, which is associated with increased expression of 5-HTT [2], is present in homozygous form in 65% of patients with IPAH compared to 27% of controls [2].

The observation of genetic mutations and polymorphisms which may identify a population at risk of developing PAH raises the possibility of early or preventive management in these patients.

Molecular and Cellular Mechanisms of Pulmonary Arterial Hypertension

Regardless of underlying cause or associations, several inter-related mechanisms play a role in the development and maintenance of PAH. These mechanisms are mediated by one or more molecular and cellular processes, including reduced prostacyclin availability due to diminished endothelial cell prostacyclin synthase activity, elevated endothelin levels resulting from enhanced production and reduced pulmonary clearance, decreased nitric oxide synthase expression, elevated plasma and low platelet 5-HTT levels, down-regulation of voltage dependent potassium (Kv1.5) channels of pulmonary vascular smooth muscle cells, activity of autoantibodies and pro-inflammatory cytokines, and prothrombotic states arising from endothelial, coagulation and fibrinolytic cascade and platelet dysfunction [2].

The result of these abnormalities gives rise to a predisposition of vasoconstriction over vasodilation of the pulmonary vasculature, to excess cellular proliferation which outpaces apoptosis and to a thrombotic diathesis. The occurrence of dynamic increase of pulmonary vascular resistance appears to be an early substrate of PAH, with intimal hyperplasia due to endothelial cell proliferation, medial thickening due to vascular smooth muscle cell proliferation, development of plexiform lesions caused by disordered endothelial proliferation, and thrombosis *in situ* becoming more prominent during the clinically apparent stages of the disease.

Appreciation of the underlying mechanisms of disease points to the means by which pharmacologic treatment can be utilized to counteract their consequences.

Diagnosis

The management of patients with PAH consists of first identifying the presence of PH and then defining the precise clinical context of the abnormal hemodynamic state, including the severity of problem, the associated or causal conditions, the functional implications, and the prognosis. This information is required in order to design the optimal therapeutic approach. The basic diagnostic strategy, therefore, is to screen for PH in symptomatic or high-risk patients, then to systematically examine potential underlying conditions with appropriate tests, delineate predictive factors, perform functional assessment, and to confirm the hemodynamic profile by invasive testing. Symptoms which require consideration of PH are shown in Table 7.2. Findings on physical examination which are important for detecting PH and guiding further evaluation are shown in Table 7.3. The algorithm for complete assessment is depicted in Figure 7.1.

Table 7.2 Symptoms requiring consideration of pulmonary hypertension in the differential diagnosis (from [3]).

Symptom	Cause

Dyspnea	Decreased oxygen transport
	  Hypoxemia
	  Low cardiac output
	Low DLCO
	Low mixed venous oxygen saturation
	Increased work of breathing

Angina	Increased myocardial oxygen demand
	  Elevated right ventricular wall stress (volume, pressure)
	Inadequate oxygen delivery
	  Reduced aorta-to-right-ventricular systolic gradient
	Left main coronary artery compression

Syncope	Hemodynamic
	  Systemic vasodilation (exertion, orthostatic, vasodepressor) and low fixed cardiac output due to high pulmonary resistance
	Arrhythmic
	  "Benign" arrhythmias (atrial fibrillation) result in loss of atrial contribution to cardiac output
	Malignant arrhythmias provoked by wall stretch, ischemia

Edema	Right ventricular failure Tricuspid regurgitation Sedentary lifestyle Chronic deep venous insufficiency

DLCO, Carbon Monoxide Diffusing Capacity

Table 7.3 Physical findings pertinent to pulmonary hypertension and their significance (from [4]).

Sign	Implication
Physical signs that indicate PH	
Accentuated pulmonary component of S2 (audible at apex in over 90%)	High pulmonary pressure increases force of pulmonary valve closure
Early systolic click	Sudden interruption of opening of pulmonary valve into high-pressure artery
Midsystolic ejection murmur	Turbulent transvalvular pulmonary outflow
Left parasternal lift	High right ventricular pressure and hypertrophy present
Right ventricular S4 (in 38%)	High right ventricular pressure and hypertrophy present
Increased jugular "a" wave	High right ventricular filling pressure

(Continued)

Table 7.3 *(Continued)*

Sign	Implication
Physical signs that indicate severity of PH	
Moderate to severe PH	
Holosystolic murmur that increases with inspiration Increased jugular v waves	Tricuspid regurgitation
Pulsatile liver	
Diastolic murmur	Pulmonary regurgitation
Hepatojugular reflux	High central venous pressure
Advanced pulmonary hypertension with right ventricular failure	
Right ventricular S3 (in 23%)	Right ventricular dysfunction
Marked distention of jugular veins	Right ventricular dysfunction or tricuspid regurgitation or both
Hepatomegaly	Right ventricular dysfunction or tricuspid regurgitation or both
Peripheral edema (in 32%)	
Ascites	
Low blood pressure, diminished pulse pressure, cool extremities	Reduced cardiac output, peripheral vasoconstriction
Physical signs that detect possible underlying cause or associations of PH	
Central cyanosis	Hypoxemia, right-to-left shunt
Clubbing	Congenital heart disease, pulmonary venopathy
Cardiac auscultatory findings, including systolic murmurs, diastolic murmurs, opening snap, and gallop	Congenital or acquired heart or valvular disease
Rales, dullness, or decreased breath sounds	Pulmonary congestion or effusion or both
Fine rales, accessory muscle use, wheezing, protracted expiration, productive cough	Pulmonary parenchymal disease
Obesity, kyphoscoliosis, enlarged tonsils	Possible substrate for disordered ventilation
Sclerodactyly, arthritis, rash	Connective tissue disorder
Peripheral venous insufficiency or obstruction	Possible venous thrombosis

PH, pulmonary hypertension.

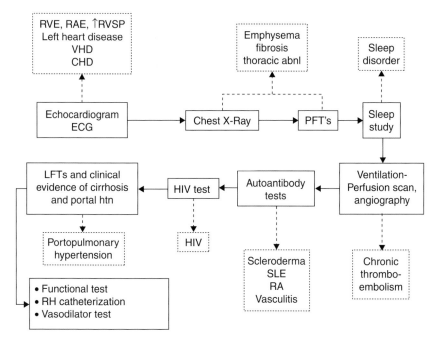

Figure 7.1 The basic diagnostic strategy for PH consists of utilizing appropriate procedures to diagnose or exclude associated underlying diseases (from [3]).

CLINICAL PEARLS

Clinical clues for diagnosis – Dyspnea, chest pain, edema and syncope are non-specific symptoms. If any are present in young or middle-aged females, however, the possibility of PAH should be *high* on the differential diagnosis – and definitely above alternative diagnoses such as deconditioning or anxiety. Further screening with Doppler-echocardiography is warranted in these patients, even if physical examination is apparently unremarkable.

Goals of Treatment

Although no current treatment of PAH can be considered curative, realistic goals of treatment are to reduce pulmonary vascular resistance and pressure, diminish symptoms and promote activity tolerance, and prolong longevity.

Available Treatment

Prior to 1996, treatment of most patients with PAH could be at best considered supportive. Supportive or adjunctive strategies remain relevant even now, when more targeted vascular treatment modalities are available. These strategies are intended to alleviate the consequences of the pulmonary hypertensive state, such as right ventricular failure with volume overload and hypoxemia.

Adjunctive Treatment

Hypoxemia results from a constellation of factors including low diffusing capacity; right-to-left shunting due to congenital heart disease (CHD), patent foramen ovale, ventilation–perfusion mismatching or frank intrapulmonary shunting; and low cardiac output resulting in low mixed venous oxygen saturation. Although supplemental oxygen administration may not totally correct low arterial oxygen saturation in all patients, it can produce sufficient improvement in many to yield a substantial functional benefit, and therefore should not be overlooked. Moreover, oxygen is a pulmonary vasodilator and may contribute to reduce pulmonary vascular resistance, though this has not been shown to be of definite long-term benefit.

Mortality related to PAH is frequently due to right ventricular failure or arrhythmias presumably related to high right ventricular wall stress. Once right ventricular failure intervenes, aggressive management is required. Sodium restriction is mandatory. Loop diuretics, supplemented by metolazone, and potassium-sparing agents are necessary in many patients but must be used judiciously in order to balance reduced intravascular volume and control of edema and ascites with adequate preload to maintain systemic arterial pressure and cardiac output. Inotropic support with digoxin, though not systematically evaluated in PAH and not recommended by all authorities, is reasonable to consider. Advanced right ventricular decompensation may require in-patient management with intravenous inotropic support using dopamine or milrinone.

Some adjunctive measures can be considered preventive or precautionary in nature. Pregnancy poses extremely high risks for the patient and fetus and should be prevented at all costs, including consideration of sterilization or dual-contraceptive measures. Oral contraceptives reportedly may provoke a prothrombotic state, but have not been unequivocally demonstrated to exacerbate the risks of thrombosis in patients with PAH, particularly when anticoagulation is used. Travel to high altitudes or air travel should be avoided for hypoxemic patients, at least unless there is near normalization of arterial oxygen saturation with supplemental oxygen. Air travel with oxygen often requires prior arrangements with the airline. While activity is encouraged to maintain fitness, attempting aggressive exercise or weight-resistance activities is inadvisable. Avoidance of pulmonary infections by influenza and pneumococcal vaccinations should be undertaken. Early antibiotic treatment of upper respiratory infections is warranted. Vasoconstrictive medications (decongestants) should be avoided.

Warfarin

Warfarin has been recommended and widely used in patients with PAH. The rationale is multifactorial: PAH patients have a prothrombotic profile, as noted above; histopathologic examination of post-mortem lungs and lungs explanted during transplantation has disclosed a high prevalence of thrombosis *in situ*; and two retrospective studies suggest a survival benefit for anticoagulated patients (Figure 7.2) [5]. An international normalized ratio (INR) of 2.0–2.5 is

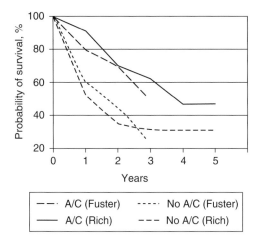

Figure 7.2 Probability of survival of patients on anticoagulation with warfarin (A/C) compared to those not treated with warfarin (No A/C) in two studies (Adapted from [6]).

the goal in patients with IPAH or associated PAH unless there is a bleeding risk or other contraindications.

Calcium Channel Blockers

Before the availability of the current armamentarium of therapeutic agents, numerous vasodilator agents were tried as treatment for pulmonary hypertensive conditions. Although anecdotal reports supported medications such as phentolamine, hydralazine, nitrates, prasozin and angiotensin-converting enzyme inhibitors, systematic scrutiny and widespread use revealed that the success rate was extremely low and compromised by adverse effects, especially systemic hypotension and reduced cardiac output. An exception was the use of calcium channel blockers, particularly nifedipine or diltiazem at high doses. An early report indicated that among patients who exhibited the ability to vasodilate in response to short-acting agents such as adenosine, the use of calcium channel blockers provided a substantial survival benefit (Figure 7.3) [7]. Unfortunately, only about 26% of patients (17 out of 64) exhibited a vasodilator response. Subsequently, acute vasodilator testing at the time of right heart catheterization has been performed to identify patients who might be adequately treated with calcium channel blockers alone (Table 7.4). However, a retrospective analysis has been recently reported of 557 IPAH patients in whom only 12.8% displayed vasoreactivity using a criteria of a >20% decrease in both mPAP and pulmonary vascular resistance [7]; of these only about half (6.8%) benefited from treatment with long-term calcium channel blockers. Those who benefited were those who tended to have a more profound acute response during invasive testing. Consequently, only patients who demonstrate a decline in mPAP of = 10 mmHg, to an mPAP = 40 mmHg while maintaining or improving cardiac output during acute testing should be treated with nifedipine, diltiazem or amlodipine. Verapamil is contraindicated because of its negatively inotropic effect.

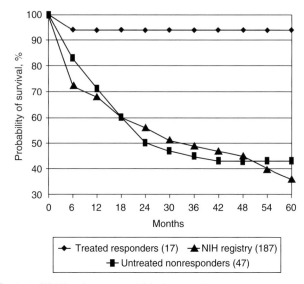

Figure 7.3 Survival of IPAH patients who exhibited a vasodilator response to adenosine and were treated with calcium channel blockers compared to untreated nonresponders and to patients in the NIH Registry (Adapted from [6]).

Table 7.4 Short-acting pulmonary vasodilators used to assess acute vasodilation during right heart catheterization (from [3]).

	Epoprostenol	Adenosine	Nitric oxide
Route of administration	Intravenous	Intravenous	Inhaled
Dose range	2–10 ng/kg/min	50–250 µg/kg/min	10–80 ppm
Dosing increments	2 ng/kg/min every 15 min	50 µg/kg/min every 2 min	10–80 ppm for 5 min
Common side effects	Headache, flushing, nausea	Chest tightness, dyspnea	None

Prostacyclin Analogues

The era of therapy targeted specifically to the correction of mechanistic aberrations underlying PAH began with FDA approval of epoprostenol sodium in 1995, and its commercial availability in 1996 for treatment of WHO III or IV patients with IPAH or PAH associated with scleroderma. The objective of treatment with epoprostenol or any of the prostacyclin analogues is to compensate for the deficiency of endogenous prostacyclin in patients with PAH. In view of its short half-life and not being absorbed through the gastrointestinal tract, epoprostenol requires continuous intravenous administration. A randomized (but open label) 12-week study of 81 IPAH patients with WHO functional class III and IV symptoms demonstrated improved six-minute walk distance (113 m compared to untreated) and pulmonary hemodynamics in treated patients, and suggested a survival benefit [7]. Subsequent clinical trials confirmed prolonged survival (with respect to historical controls in the NIH Registry) using intravenous epoprostenol [7]. Approved medical therapies for PAH are described in Table 7.5.

Table 7.5 Approved medical therapies for pulmonary arterial hypertension.

Drug class	Drug	Indications	Dosing	Main adverse effects	Major drug interactions
Calcium channel blockers	Nifedipine	PAH Positive acute vasodilator response	30–270 mg daily p.o.	Edema Palpitations Flushing Headache Hypotension	Amiodarone Atazanavir Clarithromycin Fentanyl
	Amlodipine		5–20 mg daily p.o.		Amiodarone Atazanavir Droperidol Fentanyl
	Diltiazem		180–480 mg daily p.o.	AV block Bradycardia CHF Edema Headache Hypotension	Amiodarone Aprepitant Atazanavir Cisapride (not available in US) Droperidol Erythromycin Fentanyl
Prostacyclin analogues	Epoprostenol	IPAH or PAH with sclero-derma spectrum of CTD WHO class III or IV	Begin at 2 ng/kg/min i.v. and increase by 2 ng/kg/min to target dose of 20–50 ng/kg/min after 6–12 months or until prohibitive side effects	Headache Jaw pain Flushing Skin rash Nausea Diarrhea Musculoskeletal pain Catheter infection Rebound PH if interrupted	Antihypertensives may promote hypotension when used in combination Antiplatelet agents may promote bleeding when used in combination
	Treprostinil (s.c)	PAH WHO class II, III, or IV	Begin at 1–2 ng/kg/min and increase as tolerated to target of 40–80 ng/kg/min	Injection site pain Headache Diarrhea Rash Nausea	
	Treprostinil (i.v.)	PAH WHO class II, III, IV s.c. drug not tolerated	Begin at 1–2 ng/kg/min and increase as tolerated to target of 40–80 ng/kg/min	Headache Diarrhea Rash Nausea Catheter infection	
	Iloprost	PAH WHO class III or IV	First dose 2.5 μg, then 5 μg 6–9 times daily inhaled	Cough Headache Flushing Jaw pain	
Endothelin receptor antagonist	Bosentan	PAH WHO class III or IV	62.5 mg twice daily for one month, then 125 mg twice daily p.o	Liver toxicity Headache Flushing Leg edema Anemia Teratogenicity	Cyclosporine Glyburide Ketoconazole Oral contra ceptives Tracolimus (animal studies only) Simvastatin Warfarin
Phospho-diesterase inhibitor	Sildenafil	PAH	20 mg three times daily p.o.	Headache Flushing Dyspepsia Epistaxis Abnormal vision Nasal congestion	Nitrates Atazanavir Dihydrocodeine Ritonavir

CHF, congestive heart failure; CTD, connective tissue disease; IPAH, idiopathic PAH; PAH, pulmonary arterial hypertension; PH, Pulmonary hypertension.

Evidence-based Medicine: Epoprostenol for pulmonary arterial hypertension

178 patients with PPH in New York Heart Association (NYHA) functional class III or IV were treated with epoprostenol. The 6-minute walk test (WT) and right-sided heart catheterization were performed at baseline, after three months on epoprostenol and thereafter once a year. The results showed that the overall survival rates at one, two, three, and five years were 85%, 70%, 63%, and 55%, respectively. On univariate analysis, the baseline variables associated with a poor outcome were a history of right-sided heart failure, NYHA functional class IV, 6-minute WT ≤250 m (median value), right atrial pressure ≥12 mmHg, and mean pulmonary artery pressure <65 mmHg. On multivariate analysis, including both baseline variables and those measured after three months on epoprostenol, a history of right-sided heart failure, persistence of NYHA functional class III or IV at three months, and the absence of a fall in total pulmonary resistance of >30%, relative to baseline, were associated with poor survival.

Among patients with predominantly scleroderma-associated PAH, intravenous epoprostenol significantly improved six-minute walk distance and pulmonary hemodynamics during 12 weeks of therapy, though a survival effect in this short time frame was not demonstrated [6]. Additional uncontrolled reports have indicated similarly salutary outcomes of intravenous epoprostenol in APAH related to connective tissue disease, congenital heart disease, HIV infection, and portopulmonary hypertension [8].

Administration of intravenous epoprostenol is complex, requiring that patients take an active role in their own management, including aseptic management of their indwelling central venous catheter, daily sterile preparation of the drug, use of the ambulatory infusion pump, and awareness of trouble-shooting techniques in the event of problems. Most patients experience optimal benefit at a dose of 25–40 ng/kg/min after gradual incrementation of the dose over 6–12 months following initiation at 2–6 ng/kg/min. Some patients require doses outside of this spectrum depending on level of symptomatic benefit or occurrence of adverse effects, such as flushing, rash, jaw pain, leg discomfort, loose stools or headache. Excessive dosing can produce fatigue and high output cardiac failure [8]. Additional concerns include infection of the central venous catheter, sepsis or sudden cessation of the infusion causing rebound PH and possible death.

Treprostinil

A more stable prostacyclin analogue, treprostinil has a half life of 4 hours and can be administered subcutaneously (FDA approved in 2002) or intravenously (approved in 2004). A randomized, placebo controlled study of subcutaneous treprostinil in 470 WHO class III or IV patients with IPAH, or PAH associated with connective tissue disease, or CHD demonstrated a dose-related improvement in six-minute walk distance of 16 meters in the whole treated group, and 38 meters in the quartile of patients receiving the highest dose [8]. Not all patients could be dose-increased to a high level because of pain at the infusion site in the majority, as well aside effects of headache, diarrhea, rash, and nausea.

The potential advantages of intravenous treprostinil are the absence of site pain, as well as easier preparation and administration and less rebound compared to epoprostenol. An open label study of intravenous treprostinil in 16 symptomatic PAH patients showed an 82 meter increase in six-minute walk distance after 12 weeks, and improved pulmonary hemodynamics [9]. Most patients originally treated with epoprostenol can be switched over to intravenous treprostinil with maintenance of six-minute walk distance, though at a larger dose [10]. Studies of inhaled and oral administration of treprostinil are underway.

Iloprost

The prostacyclin analogue iloprost is an inhaled aerosol approved for use in 2004. In a randomized, placebo-controlled 12 week study, iloprost produced a placebo-corrected improvement in six-minute walk distance by 36 meters in 207 patients with symptomatic IPAH, PAH associated with connective tissue disease or appetite suppressants, or PH related to inoperable chronic thromboembolic disease [11]. Long-term maintenance of beneficial effects of exercise capacity and hemodynamics have been observed [11]. Iloprost may cause side effects common to prostacyclin analogues including headache, flushing, and jaw pain, and also may cause cough.

Endothelin Receptor Antagonism

The objective of treatment with an endothelin receptor antagonist is to minimize the impact of excessive endothelin effects in the pulmonary vasculature in patients with PAH (see Table 7.5). Bosentan is a non-selective, or dual, A and B-endothelin receptor antagonist available in oral form. Placebo-controlled randomized drug trials have shown a relative improvement in six-minute walk distance ranging from 36 to 76 meters, an improvement in pulmonary hemodynamics, and a delay in clinical worsening, defined as any occurrence of death, initiation of intravenous epoprostenol, hospitalization for worsening PAH, lung transplantation, or atrial septostomy [11]. Survival of patients with IPAH treated with bosentan is prolonged compared to expected survival based on historical controls [11].

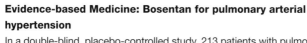

Evidence-based Medicine: Bosentan for pulmonary arterial hypertension

In a double-blind, placebo-controlled study, 213 patients with pulmonary arterial hypertension (primary or associated with connective-tissue disease) randomly assigned to receive placebo or 62.5 mg of bosentan twice daily for 4 weeks, followed by either of two doses of bosentan (125 mg or 250 mg twice daily) for a minimum of 12 weeks. The primary end point was the degree of change in exercise capacity. Secondary end points included the change in the Borg dyspnea index, the change in the WHO functional class, and the time to clinical worsening. The results showed that at week 16, patients treated with bosentan had an improved six-minute walking distance; the mean difference between the placebo group and the combined bosentan groups was 44 m (95% CI 21–67; $P < 0.001$). Bosentan also improved the Borg dyspnea index and WHO functional class and increased the time to clinical worsening.

Increases in hepatic enzymes to greater than three times the upper limit of normal have been observed in approximately 11% of patients treated with bosentan in clinical trials. Other side effects include headache, flushing, lower extremity edema, and rarely anemia. Bosentan is teratogenic. Bosentan has been approved by the FDA for treatment of WHO functional class III and IV PAH. Careful monitoring of therapy is required with liver function tests on a monthly basis, hemoglobin/hematocrit on a quarterly basis, and pregnancy test in women of child bearing potential on a monthly basis. Patients and prescribing physicians should be aware of the potential side effect of lower extremity edema, particularly within the first several weeks after initiation of therapy, and be prepared to adjust diuretics as needed. Ongoing investigational trials with bosentan include studies in patients with WHO functional class II symptoms, sickle cell disease, and chronic thrombotic and/or embolic diseases (CTEPH).

Phosphodiesterase-5 Inhibition

The rationale for treatment of PAH with phosphodiesterase-5 inhibition is to compensate for the relative deficiency of nitric oxide production, by preventing the metabolism of cyclic guanasine $3',5'$ monophosphate (cGMP) and therefore promoting the availability of this second messenger in the pathway leading to vasodilation and control of cellular proliferation. Sildenafil, which was approved for use in 2005, has been shown to improve six-minute walk distance by 45 meters compared to control when a dose of 20 mg three times daily was used in a study of patients with IPAH or PAH associated with connective tissue disease or surgically corrected congenital heart disease [12] (see Table 7.5).

Evidence-based Medicine: Phosphodiesterase-5 inhibition for pulmonary arterial hypertension

In a double-blind, placebo-controlled study, 278 patients with symptomatic PAH (either idiopathic or associated with connective-tissue disease or with repaired congenital systemic-to-pulmonary shunts) were randomized to placebo or sildenafil (20 mg, 40 mg, or 80 mg) orally three times daily for 12 weeks. The primary end point was the change from baseline to week 12 in the distance walked in six minutes. The change in mean pulmonary-artery pressure and WHO functional class and the incidence of clinical worsening were also assessed, but the study was not powered to assess mortality. Patients completing the 12-week randomized study could enter a long-term extension study. The results showed that the distance walked in six minutes increased from baseline in all sildenafil groups; the mean placebo-corrected treatment effects were 45 m (+13.0%), 46 m (+13.3%), and 50 m (+14.7%) for 20 mg, 40 mg, and 80 mg of sildenafil, respectively ($P < 0.001$ for all comparisons). All sildenafil doses reduced the mean pulmonary-artery pressure ($P = 0.04$, $P = 0.01$, and $P < 0.001$, respectively), improved the WHO functional class ($P = 0.003$, $P < 0.001$, and $P < 0.001$, respectively), and were associated with side effects such as flushing, dyspepsia, and diarrhea. The incidence of clinical worsening did not differ significantly between the patients treated with sildenafil and those treated with placebo. Among the 222 patients completing one year of treatment with sildenafil monotherapy, the improvement from baseline at one year in the distance walked in six minutes was 51 m.

Treatment Algorithm

The selection of appropriate treatment for patients with PAH is hampered by the absence of head-to-head trials of different agents among various patient categories based on severity of PH, specific type of PAH, exercise capacity, or symptomatic status. In general, most experienced investigators and clinicians agree that more advanced PAH should be treated initially with parenteral prostacyclin analogues, especially in the setting of right ventricular failure. Figure 7.4 depicts a suggested algorithm utilizing assessment of disease severity.

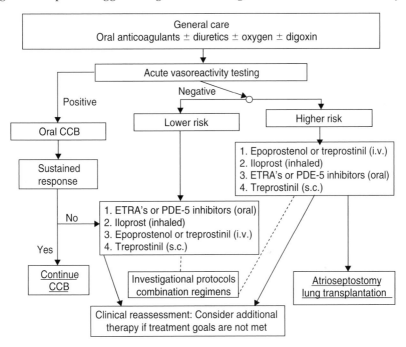

Lower	Determinants of risk	Higher
No	**Clinical evidence of RV failure**	Yes
Gradual	**Progression**	Rapid
II, III	**WHO class**	IV
Longer (>400 m)	**6 Minute walk distance**	Shorter (<300 m)
Minimally elevated	**BNP**	Very elevated
Minimal RV dysfunction	**Echocardiographic findings**	Pericardial effusion Significant RV dysfunction
Normal/Near normal RAP and CI	**Hemodynamics**	High RAP, Low CI

Figure 7.4 Suggested algorithm for determining treatment approach based on parameters of severity of disease. Acute vasoreactivity testing is conducted at the time of right heart catheterization using a short acting pulmonary vasodilator (epoprostenol or nitric oxide). A positive response is considered to be a decrease in mean pulmonary artery pressure of at least 10 mmHg to a value of less than 40 mmHg without a reduction in cardiac output (from [3]). RAP, right atrial pressure; CI, cardiac index.

Future Potential Treatment

Some experts hypothesize that the beneficial effect of endothelin receptor antagonists are predominantly mediated via the endothelin A receptor. Two endothelin receptor antagonists with more A-receptor selectivity have been studied (sitaxsentan) or are under investigation (ambrisentan). Two studies of sitaxsentan [10] in patients with IPAH or PAH associated with CHD or connective tissue disease and WHO class II–IV symptoms have shown an improvement in six-minute walk distance of 31–34 meters compared to placebo (but not in cardiopulmonary exercise test parameters) and in pulmonary hemodynamics. Adverse effects included headache, edema, nausea, nasal congestion, dizziness, potentiation of the anticoagulant effect of warfarin, and elevation of hepatic enzymes in 5% patients using a dose of 100 mg daily (and in 21% of patients on 300 mg daily).

Early investigational results of ambrisentan demonstrate improved six-minute walk distance (36 meters compared to baseline) and pulmonary hemodynamics in patients with IPAH or PAH associated with connective tissue disease, diet pill use, or HIV infection [13]. The occurrence of hepatic transaminase elevation greater than three times the upper limit of normal was 3.1%. Randomized placebo-controlled trials are underway.

Difficult Situations and Suggested Solutions

Although diagnostic and treatment algorithms are useful for guiding a general approach to the management of PAH, the clinician is more often confronted by deviations from the norm than by patients who present with typical findings and responses to therapy. Unfortunately, there are seldom clear-cut evidence-based strategies to provide guidance under these circumstances. Nevertheless accrued experience, consensus opinion, and sound reasoning can often yield a rational course of action. Below issues which should be considered in problematic situations of PAH management are discussed.

Real World Question Do We Need Diagnostic Consistency in Long-term Monitoring?

An important benchmark of therapeutic success is the degree to which an indicator of disease severity changes over time. Among clinical trial populations, a beneficial drug effect has often been identified on the basis of an improvement in six-minute walk distance in the range of 16–50 meters compared to placebo or historical controls, or to baseline walk distance. However, in an individual patient, does an improvement of 20 meters in six-minute walk distance after 3 months of treatment constitute a positive outcome? The answer depends on several factors, including: (1) whether this change exceeds random variation of distance walked during multiple tests; (2) whether the change corresponds with changes in other parameters of disease severity; (3) whether the patient perceives a functional benefit of that degree to have value; (4) whether the change proves ultimately to be part of a longer-term trend in a consistent direction; and (5) whether factors unrelated to disease severity are having an impact on six-minute walk distance, such as orthopedic limitations. While no specific cut-off for a clinically significant change in individual walk distance can be specified, it is important for the clinician to recognize these ambiguities when assessing treatment outcome.

Periodic non-invasive or invasive hemodynamic studies are generally performed as part of the ongoing evaluation of treatment effectiveness in PAH patients. Although Doppler-echocardiographically estimated pulmonary artery systolic pressure (PASP) correlates closely with simultaneous direct catheter measurements [14], the difference between the two techniques may be substantial for an individual patient. Thus, how much difference in Doppler-echocardiographic measurements before and after treatment can be reliably attributed to the intervention? A reliable value of PASP determined by Doppler-echocardiography requires a suitable tricuspid regurgitant flow velocity signal, careful measurement and an accurate estimation of right atrial pressure. As a rule, a reported value of PASP should be interpreted as having a "confidence range" of plus or minus 5 mmHg. Thus measurements on two occasions that are no more than 10 mmHg different may not represent any actual change whatsoever. Similarly, misapplication of right atrial pressure estimation may affect whether a patient is felt to have pulmonary hypertension or not. For example, a tricuspid regurgitant velocity of 2.9 m/sec in a patient with a right atrial pressure of 5 mmHg reflects an estimated PASP of 38 mmHg – a value that suggests minimal, if any, PH. However, if the right atrial pressure was assumed to be 20 mmHg, the resulting PASP estimate would be 53 mmHg, a value which would "confidently" but erroneously suggest PH in a moderate range. Finally, the presence of coexisting pulmonic valve stenosis renders the right ventricular systolic pressure inaccurate in estimating PASP unless the valvular gradient is taken into account.

Although right heart catheterization is considered to be the definitive measurement of pulmonary hemodynamics, it too must be interpreted with some caution. Even during short-term continuous monitoring, catheter-measured pulmonary artery pressure can vary significantly in the absence of any interventions [14]. Thus, brief repeat measurements at intervals of months to years risk superimposing spontaneous variation (plus effects of hydration status, anxiety, etc) on any changes due to either progression of disease or response to therapy. Inaccuracy can be further compounded by errors in technique: imprecise pulmonary capillary wedge pressures due to failure to confirm position with a wedged blood saturation, or relying on thermodilution cardiac output measurement in the setting of tricuspid regurgitation or intracardiac shunt.

The problems caused by inaccuracy and "random sampling" during follow-up has led to the concept that continuous ambulatory hemodynamic monitoring may provide more reliable data about trends and responses of pulmonary hemodynamics over time, and may identify more precise predictors of outcome. In the meantime, judgments about disease progression must incorporate all information about a patient's status, rather than a single set of numbers about hemodynamics, even if obtained invasively. This body of information should include (but not be limited to) symptomatic status, physical examination, formal functional assessment, morphology and function of the right ventricle, and brain natriuretic peptide level.

Real World Question Do All Patients with Mild Pulmonary Hypertension have Pulmonary Arterial Hypertension?

A policy of screening high risk populations, such as members of a family with known familial PAH or patients with limited scleroderma, or of obtaining Doppler-echocardiographic studies in patients with any symptoms or findings that may have a cardiac basis, results in numerous patients identified with an estimated PASP above the standard upper limit of normal. The question then arises about how much significance to attach to this finding. A number of issues impact on the answer for any given patient, and should be systematically addressed (discussed below).

Real World Question What are the Presenting Symptoms?

Symptoms of dyspnea or fatigue presumably raise the probability that PH may be a valid cause, though this does not constitute a confirmation since such symptoms are highly non-specific. Perhaps more importantly, atypical symptoms should raise wariness that either the measurement is erroneous, or even if accurate does not explain the symptoms which therefore may need further evaluation in any event.

Real World Question Are There Other Problems Which are More Likely to Explain the Symptoms?

The preliminary observation of possible mild PH should not distract the clinician from an appropriate search for more likely substrates. Dyspnea, for example, in a 68 year-old man with a smoking history and hyperlipidemia, is more likely to be an anginal equivalent suggestive of coronary artery disease than due to the finding of an estimated right ventricular systolic pressure of 41 mmHg on Doppler-echocardiographic study.

Real World Question What is the Reliability of the Echocardiography Laboratory and Sonographer?

Clearly the skills and interpretive ability of the echocardiographer determine to some extent the degree to which a particular value of right ventricular systolic pressure should be accepted at face value, since visualization of a distinct tricuspid regurgitant velocity signal is operator dependent. In addition, the more technically difficult the examination, either due to body habitus or to coexisting factors such as lung disease, the more suspect the results may be.

Real World Question What is the Expected Normal Pulmonary Arterial Systolic Pressure for the Patient?

It is incorrect to assume that a single value represents the cut-off between normal and abnormal pulmonary pressures. Firstly, the commonly used point of reference (PASP > 35 mmHg) is based on a combination of a population average and expert consensus; unlike systemic hypertension, pulmonary measures have not been subjected to long-term outcome studies to determine which values in otherwise asymptomatic patients are related to worse outcomes. Secondly, older or more overweight individuals tend to have higher estimated PASP's on echocardiographic assessment (Figure 7.5) [15] and the clinical or predictive significance is unknown.

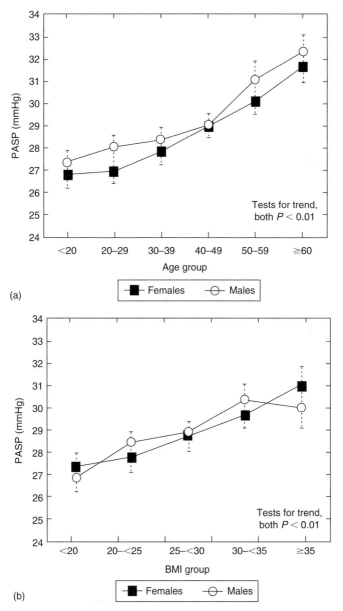

(a)

(b)

Figure 7.5 Pulmonary arterial systolic pressure in otherwise normal echocardiograms from people without clinical evidence of PH [18].

Real World Question Do Other Findings Corroborate a Finding of Pulmonary Hypertension of Any Degree?

The presence of right cardiac chamber enlargement, right ventricular dysfunction, physical findings, right axis deviation or right ventricular hypertrophy on electrocardiogram, or prominent hilar vessels on chest X-ray increases the probability that an elevated estimated pulmonary artery pressure is valid. However, the absence of these findings does not exclude the possibility of mild or early pulmonary vascular disease.

The approach to the discovery of potential mild PH depends upon the context. In symptomatic patients in whom no other explanation is apparent, exploration to identify a cause of PH is warranted, and verification and characterization with right heart catheterization is required. Coupling the right heart catheterization with exercise is advisable if resting pressures are near normal. Conversely, if the finding of mild PH occurs in a low risk patient without symptoms, a more conservative approach is appropriate and includes repeating a directed echocardiographic study in three months to determine if the result is consistent. If it is, then a search for a treatable underlying cause is justified. However, even if mild asymptomatic or minimally symptomatic PH is confirmed by right heart catheterization, none of the currently available therapies have been shown to have a favorable risk- or cost-to-benefit outcome in this population.

Real World Question How to Make a Diagnosis of Pulmonary Hypertension in the Setting of Comorbidities?

PH is often recognized in the setting of other factors which technically disallow the diagnosis of PAH, but do not in themselves explain the presence of PH or symptoms. Examples are mild to moderate left ventricular diastolic dysfunction, systemic hypertension, mild to moderate left sided valvular heart disease, obstructive sleep apnea, mild to moderate chronic obstructive pulmonary disease, or mild to moderate pulmonary fibrosis. Since these conditions usually excluded patients from clinical drug studies, evidence-based treatment recommendations do not exist, and pulmonary vascular targeted medications are not labeled for use in any of these populations. Consequently, health plans often do not provide medical coverage for treatment of these conditions with expensive medications labeled for PAH. Nevertheless, pending initiation and completion of studies of these disease categories, treatment of patients whose symptoms or longevity are related to PH is clearly warranted.

The initial step in treatment is to treat any contributing causes such as afterload reduction, volume management with diuretics and sodium restriction for control of elevated left sided filling pressures, aggressive control of systemic hypertension, polysomnography in suspected sleep apnea and consideration of continuous positive airway pressure nocturnal breathing assistance if appropriate, or bronchodilators and oxygen in reactive airways disease.

Only after such factors have been addressed should treatment with targeted pulmonary vascular therapy be considered. Empiric treatment, however, requires a careful treatment plan and a commitment to reassess to determine whether treatment goals have been achieved and whether adverse effects may be occurring. It is especially important to make sure that there are not contraindications to using any of the available medications. For example, epoprostenol administered to patients with pulmonary venous hypertension due to high left heart filling pressures, mitral stenosis, or pulmonary vein obstruction can result in pulmonary edema; the same may be true for other drugs with pulmonary vasodilating capabilities.

Both physicians and patients must understand that unless symptoms are predominantly occurring from the pulmonary hypertension and right heart dysfunction, rather than from the comorbid condition, even aggressive vascularly directed treatment will be unlikely to produce subjective benefit.

Real World Question How to Assess the Treatment Goals?

The intention of treatment is to reduce symptoms, increase six-minute walk distance and improve pulmonary hemodynamics. Reasonable specific benchmarks are an improvement in WHO functional status by 1 class, extension of six-minute walk distance by 10% or more, and/or reduction of mean pulmonary artery pressure by at least 10 mmHg to less than 40 mmHg while maintaining or increasing pulmonary blood flow. These goals should be considered guidelines, but do provide a means by which to determine whether a given treatment strategy can be considered effective. In evaluating outcomes, one must keep in mind the potential inaccuracies and variations in outcome measurements outlined above. Seldom can an effective approach be documented immediately; a period of dose optimization and allowance for the effects of reverse vascular remodeling is necessary before a therapy is deemed unsuccessful. A minimum of three months of treatment in a reasonably stable patient should be undertaken before re-evaluation, and in many patients a duration of one year or more may be needed to see appreciable benefit.

Real World Question Which is Better? Monotherapy vs. Combination Therapy

Only single drug regimens have been formally evaluated in appropriately designed studies. Many patients, however, fail to achieve treatment objectives on monotherapy. Consequently, various combinations and sequences of drugs are currently under evaluation, and experience is also accruing with the empiric use of dual or triple therapy. From a theoretical standpoint, multidrug approaches are attractive since the three major classes of medications exert their effects by different mechanisms which may be additive or complementary. Thus, two or more drugs may have an augmented effect, or may allow for dosing below the level of side effects. However, at present this supposition has not been rigorously confirmed, so again careful ongoing re-assessment is mandated.

For stable WHO class III patients who have been started on an oral agent (sildenafil or bosentan) and failed to improve, addition of the other oral agent may be explored. If the patient deteriorates despite use of one oral agent, consideration should be given to transitioning to or adding a prostacyclin analogue (epoprostenol, treprostinil or iloprost).

Patients who are unstable or have WHO class IV symptoms should be started on a prostacyclin analogue, preferably epoprostenol. If improvement does not occur in 3 months or less (depending on level of urgency), one of the oral agents can be added. Once improvement and stability is achieved, simplification of the regimen can be done by transitioning to oral agents alone or in combination with a more tolerable form of prostacyclin, such as iloprost.

The importance of monitoring cannot be over-emphasized. The need for systematic re-evaluation of patients using a reproducible protocol is a compelling argument for managing these patients in a higher volume referral center with expert physician and nursing staff.

Real World Question When Does the Patient Need Surgical Intervention?

Failure of medical treatment should lead to consideration of possible surgical intervention, either lung transplantation or balloon atrial septostomy. Patients should be evaluated for transplant candidacy at the time they are started on an intravenous prostacyclin analogue, even before their response to medications is established, because of the expected waiting period before a donor organ is available after the patient is listed.

Patients with advanced right ventricular failure who have failed medical treatment and who have arterial oxygen saturations within an acceptable range should be considered for percutaneous balloon atrial septostomy at experienced centers [16].

Real World Question How to Treat Angina in Patients with Pulmonary Arterial Hypertension?

Symptoms of angina occur in up to one-third of patients with PAH. The cause is most often attributable to increased right ventricular myocardial oxygen demand due to high wall stress, coupled with a decreased aortic-to-right-ventricular endocardial gradient leading to decreased coronary blood flow. Treatment directed to improvement of pulmonary vascular hemodynamics would be expected to benefit both sides of the coronary blood flow/myocardial oxygen demand imbalance. Among patients who fail to improve, alternative explanations should be sought. Atherosclerotic coronary artery disease can coexist with PAH, though the typical IPAH population usually has a low risk profile for coronary artery disease. A greater concern, which is being increasingly recognized as a cause of angina or asymptomatic ischemia in patients with severe PAH, is compression of the left main coronary artery by the dilated left main pulmonary artery. A low threshold for performing coronary angiography should be maintained; successful stenting of a compressed left main coronary artery under these circumstances has been reported [17].

Take Home Message

PAH, while not curable, is clearly treatable. Effective treatment improves symptoms, functional status, exercise tolerance, pulmonary hemodynamics and survival. Optimal management requires timely and accurate diagnosis with appropriately tailored therapy.

Diagnostic suspicion of PAH is raised by symptoms of fatigue, dyspnea, chest pain, syncope or edema. Suspicion is heightened in patients with associated risks or conditions such as connective tissue disease, HIV infection, prior exposure to known toxins, cirrhotic liver disease with portal hypertension, congenital heart disease, or family history of PAH. Symptoms in a patient in whom other causes are less likely (such as middle-aged women) or have been ruled-out (such as obstructive pulmonary disease, heart failure or ischemic heart disease) raise further warning signs.

A basic cardiovascular physical examination and screening laboratory assessment will direct further evaluation if any of these indicators are present: loud P2, right ventricular lift, right ventricular hypertrophy on ECG, and/or central pulmonary artery prominence on chest x-ray. The Doppler – echocardiographic examination can be confirmatory if a high right ventricular systolic pressure is detected, especially if coupled with right ventricular enlargement or dysfunction, and can suggest underlying substrates. Hemodynamic catheterization is required to fully characterize pulmonary arterial hemodynamics, including response to vasoactive agents (nitric oxide or epoprostenol).

Treatment is typically complex and intense, requiring careful monitoring and follow-up, preferably in a dedicated facility with expert nursing and physician staff with access to multidisciplinary consultation and participation in clinical studies. Currently treatment utilizes prostacyclin derivatives, endothelin receptor antagonism, or phosphodiesterase-5 inhibition. Although these agents have potent vasodilatory characteristics, their main mode of action may be through vascular remodeling mechanisms. Consequently, clinical effects may be gradual and progressive.

References

1 Barst RJ, McGoon MD, Torbicki A *et al.* Diagnosis and differential assessment of pulmonary arterial hypertension. Journal of American College of Cardiology 2004;43:40S–47S.
2 Yuan JXJ, Rubin LJ. Pathogenesis of pulmonary arterial hypertension. The need for multiple hits. Circulation 2005;111:534–538.
3 Channick RN, Simonneau G, Sitbon O *et al.* Effects of the dual endothelin-receptor antagonist bosentan in patients with pulmonary hypertension: a randomised placebo-controlled study. Lancet 2001;358(9288):1119–1123.
4 Giaid A, Yanagisawa M, Langleben D, *et al.* Expression of endothelin-1 in the lungs of patients with pulmonary hypertension. NEJM 1993;328:1732–1739.
5 Rich S, Dantzker DR, Ayres SM *et al.* Primary pulmonary hypertension: A national prospective study. Ann Int Med 1987;107:216–223.

6 Tuder RM, Groves BM, Badesch DB, Voelkel NF. Exuberant endothelial cell growth and elements of inflammation are present n plexiform lesions of pulmonary hypertension. Am J Path 1994;144:275–285.

7 Lane KB, Machado RD, Pauciulo MW *et al.* Heterozygous germline mutations in BMPR2, encoding a TGF-beta receptor, cause familial primary pulmonary hypertension. The International PPH Consortium.[see comment]. Nature Genetics 2000;26:81–84.

8 Deng Z, Morse JH, Slager SL *et al.* Familial primary pulmonary hypertension (gene PPH1) is caused by mutations in the bone morphogenetic protein receptor-II gene. American Journal of Human Genetics 67:electronically published, 2000.

9 Tapson VF, Gomberg-Maitland M, Mclaughlin V *et al.* Safety and Efficacy of Intravenous Treprostinil for Pulmonary Arterial Hypertension: A Prospective, Multicenter, Open-Label 12-Week Trial. Chest 2006;In press.

10 Gomberg-Maitland M, Tapson VF, Benza RL *et al.* Transition from intravenous epoprostenol to intravenous treprostinil in pulmonary hypertension. American Journal of Respiratory and Critical Care Medicine 2005;172(12):1586–1589.

11 Newman JH, Trembath RC, Morse JA *et al.* Genetic basis of pulmonary arterial hypertension:current understanding and future directions. Journal of the American College of Cardiology 2004;43:33S–39S.

12 Loyd JE, Butler MG, Foroud TM, Conneally PM, Phillips JA, Newman JH. Genetic anticipation and abnormal gender ratio at birth in familial primary pulmonary hypertension. American Journal of Respiratory and Critical Care Medicine 1995;152:93–97.

13 Galie N, Badesch DB, Oudiz R *et al.* Ambrisentan therapy for pulmonary arterial hypertension. Journal of American College of Cardiology 2005;46(3):529–535.

14 Harrison R, Flanagan JA, Sankelo M *et al.* Molecular and functional analysis identifies ALK-1 as the predominant cause of pulmonary hypertension related to hereditary haemorrhagic telangiectasia. Journal of Medical Genetics 2003;40:865–71.

15 Marcos E, Fadel E, Sanchez O et al. Serotonin-induced smooth muscle hyperplasia in various forms of human pulmonary hypertension.[see comment]. Circulation Research 2004;94:1263–1270.

16 Christman BW, McPherson CD, Newman JH *et al.* An imbalance between the excretion of thromboxane and prostacyclin metabolites in pulmonary hypertension. NEJM 1992;327:70–75.

17 Cacoub P, Dorent R, Maistre G *et al.* Endothelin-1 in primary pulmonary hypertension and the Eisenmenger syndrome. American J Cardiol 1993;71:448–450.

18 Altman R, Scazziota A, Rouvier J *et al.* Coagulation and fibrinolytic parameters in patients with pulmonary hypertension. Clinical Cardiology 1996;19:549–554.

Further Reading

Aguilar RV, Farber HW:Epoprostenol (prostacyclin) therapy in HIV–associated pulmonary hypertension. American Journal of Respiratory & Critical Care Medicine 162:1846–50, 2000.

Badesch DB, Tapson VF, McGoon MD, Brundage BH, Rubin LJ, Wigley FM, Rich S, Barst RJ, Barrett PS, *et al.* Continuous intravenous epoprostenol for pulmonary hypertension due to the scleroderma spectrum of disease. Annals of Internal Medicine 132:425–34, 2000.

Barst R, D. L, Badesch D, Frost A, Clinton L, Shapiro S, Naeije R, Simmoneau G, Galie N: Sitaxsentan Therapy for Pulmonary Arterial Hypertension. Journal of American College of Cardiology In Press, 2006.

Barst RJ, Langleben D, Frost A, Horn EM, Oudiz R, Shapiro S, McLaughlin VV, Hill N, Tapson VF, Robbins IM, Zwicke D, Duncan B, Dixon RA, Frumkin LR:Sitaxsentan therapy for pulmonary arterial hypertension. American Journal of Respiratory and Critical Care Medicine 169:441–447, 2004.

Barst RJ, Rubin LJ, Long WA, McGoon MD, Rich S, Badesch DB, Groves BM, Tapson VF, Bourge RC, Brundage BH, Koerner SK, Langleben D, Keller CA, Murali S, Uretsky BF, Clayton LM, Jobsis MM, Blackburn Jr. SD, Shortino D, Crow JW: A comparison of continuous intravenous epoprostenol (prostacyclin) with conventional therapy for primary pulmonary hypertension. New England Journal of Medicine 334:296–301, 1996.

Bonderman D, Fleischmann D, Prokop M, Klepetko W, Lang IM:Left main coronary artery compression by the pulmonary trunk in pulmonary hypertension. Circulation 105:265, 2002.

Channick RN, Rubin LJ, Simonneau G, Robbins IM, Tapson VF, Frost A, Badesch DB, Bodin F, Roux S:Bosentan, a dual endothelin receptor antagonist, improves exercise capacity and hemodynamics in patients with pulmonary arterial hypertension:results of a double blind, randomized, placebo-controlled trial [abstr]. Circulation 102 (Suppl II):II–100, 2000.

Currie PJ, Seward JB, Chan KL:Continuous wave Doppler determination of right ventricular pressure: A simultaneous Doppler–catheterization study in 127 patients. J Am Coll Cardiol 6:750–6, 1985.

D' Alonzo GE, Barst RJ, Ayres SM, Bergofsky EH, Brundage BH, Detre KM, Fishman AP, Goldring RM, Groves BM, Kernis JT:Survival in patients with primary pulmonary hypertension:results from a national prospective registry. Annals of Internal Medicine 115: 343–349, 1991.

Decuypere V, Delcroix M, Budts W:Left main coronary artery and right pulmonary vein compression by a large pulmonary artery aneurysm. Heart 90, 2004.

Demoncheauxa EAG, Higenbottamc TW, Kielyb DG, Wonga JM, Whartona S, Varcoea R, Siddonsa T, Spiveyd AC, Halle K, Gizee AP: Decreased whole body endogenous nitric oxide production in patients with primary pulmonary hypertension. Journal of Vascular Research 42:133–136, 2005.

Dorfmuller P, Perros F, Balabanian K, Humbert M:Inflammation in pulmonary arterial hypertension. European Respiratory Journal 22:358–63, 2003.

Eddahibi S, Humbert M, Fadel E, Raffestin B, Darmon M, Capron F, Simonneau G, Dartevelle P, Hamon M, Adnot S: Hyperplasia of pulmonary artery smooth muscle cells is causally related to overexpression of the serotonin transporter in primary pulmonary hypertension. Chest 121:97S–98S, 2002.

Eddahibi S, Humbert M, Fadel E, Raffestin B, Darmon M, Capron F, Simonneau G, Dartevelle P, Hamon M, Adnot S: Serotonin transporter overexpression is responsible for pulmonary artery smooth muscle hyperplasia in primary pulmonary hypertension. Journal of Clinical Investigation 108:1141–50, 2001.

Fuster V, Frye RL, Gersh BJ, McGoon MD, Steele PM: Primary pulmonary hypertension:natural history and the importance of thrombosis. Circulation 70:580–7, 1984.

Galie N, Ghofrani HA, Torbicki A, Barst RJ, Rubin LJ, Badesch D, Fleming T, Parpia T, Burgess G, Branzi A, Grimminger F, Kurzyna M, Simmoneau G: Sildenafil citrate therapy for pulmonary arterial hypertension. New England Journal of Medicine 353:2148–57, 2005.

Giaid A, Saleh D:Reduced expression of endothelial nitric oxide synthase in the lungs of patients with pulmonary hypertension. New England Journal of Medicine 333:214–21, 1995.

Hassell KL: Altered hemostasis in pulmonary hypertension. Blood Coagulation & Fibrinolysis 9:107–17, 1998.

Herve P, Launay JM, Scrobohaci ML, Brenot F, Simmoneau G, Petitpretz P, Poubeau P, Cerrina J, Duroux P, Drouet L: Increased plasma serotonin in primary pulmonary hypertension. American Journal of Medicine 99:249–54, 1995.

Hoeper MM, Schwarze M, Ehlerding S, Adler–Schuermeyer A, Spiekerkoetter E, Niedermeyer J, Hamm M, Fabel H:long-term treatment of primary pulmonary hypertension with aerosolized iloprost, a prostacyclin analogue. New England Journal of Medicine 342:1866–70, 2000.

Hoeper MM, Sosada M, Fabel H:Plasma coagulation profiles in patients with severe primary pulmonary hypertension. European Respiratory Journal 12:1446–9, 1998.

Kawut S, F. S, Ferrari V, DeNofrio D, Axel L, Loh E, Palevsky HI:Extrinsic compression of the left main coronary artery by the pulmonary artery in patients with long-standing pulmonary hypertension. American Journal of Cardiology 83:984–6, 1999.

Kuhn KP, Byrne DW, Arbogast PG, Doyle TP, Loyd JE, Robbins IM:Outcome in 91 consecutive patients with pulmonary arterial hypertension receiving epoprostenol. American Journal of Respiratory and Critical Care Medicine 167:580–583, 2002.

Kuo PC, Johnson LB, Plotkin JS, Howell CD, Bartlett ST, Rubin LJ:Continuous intravenous infusion of epoprostenol for the treatment of portopulmonary hypertension. Transplantation 63:604–16, 1997.

Langleben D, Dupuis J, Hirsch A, Giovinazzo M, Langleben I, Khoury J, Ruel N, Caron A: Pulmonary endothelin–1 clearance in human pulmonary arterial hypertension. Chest 128:622S, 2005.

Machado RD, James V, Southwood M, Harrison RE, Atkinson C, Stewart S, Morrell NW, Trembath RC, Aldred MA:Investigation of second genetic hits at the BMPR2 locus as a modulator of disease progression in familial pulmonary arterial hypertension. Circulation 111:607–613, 2005.

McGoon MD, Fuster V, Freeman WK, Edwards WD, Scott JP: The heart and the lungs:pulmonary hypertension. In Mayo Clinic Practice of Cardiology. Edited by ER Guiliani, BJ Gersh, MD McGoon, DL Hayes and HV Schaff, 3rd edition. New York, Mosby Yearbook, 1996, pp 1815–36.

McLaughlin V, Sitbon O, Badesch DB, Barst RJ, Black C, Gailie N, Rainisio M, Simonneau G, Rubin L:Survival with firST-line bosentan in patients with primary pulmonary hypertension. European Respiratory Journal 25:244–249, 2005.

McLaughlin VV, Genthner DE, Panella MM, Hess DM, Rich S:Compassionate use of continuous prostacyclin in the management of secondary pulmonary hypertension: A case series. Annals of Internal Medicine 130:740–3, 1999.

McLaughlin VV, Shillington A, Rich S:Survival in primary pulmonary hypertension: The impact of epoprostenol therapy. Circulation 106:1477–82, 2002.

McQuillan BM, Picard MH, Leavitt M, Weymann AE:Clinical correlates and reference intervals for pulmonary artery systolic pressure among echocardiographically normal subjects. Circulation 104:2797–2802, 2001.

Mesquita S, Castro C, Ikari N, Oliveira S, Lopes A:Likelihood of left main coronary artery compression based on pulmonary trunk diameter in patients with pulmonary hypertension. American Journal of Medicine 116:369–374, 2004.

Olschewski H, Simonneau G, Galie N, Higenbottam T, Naeije R, Rubin LJ, Nikkho S, Speich R, Hoeper MM, Behr J, Winkler J, Sitbon O, Popov W, Ghofrani HA, Manes A, Kiely DG, Ewert R, Meyer A, Corris PA, Delcroix M, Gomez–Sanchez M, Siedentop H, Seeger W: Inhaled iloprost for severe pulmonary hypertension. New England Journal of Medicine 347:322–9, 2002.

Reichenberger F, Popke–Zaba J, McNeil K, Parameshwar J, Shapiro LM: Atrial septostomy in the treatment of severe pulmonary arterial hypertension. Thorax 58:797–800, 2003.

Rich S, Brundage BH:high-dose calcium channel–blocking therapy for primary pulmonary hypertension:evidence for long-term reduction in pulmonary arterial pressure and regression of right ventricular hypertrophy. Circulation 76:135–41, 1987.

Rich S, D'Alonzo GE, Dantzker DR, Levy PS:Magnitude and implications of spontaneous hemodynamic variability in primary pulmonary hypertension. American Journal of Cardiology 55:159–63, 1985.

Rich S, Kaufmann E, Levy PS: The effect of high doses of calcium–channel blockers on survival in primary pulmonary hypertension. N Engl J Med 327:76–81, 1992.

Rich S, McLaughlin VV, O'Neill W:Stenting ito reverse left ventricular ischemia due to left main coronary artery compression in primary pulmonary hypertension. Chest 120:1412–5, 2001.

Rich S, McLaughlin VV: The effects of chronic prostacyclin therapy on cardiac output and symptoms in primary pulmonary hypertension. Journal of the American College of Cardiology 34:1184–7, 1999.

Rosenzweig EB, Kerstein D, Barst RJ:long-term prostacyclin for pulmonary hypertension with associated congenital heart defects. Circulation 99:1858–65, 1999.

Rubin LJ, Badesch DB, Barst RJ, Galie N, Black CM, Keogh A, Pulido T, Frost A, Roux S, Leconte I, Landzberg M, Simonneau G:Bosentan therapy for pulmonary arterial hypertension. New England Journal of Medicine 346:896–903, 2002.

Sandoval J, Gaspar J, Pulido T, Bautista E, Martinez–Guerra ML, Zeballos M, Palomar A, Gomez A:Graded balloon dilation atrial septostomy in severe primary pulmonary hypertension. Journal of the American College of Cardiology 32:297–304, 1998.

Simonneau G, Barst RJ, Galie N, Naeije R, Rich S, Bourge RC, Keogh A, Oudiz R, Frost A, Blackburn SD, Crow JW, Rubin LJ:Continuous subcutaneous infusion of treprostinil, a prostacyclin analogue, in patients with pulmonary arterial hypertension. American Journal of Respiratory and Critical Care Medicine 165:800–4, 2002.

Simonneau G, Galie N, Rubin L, Langleben D, Seeger W, Domenighetti G, Gibbs S, Lebrec D, Speich R, Beghetti M, Rich S, Fishman A:Clinical classification of pulmonary hypertension. Journal of American College of Cardiology 43, Supplement 1:S5–S12, 2004.

Sitbon O, Humbert M, Jais X, Ioos V, Hamid A, Provencher S, Garcia G, Parent F, Herve P, Simonneau G:long-term response to calcium channel blockers in idiopathic pulmonary arterial hypertension. Circulation 111:3105–3111, 2005.

Sitbon O, Humbert M, Nunes H, Parent F, Garcia G, Herve P, Rainisio M, Simonneau G:long-term intravenous epoprostenol infusion in primary pulmonary hypertension:prognostic factors and survival. Journal of the American College of Cardiology 40:780–8, 2002.

Trembath R, Thomson J, Machado R, Morgan NV, Atkinson C, Winship I, Simonneau G, Galie N, Loyd JE, Humbert M, Nichols WC, Morrell N:Clinical and molecular genetic features of pulmonary hypertension in patients with hereditary hemorrhagic telangiectasia. New England Journal of Medicine 345:325–34, 2001.

Weir EK, Reeve HL, Huang JM, Michelakis E, Nelson DP, Hampl V, Archer SL: Anorexic agents aminorex, fenfluramine, and dexfenfluramine inhibit potassium current in rat pulmonary vascular smooth muscle and cause pulmonary vasoconstriction. Circulation 94:2216–20, 1996.

Welsh C, Hassell KL, Badesch DB:Coagulation and fibrinolytic profiles in patients with severe pulmonary hypertension. Chest 110:710–7, 1996.

Yuan JJ, Aldinger AM, Juhaszova M, Wang JK, Conte JV, Gaine SP, Orens JB, Rubin LJ:Dysfunctional voltage–gated K + channels in pulmonary artery smooth muscle cells of patients with primary pulmonary hypertension. Circulation 98:1400–6, 1998.

CHAPTER 8

Heart Failure

Thach N. Nguyen, Loan T. Pham, Pham Nguyen Vinh, Norbert Lingling D. Uy, Gaurav Kumar and Hoang Pham

Introduction

Heart failure (HF) is a common clinical syndrome resulting from any structural and functional cardiac disorders that impairs the capacity of the ventricle to fill or to eject the appropriate amount of blood [1]. The most common causes of HF are coronary artery disease (CAD), long standing uncontrolled hypertension (HTN), dilated cardiomyopathy, valvular heart disease and diastolic dysfunction due to age, etc. In the examination of a patient at high risk for HF or with HF, it is important to investigate by echocardiography, stress testing, coronary angiography or blood test for any possible treatable underlying causes. Many details in the family history could point toward a genetic predisposition such as family history of sudden cardiac death (SCD), CAD, dilated or hypertrophic cardiomyopathy, skeletal myopathies, etc. The list of predisposing causes of HF is shown in Table 8.1.

Table 8.1 Predisposing causes of heart failure.

1. Hypertension
2. Diabetes mellitus
3. Dyslipidemia
4. Valvular heart disease
5. CAD
6. Myopathy
7. Rheumatic fever
8. Mediastinal radiation
9. Sleep apnea disorders
10. Exposure to cardiotoxin agents
11. Alcohol abuse
12. Smoking
13. Collagen vascular disease
14. Thyroid disorder
15. Pheochromocytoma
16. Old age
17. Metabolic syndrome

CAD, coronary artery disease.

Target Patient Populations

According to the new ACC/AHA classification, in stage AHF, the patient is totally asymptomatic without structural abnormality. In stage B, the patient has left ventricle (LV) remodeling without symptom or sign of HF. In stage C, the patient had or has the conventional symptoms and signs of HF. At stage D, the patients have refractory end-stage HF [1]. However, in clinical practice, patients with HF can present with an ejection fraction (EF) ranging from 20% to 65%, level of congestion ranging from dry to wet or nearly drowned from pulmonary edema, and prognosis from excellent to dying. So they are to be classified under separate subsets requiring different strategies according to various phases or stages of HF (Table 8.2).

Table 8.2 Classification of Heart Failure patients.

1. Stage A	Patient with high risks for HF
2. Stage B	Asymptomatic patients with LV dysfunction
3. Well compensated Stage C	Patients with minimal symptom treated as outpatient in office
4. Early decompensated Stage C	Patient with first hospitalization because of decompensated HF
5. Recurrent decompensated Stage C	Patients with recurrent hospitalizations because of frequent relapse of decompensated HF
6. Stable very low EF, Stage C	Patients with multiple previous hospitalizations now followed-up at a dedicated HF clinic

HF, heart failure; LV, left ventricle.

Management Strategies

In principle, every management plan for HF would include treatment and prevention of risk factors, administration of outcome-proven medications and prevention of clinical deterioration. The main strategies are outlined in Table 8.3.

Table 8.3 Main strategies for patients with heart failure.

1. Lifestyle modification
2. Prevent precipitating and aggravating factors
3. Essential pharmacologic management with BB, ACEI/ARB
4. Complimentary treatment with diuretics or vasodilators
5. Reverse structural abnormalities (remodeling with hypertrophy or dilation)
6. Device therapy including implantable cardioverter defibrillators, bi-ventricular pacing

ACEI, angiotensin converting enzyme inhibitors; ARB, angiotensin II receptor blockers; BB, β-blockers.

The prevention of risk factors and lifestyle modifications are the cornerstones in any management plan. They are the main treatment for early stages HF (A and B), while at the late stages (C and D), prevention is secondary because the main focus is to urgently control the severely symptomatic manisfestations and complications of decompensated HF. All medications or situations which can precipitate or aggravate HF should be clearly identified so they can be effectively prevented. Between all medications, β-blockers (BB), angiotensin converting enzyme inhibitors (ACEI) or angiotensin receptor blockers (ARB) are the absolutely essential medications. Without them, the patient does not *yet* receive basic treatment for HF. The complimentary medications include diuretics, digoxin, aldosterone antagonists, and vasodilators (hydralazine and isosorbide). These medications are optional for patients who have fluid retention or remain symptomatic despite maximal medical therapy with BB and ACEI/ARB. As the disease progresses, more diuretics are used if the patients have more relapses of excessive fluid retention. Then BB and ACEI/ARB are given more frequently, even for patients with relative contra-indications, and at higher doses in an effort to control more severe HF. More comorbidities and side-effects, e.g. renal insufficiency, liver dysfunction or orthostatic hypotension occur, so BB, ACEI or ARB and all medications are more likely to be challenged for dosage decrease or discontinuation. At this stage, the device therapy includes implantable cardioverter defibrillator (ICD) and chronic resynchronization therapy (CRT). Finally, in the long term strategic plan, any modality of treatment that can reverse the cardiac structural abnormality should be pursued aggressively at the earliest.

CLINICAL PEARLS

What to focus on in the management of HF? In stage A, it is *prevention* and treatment of risk factors. In stage B, it is the same: *prevention* of clinical deterioration (advance to stage C) and treatment of risk factors. In stage C, the main and most frequent cause of multiple relapses of acute decompensation is *fluid overload*. Fluid restriction and diuretics are the main treatment, they do not prolong life: they cause complications. However, without them, without judicious use of diuretics, and without intelligent and disciplined fluid restriction regimen, all patients with HF stage C will have frequent relapses. Low cardiac output is a big problem, but it is not so prominent until near the end of HF (end of stage C and stage D).

In general, all preventive and therapeutic modalities of treatment for HF mentioned above are applied to all patients however at various extent because each stage requires different level of intensive or preventive care.

Stage A: High Risk for HF Without Structural Abnormality

At this stage, the patients are healthy without any cardiovascular structural abnormalities. The only problem is that they are at high risk of developing HF. The main management is to screening asymptomatic patients at high risk for ventricular remodeling, to treating any underlying clinical diseases (hypertention, diabetes, hypercholesterolemia, alcohol abuse, tobacco addiction, obesity, etc.), while applying all generic preventive measures (lifestyle change, low sodium, low cholesterol diet, exercise and education). The end goal of treatment in this stage is to prevent the LV remodeling and forestall the rise of symptoms of HF.

The pathologic targets of the prevention for heart disease in patients at stage A are to prevent the occurrence of any atrial or ventricular hypertrophy or dilation or diastolic dysfunction. The ultimate goal is to protect the LV and to prevent any remodeling of any cardiac chamber or of the LV which is the most important and clinically relevant end result of any cardiac injury. The strategy is to prevent any remodeling in the right and left atrium, right ventricle, the pulmonary vasculature and flow and the systemic flow. The reason is because that the LV systolic and diastolic function is directly influenced by any persistently abnormal decrease or increase flow or pressure from the systemic circulation or the pulmonary system or the left or right side chambers. By that understanding, is mitral regurgitation (MR), a very common finding in routine echocardiography, or left bundle branch block (LBBB), a structural abnormality? Technically, the answer is yes. By that, all patients with MR are considered stage B HF. Any entity which can lead to the end result of LV remodeling and its preventive or corrective measures are listed in Table 8.4.

Table 8.4 shows that the general measures in the management of stage A include the lifestyle change and treatment of any clinical entities which lead to LV remodeling. Detailed instructions on diet, control of blood pressure (BP), high cholesterol level, prevention of diabetes or CKD, are discussed in chapter 6: Integrated prevention of cardiovascular disease.

Table 8.4 Entities Leading to Ventricular Remodeling and Preventive Measures.

Clinical entity	Pathology	Preventive measure
Diabetes	Dilated cardiomyopathy	Diet
Uncontrolled HTN	LV hypertrophy, dilation	Drug
CKD	LV hypertrophy, dilation	Diet
CAD	Ischemic cardiomyopathy	Drug
Valvular stenosis		
Mitral stenosis	Pulmonary HTN, right HF	Valvuloplasty
Aortic stenosis	LV hypertrophy	Valve change
Valvular insufficiency		
Aortic insufficiency	LV dilation	Medicine and Surgery
Mitral regurgitation	Left atrial and LV dilation	Surgery
Toxin (ETOH, drugs)	Dilated cardiomyopathy	Treat cause
Aging	Diastolic dysfunction	Diet?
Viral infection	Dilated cardiomyopathy	?
Obesity	Diastolic dysfunction	Weight loss
Post partum cardiomyopathy	Dilated cardiomyopathy	?
Uncontrolled arrhythmias	Dilated cardiomyopathy	Treat cause

CAD, coronary artery disease; CKD, chronic kidney disease; ETOH, alcohol; HF, heart failure; HTN, hypertension; LV, left ventricle.

Stage B: Asymptomatic Left Ventricular Remodeling

In stage B, the patient has low EF (<50%) while being asymptomatic. It is not rare to see asymptomatic patient with prior myocardial damage and low EF. More patients with acute myocardial infarction (MI) aborted by expedite percutaneous coronary interventions (PCI) or having CAD lesion opened by drug-eluting stent (DES), these patients with low EF can still enjoy a highly active lifestyle. Because the patients are asymptomatic, the management strategies are for: (1) prevention of clinical worsening; (2) reduction of morbidity and mortality; and (3) reversal of ventricular remodeling (Table 8.5).

Table 8.5 Management strategies for asymptomatic heart failure stage B patients.

1. Detect and treat the causes of HF
2. Maintain asymptomatic status by diet, exercise and medications
3. Prevent and treat precipitating and exacerbating factors
4. Prevent progression of HF at the cellular level
5. Prevent SCD with ICD
6. Reverse ventricular remodeling by diet, exercise and medications

HF, heart failure; ICD, implantable cardioverter defibrillator;
SCD, sudden cardiac death.

Initial Evaluation

In the first visit, the patient with HF is evaluated for causes, extent of LV dysfunction, risk of severe arrhythmias and sudden death or chance for relapse (Table 8.6). In developed countries, especially in the US and Europe, the most common cause of HF is CAD, while in developing countries, it can be long standing uncontrolled HTN, infection (Chaga's disease) or rheumatice fever, etc. [2]. This is why the US or European patients should undergo stress test to find out whether they have CAD. If the patients have reversible ischemia, an angiogram should be done and revascularization performed if indicated [2].

Table 8.6 Initial evaluation of patients with heart failure.

1. Assess clinical severity of HF by history and physical examination
2. Assess cardiac structure and function
3. Determine the etiology of HF
4. Evaluate for coronary disease and myocardial ischemia
5. Evaluate the risk of life-threatening arrhythmia
6. Identify any exacerbating factors for HF
7. Identify comorbidities which influence therapy
8. Identify barriers to adherence and compliance

HF, heart failure.

Life-Style Change and Education

The first step in the treatment plan for asymptomatic HF patients is life-style change: low sodium, low cholesterol diet, fluid restriction ($<$2000 cc/day), no smoking and exercise. Because the patient is asymptomatic, the main focus is prevention and education of the patient about the disease, disease process, worsening of symptoms and signs. The instructions for HF are listed in Table 8.7.

Table 8.7 Instructions for patients with heart failure.

1. Rationale and practical tips for compliance with low sodium, low cholesterol diet
2. Rationale and practical tips for compliance of fluid restriction
3. Rationale and practical tips for compliance with medication, office visit and blood testing
4. Rationale and practical tips for low calorie diet and losing weight
5. Rationale and practical tips for regular exercise
6. Keep a daily log of blood pressure and weight
7. Explanation of signs and symptoms of HF and change due to worsening HF

HF, heart failure.

Pharmacologic Therapy

ACEI and BB are the main treatment and should be given to patients with asymptomatic LV dilation or hypertrophy, especially in patients with prior MI even with normal EF. ACEI and BB are to reduce mortality, prevent, delay or reverse LV remodeling. With appropriate treatment against congestion and low cardiac output, the HF patient can be asymptomatic and function normally for a long time, especially the patients who did exercise well and regularly before the onset of cardiomyopathy. The benefits of ACEI were proved by the SOLV trial detailed below.

So the ACEI enalapril significantly reduced the incidence of HF and the rate of related hospitalizations, as compared with the rates in the group given placebo, among patients with asymptomatic LV dysfunction [3]. Besides ACEI or on top of a background of ACE inhibition, BB is also the second most important drug for HF. The evidence which proved the benefits of BB on HF stage B was in the Carvedilol US Heart Failure trial which randomized a large group of patients with mild, moderate and severe HF.

Evidence-based Medicine: The SOLV trial

At the beginning of the nineties, it was not known whether the treatment of patients with asymptomatic LV dysfunction with ACEI reduces mortality and morbidity. 4228 patients with EF of 0.35 or less who were not receiving drug treatment for HF, were randomly assigned to receive either placebo ($n = 2117$) or enalapril ($n = 2111$) at doses of 2.5–20 mg/day in a double-blind fashion. After a follow-up at an average of 37.4 months, there were 334 deaths in the placebo group, as compared with 313 in the enalapril group (reduction in risk, 8%, $P = 0.30$). The reduction in mortality from cardiovascular causes was larger but was not statistically significant (298 deaths in the placebo group vs. 265 in the enalapril group; risk reduction, 12%; $P = 0.12$). When the numbers of patients in whom HF developed and those who died were combined, the total number of deaths and cases of HF was lower in the enalapril group than in the placebo group (630 vs. 818; risk reduction, 29%; $P < 0.001$). In addition, fewer patients given enalapril died or were hospitalized for HF (434 in the enalapril group; vs. 518 in the placebo group; risk reduction, 20%; $P < 0.001$) [3].

Evidence-based Medicine: The US carvedilol heart failure trial

1094 patients with mild, moderate, or severe heart failure and an EF ≤ 0.35 were enrolled. The mild patients are the patients of today stage B HF. They were randomly assigned to receive either placebo ($n = 398$) or carvedilol ($n = 696$) on a background therapy with digoxin, diuretics, and an ACEI. After 12 months observation (for the group with mild heart failure), the overall mortality rate was 7.8% in the placebo group and 3.2% in the carvedilol group; the reduction in risk attributable to carvedilol was 65% (95% CI, 39–80%; $P < 0.001$). In addition, as compared with placebo, carvedilol therapy was accompanied by a 27% reduction in the risk of hospitalization for cardiovascular causes (19.6% vs. 14.1%, $P = 0.036$), as well as a 38% reduction in the combined risk of hospitalization or death (24.6% vs. 15.8%, $P < 0.001$) [4].

With evidence from the trial above, BB therapy is recommended even if there is concomitant diabetes, chronic obstructive lung disease, or peripheral vascular disease. BB therapy should be used with caution in patients with asthma, resting limb ischemia or diabetes with recurrent hypoglycemia. Considerable caution should be exercised if BBs are initiated in patients with marked bradycardia (<55 beats/min) or marked hypotension (systolic blood pressure <80 mmHg). BBs are not recommended in patients with asthma with active bronchospasm [4].

Diuretics are not the first line drug treatment in stage B because the patient has no sign of fluid retention. If fluid overload is to be prevented, low sodium diet and fluid restriction is the first line of therapy. Low dose diuretics can be used intermittently or as needed. Digoxin is not indicated either unless there are atrial arrhythmias. As the benefits of BB or ACEI are supported by reduction of mortality and morbidity from randomized clinical trials (RCT), the patients should be given the same dosage at which the benefits were proven (Table 8.8).

Table 8.8 Dosage of medications in clinical trials of heart failure.

Medication	Starting dose	Target dose	Clinical trial
Captopril	6.25–12.5 mg TID	50 mg TID	SAVE [5]
Enalapril	2.5–5 mg BID	10–20 mg BID	SOLV [3]
Ramipril	2.5 mg BID	5 mg BID	AIRE [6]
Trandolapril	1 mg/day	4 mg/day	TRACE [7]
Carvedilol	3.125 mg BID	25 mg BID	Carvedilol HF [4]
		50 mg BID for >187 lbs	
Metoprolol succinct	12.5–25 mg/day	200 mg/day	MERIT-HF [8]
Candesartan	4–8 mg/day	32 mg/day	RESOLVD [9]
Losartan	12.5 mg/day	50 mg/day	ELITE [10]
Valsartan	20 mg/day	160 mg BID	CHARM [11]
Spirinolactone		25 mg QD	RALES [12]
Isosorbide		120 mg	Aheft [13]
Hydralazine		225 mg	Aheft [13]

Revascularization for Heart Failure Patients

CAD is manifested as localized wall motion abnormalities on echocardiography. Dysfunctional segments with normal perfusion and normal glucose utilization are considered to be stunned, and dysfunctional segments with reduced perfusion and preserved glucose utilization are considered to be hibernated. Patients with LV dysfunction have higher mortality during open heart surgery (coronary artery bypass grafting, CABG), therefore, there is a need to assess myocardial perfusion, myocardial viability in order to select

CLINICAL PEARLS

Which test is best for detecting myocardial viability? There are three ways to test the viability of myocardium: Myocardial contrast echocardiography (MCE), dobutamine echocardiography (DE) and thallium scintigraphy (T1-201). The best concordance was found with MCE and TI-201; for detecting myocardial hibernation, both methods had similar high sensitivity but a low specificity for predicting recovery of function [14]. Importantly, the three techniques identified all patients who had significant improvement in global ventricular function. Using a biphasic response during DE, concordance between TI-201 scintigraphy and DE was 56%, and between MCE and DE 67%. While any improvement during dobutamine infusion was considered an indicator of viability, concordance increased between DE and both TI-201 scintigraphy and MCE (66% and 72%, respectively) [15]. Recently, separate studies reported that assessing end-diastolic wall thickness (EDWT) via DE can be useful in predicting recovery. If a patient had EDWT <5–6 mm [16], the chance of recovering function is minimal; conversely, if wall thickness is assessed to be greater or equal to 5–6 mm, there is a 50% or greater chance of wall motion improvement after CABG [17].

the patients who would survive, have the function of the myocardium recovered so to benefit from CABG.

Overall, there is a strong association between myocardial viability on non-invasive testing and improved survival after revascularization in patients with chronic CAD and LV dysfunction. For patients with defined myocardial viability, annual mortality was 16% in medically treated patients versus only 3.2% for revascularized patients ($P < 0.0001$). This represents a 79.6% relative reduction in risk of death associated with revascularization. For patients without viability, annual mortality was not significantly different according to treatment method: 7.7% with revascularization vs. 6.2% for medical therapy ($P =$ ns) [17].

CRITICAL THINKING

Revascularization for patients with severe HF. 765 consecutive patients (age 64 ± 11 years, 80% men) with advanced LV dysfunction (EF ≤35%) and without significant valvular heart disease who underwent PET/FDG study at the Cleveland Clinic between 1997 and 2002 were followed-up. Early intervention was defined as any cardiac intervention (surgical or percutaneous) within the first 6 months of the PET/FDG study. In the entire cohort, 230 patients (30%) underwent early intervention (188 [25%] had open heart surgery, most commonly coronary artery bypass grafting, and 42 [5%] had percutaneous revascularization); 535 (70%) were treated medically. Using 39 demographic, clinical and PET/FDG variables, it was possible to propensity-match 153 of the 230 patients with 153 patients who did not undergo early intervention. Among the propensity-matched group, there were 84 deaths during a median of 3 years follow-up. Early intervention was associated with a markedly lower risk of death (3-year mortality rate of 15% versus 35%, propensity adjusted hazard ratio 0.52, 95%CI 0.33–0.81, $P = 0.0004$) [18].

While revascularization can potentially reverse LV function, it has been less clear if this outweighs the perioperative risks and whether the long-term outcomes actually improve [2,18]. Besides improving the symptoms and prevent clinical deterioration, another problem facing the HF stage B patients is severe or possibly fatal arrhythmias. What we can do to solve the problem?

Primary Prevention of Sudden Cardiac Death in Ischemic Cardiomyopathy

At first, for patients with recent MI and CABG, findings from the Defibrillator in Acute Myocardial Infarction Trial (DINAMIT) [19] and the Coronary Artery Bypass Graft Patch (CABG-Patch) [20] trial did not find statistically significant benefits of ICDs on survival of these patients. However, in the MADITT 2 trial, benefits were found in patient with low EF, more than one month after the index MI.

So, in patients with a prior MI and advanced LV dysfunction, prophylactic implantation of an ICD improves survival [21]. The number needed to treat (NNT) to avoid one death was 18. Patients with MI within 1 month of enrollment

Evidence-based Medicine: The MADITT II trial

Over the course of four years, 1232 patients with a prior MI and a left ventricular ejection fraction (LVEF) of 0.30 or less were randomly assigned in a 3:2 ratio to receive an ICD or conventional medical therapy. Death from any cause was the end point. The results showed after an average follow-up of 20 months, the mortality rates were 19.8% in the conventional-therapy group and 14.2% in the ICD group (P = 0.016). The effect of ICD therapy on survival was similar in subgroup analyses stratified according to age, sex, EF, NYHA class, and the QRS interval [21].

or with coronary revascularization within the prior 3 months were excluded because the negative results of the DANAMIT and CABG-Patch trials. The findings in the MADITT 3 trial suggested that abolition of malignant ventricular arrhythmias by ICD reduced mortality and prevent further worsening of HF. However, recurrent ICD discharge might contribute to the higher rate of rehospitalization [21]. Does ICD prevent SCD in stage B HF patients with non-ischemic dilated cardiomyopathy?

Primary Prevention of Sudden Death in Non-Ischemic Cardiomyopathy

The evidence of prevention of SCD in non-ischemic HF patients is seen in the SCD-HeFT trial, detailed below [22].

Evidence-based Medicine: The SCD-HeFT trial

In the Sudden Cardiac Death-Heart Failure trial, 2521 patients with NYHA class II or III and a LVEF of 35% or less were randomized to conventional therapy for CHF plus placebo (847 patients), conventional therapy plus amiodarone (845 patients), or conventional therapy plus a conservatively programmed, shock-only, single-lead ICD (829 patients) (no pacing for bradycardia). The primary end point was death from any cause. The cause of cardiomyopathy was ischemic in 52% and non-ischemic in 48%. The median follow-up was 45.5 months. The results showed that there were 29% mortality in the placebo group, 28% in the amiodarone group, and 22% in the ICD group. The NNT to prevent one death was 14. The results did not vary according to either ischemic or non-ischemic causes however, the benefits of ICD were more marked (and significant only) among patients in NYHA FC II, with an absolute reduction in mortality of 11.9% (NNT = 8) [22].

Guidelines

For stage B HF patients, because they are asymptomatic, so the goal of ICD is to prevent SCD (primary prevention). ICD is indicated in patients with ischemic cardiomyopathy, at least 40 days post-MI, with EF of 30% or less, NYHA FC class I on chronic optimal medical therapy (OMT). (Class IIa recommendation; B level evidence) ICD might be considered in patients who have nonischemic cardiomyopathy and an EF of 30% or less, in NYHA FC I with OMT (Class IIb recommendation; C level evidence) [1]. Even the patient is asymptomatic and stable, even at low EF, the patients are under tremendous pressure and risk of clinical deterioration or decompensation when any precipitating factor strucks.

Prevention and Treatment of Precipitating Factors

The compensated condition in stage B or C can change quickly when any precipitating factor tips over the precarious clinical balance (Table 8.9). This is why prevention of any precipitating or aggravating factor is the second most important strategy in this group of asymptomatic patients. The goal is to keep the patient asymptomatic as long as possible and it is an achievable goal.

Table 8.9 Precipitating factors of heart failure.

1. Infection
2. Brady- or tachyarrhythmia
3. Myocardial ischemia or MI
4. Physical or emotional stress
5. Pulmonary embolism
6. High-output states such as anemia, thyrotoxicosis, Paget's disease, pregnancy, Beriberi and arteriovenous fistula
7. Cardiac infection and inflammation (myocarditis, infective endocarditis)
8. Comorbidities (renal, liver, thyroid, respiratory insufficiency)
9. Cardiac toxin (chemotherapy, cocaine, alcohol etc.)

MI, myocardial infarction.

Reversal of Cardiac Structural Abnormalities

It is important to correct the underlying disease which causes ventricular remodeling such as CAD, arrhythmias, ETOH, etc, because the LV remodeling could be reversed and the disease progression stopped. The evidence that treatment with BB reversed the LV remodeling is shown in the REVERT trial [23]. Can cardiac resynchronization therapy (CRT) delay the progression of HF?

Evidence-based Medicine: The REVERT trial

In the Reversal of Ventricular Remodeling With Toprol-XL trial, asymptomatic patients with LV systolic dysfunction were randomized to metoprolol 25 mg titrated over 2 months to a target dose of 50 mg or 200 mg or to placebo. With treatment, metoprolol succinate produced dose-dependent decrease in heart rate but no consistent changes in systolic blood pressure. At 12 months, the results showed that the mean change (mL/m^2) of the LV end-systolic volume index was −14.5% and LV EF + 6% from baseline. They were dose-dependent and greatest with 200 mg metoprolol [23].

LV remodeling (dilation or hypertrophy) is considered detrimental; this is why reversal of LV dilation is an ideal goal and concrete evidence of treatment success. The LV dilation can be transient or disappears after a few months. The list of conditions in which remodeling can be reversed is in Table 8.10.

Table 8.10 Conditions in which ventricular remodeling could be reversed.

1. Viral cardiomyopathy
2. Post partum cardiomyopathy
3. Atrial fibrillation induced cardiomyopathy
4. Aortic stenosis with LV hypertrophy
5. Mitral regurgitation with dilated left ventricle
6. ETOH induced dilated cardiomyopathy
7. Dilated left ventricle from metabolic syndrome
8. LV hypertrophy after long standing uncontrolled HTN
9. Stress-induced cardiomyopathy
10. Tachycardia mediated-cardiomyopathy
11. Nutritional deficiency: beriberi, selenium deficiency
12. Metabolic causes: hypocalcemia, hypophosphate
13. Endocrine disorders: hypo- and hyperthyroidism

ETOH, alcohol; HTN, hypertension; LV, left ventricular.

Stage C: Patient With Symptomatic Heart Failure

In this stage C, patients had or have clinical symptoms and signs of HF. The goal of management is to ameliorating the symptoms, preventing deterioration and reducing mortality by treating underlying diseases, and eliminating any exacerbation factors. The patients in stage C can be: (1) an minimally symptomatic, well compensated HF patient who is being followed up at the office; (2) a hospitalized patient with a first acute decompensated HF (ADHF); (3) a patient with frequent relapses of decompensated HF (acute on chronic HF); or (4) a patient with chronic compensated HF and very low EF in the outpatient setting of a dedicated HF clinic (see Table 8.2).

Management of Stage C Well Compensated Heart Failure Patients in Office

In the history and physical examination, the symptoms and signs of HF are observed to be clustered into two groups due to: (1) fluid retention; or (2) low cardiac output (hypoperfusion). Fluid retention is frequently the earliest sign or symptom of HF prompting the patient to seek medical attention. Fluid retention in different organs gives out different signs and symptoms such as shortness of breath (lungs congestion and edema), fullness or pain in the right upper quadrant, no energy (liver congestion), fullness or pain in the left upper quadrant (spleen congestion), bloating sensation (mesenteric edema), easy fullness after a small meal (edema in the stomach), heaviness in the abdomen area (thickening of the abdominal wall due to fluid infiltration), etc.

Inappropriate low cardiac output or hypoperfusion would present as decreased exercise tolerance, easy fatigue, sleepiness, lack of energy (no pep) or poor sense of well-being (don't feel good) due to generalized hypoperfusion. Hypoperfusion can aggravate angina (due to myocardial hypoperfusion) or cause syncope, presyncope, or lightheadness due to cerebral hypoperfusion.

CLINICAL PEARLS

How to detect fluid retention in patients without rales or leg edema?

In a well managed patient with HF or in patient with HF at early stage, it is rare to see the conventional signs of HF: rales in lungs and leg edema. The earliest sign predicting decompensated HF is the increase of international normalized ratio (INR) in a patient on maintenance dose of coumadin. It can happen in 2–3 days while the patient is totally asymptomatic, before the development of ADHF requiring hospitalization. Then the patient needs to retain 5 liters of fluid in the abdominal cavity or wall before the development of ankle edema. At that time, the abdominal wall is thicker and harder because it is infiltrated with fluid. At any phase of HF, there is a need evaluate the status of fluid congestion in different organs or areas in order to assess the extent of fluid retention or the success of fluid removal following treatment (Table 8.11).

Table 8.11 Earliest symptoms of fluid retention.

Is the appetite bad?
  If it is bad, then there is enough *liver congestion* (differential diagnoses: prerenal azotemia, renal failure, etc.)
Does the patient feel bloated or full quickly after a small meal?
  Mesenteric edema with poor absorption of foods and medication
Does the patient feel lack of energy?
  Liver congestion (differential diagnoses: renal failure, hypothyroidism, low cardiac output, mental depression)
Is the patient aware that he or she has to make an effort to breathe?
  The lungs are stiffer because they begins to be filled with fluid

There is another set of symptoms due to embolic events in the presence of ventricular thrombus.

In the early stage of HF, the signs and symptoms of fluid retention are predominant, while at the later stage, the signs and symptoms of low cardiac output or hypoperfusion are more prominent, especially in patients who are well treated and had no excessive fluid retention.

The management of an asymptomatic or mildly symptomatic, well compensated, first time diagnosed HF patient while being followed up at the doctor's office consists of life style change, reinforcement of patient instruction and medications (Table 8.12).

At this stage the patient needs to understand the importance and priority rank of each modality of treatment or medications, to understand the signs and symptoms of worsening or improving HF and to be able to modify the components of the treatment regimen accordingly. Many patients with the first occurrence of HF have to decrease their level of activities, do not realize the severity of their HF or due to psychological denial, could rebel against medical advices and stop some or all medications. So the focus of this stage is to educate the patient on the cause and treatment of HF, start lifestyle change, treat risk factors and reinforce medical treatment regimen.

Table 8.12 Management of patients with heart failure (Stage C).

1. Treat underlying etiologies
   Treat underlying disease: HTN, DM, CAD, cardiomyopathy
   Eliminate exacerbating factors: ETOH, smoking, salty foods, high fluid intake, uncontrolled atrial or ventricular arrhythmias
   Lifestyle change: No alcohol, no cigarette, exercise, low sodium, low cholesterol diet, fluid restriction, weight loss program
2. Medications to prevent functional deterioration
   ACEI, BB
3. Medications to reduce mortality
   ACEI, BB, ARB, hydralazine-ISDN, aldosterone antagonists
4. Medications to control symptoms
   ACEI, BB, ARB, digoxin, diuretics
5. Medications to avoid
   Most antiarrhythmic drugs, most calcium channel blocker, thiazolidinediones, non-steroidal anti-inflammatory drug, tri-cyclic antidepressant, antihistamines, herbal medicine (ephedrine, Ma huang)

ACEI, angiotensin converting enzyme inhibitors; ARB, angiotensin II receptor blockers; BB, β-blockers; CAD, coronary artery disease; DM, diabetes mellitus; ETOH, alcohol; HTN, hypertension; ISDN, isosorbide dinitrate.

Table 8.13 Performance indicators of comprehensive care in the office setting.

1. LV systolic function assessment and documentation in chart
2. Change of body weight at each visit
3. Blood pressure measurement at each visit
4. Completion of a physical examination pertaining to volume status
5. Assessment of functional capacity and activity level
6. Presence or absence of exacerbating factor: unstable CAD, uncontrolled HTN, new or worsening valvular disease
7. Patient understanding of and compliance with sodium restriction
8. Patient understanding of and compliance with medical regimen
9. History of arrhythmia, syncope, presyncope, or palpitation
10. β-blockers
11. ACEI or ARB
12. Implantable cardiovert defibrillator if EF <35% or indicated when symptomatic
13. CRT in patient with ventricular dysynchrony
14. Warfarin for atrial fibrillation

ACEI, angiotensin converting enzyme inhibitor; ARB, angiotensin receptor blocker; CAD, coronary artery disease; CRT, cardiac resynchronization therapy; EF, ejection fraction; HTN, hypertension; LV, left ventricular.

Performance Assessment

As HF is the manifestation of a long and complex process, the management of these patients needs also to be comprehensive. In order to guarantee the best care for these HF patients, the ACC and the Heart Failure Society of America (HFSA) guidelines suggested a check list of essential steps assuring the completeness of treatment. It is shown in Table 8.13 [24].

Management of Stage C Heart Failure Patients in the First Few Hospitalizations

Any patients with HF for whom the symptoms or signs could not be corrected safely in an outpatient setting, and monitored on the phone, should be hospitalized. Once the patient is admitted, besides the mandatory investigation of precipitating events, the patients with high mortality risk should be identified so the management could be more focused on these patients for better reduction in morbidity and mortality.

CRITICAL THINKING

Identification of the high mortality patient by the ADHERE registry.
The Acute Decompensated Heart Failure National Registry analyzed data of patients hospitalized with ADHF. The first 33,046 hospitalizations (derivation cohort) were analyzed to develop the model and then the validity of the model was prospectively tested using data from 32,229 subsequent hospitalizations (validation cohort). The main outcome measures are variables predicting mortality in ADHF. The results indicated that the best single predictor for mortality was high admission levels of blood urea nitrogen (BUN) ($\geq$43 mg/dL) followed by low admission systolic BP ($<$115 mmHg) and then by high levels of serum creatinine ($\geq$2.75 mg/dL). A simple risk tree identified patient groups with mortality ranging from 2.1% to 21.9% [25].

The reason for high mortality in patients with high BUN and creatinine is probably because the compensatory mechanism of the cardiovascular system in maintaining a balanced fluid status is overwhelmed. This failure is manifested as clinical decompensation (reason for hospitalization) at the expense of decreased renal function even on maximal dose of diuretics. This increased BUN and creatinine is also a sign of severe or advanced HF.

Urgent Therapy

As the patient is admitted to the emergency room or the intermediate cardiac care unit due to ADHF, early edema or frank pulmonary edema, the patients should be given intravenous (IV) diuretics to relieve the lung congestion and shortness of breath (SOB). If the patient does not respond quickly and completely to IV diuretics, then IV nesiritide would help to decrease the pulmonary artery pressure and relieve the SOB within a few hours of infusion.

CRITICAL THINKING

The VMAC trial. The Vasodilation in the Management of Acute CHF trial is a multicenter, randomized, controlled evaluation of nesiritide in 489 hospitalized patients with ADHF. Patients were randomized to one of three treatment groups (placebo, nesiritide, nitroglycerin). The primary end points included pulmonary capillary wedge pressure and dyspnea evaluation at 3 hours. Patients receiving nesiritide, but not IV nitroglycerin, had significantly reduced pulmonary capillary wedge pressure vs. placebo at 3 hours regardless of β-blocker use [26].

Guidelines of the Heart Failure Society of America About Short Term Vasodilator

In the absence symptomatic hypotension, IV nitroglycerin, nitroprusside, or nesiritide may be considered as an addition to diuretic therapy for rapid improvement of congestive symptoms in patients admitted with ADHF. Frequent blood pressure monitoring is recommended with these agents (strength of evidence: B).

These agents should be decreased in dosage on discontinued if symptomatic hypotension develops (strength of evidence: B). Reintroduction in increasing doses may be considered once symptomatic hypotension is resolved (strength of evidence: C).

Intravenous vasodilators (nitroprusside, nitroglycerin, or nesiritide) may be considered in patients with ADHF and advanced HF who have persistent severe HF despite aggressive treatment with diuretics and standard oral therapies (strength of evidence: C) [24].

CRITICAL THINKING

A pooled analysis of RCTs on Nesiritide. This is a retrospective meta-analysis of data collected from primary reports of completed clinical trials obtained from the US Food and Drug Administration (FDA), the study sponsor (Scios Inc), a PubMed literature search using the terms nesiritide, clinical trials, and humans, and a manual search of the data presented at the annual meetings of 3 heart associations. Of 12 randomized controlled trials evaluating nesiritide, three were selected because they met all inclusion criteria of this review: randomized double-blind study of patients with acutely decompensated HF, therapy administered as single infusion ($\geq$6 hours), inotrope not mandated as control, and reported 30-day mortality. In these three trials, 485 patients were randomized to nesiritide and 377 to control therapy. Death within 30 days tended to occur more often among patients randomized to nesiritide therapy (35 [7.2%] of 485 vs. 15 [4.0%] of 377 patients; risk ratio from meta-analysis, 1.74; 95%CI, 0.97–3.12; P = 0.059; and hazard ratio after adjusting for study, 1.80; 95%CI, 0.98–3.31; P = 0.057). The conclusions speculated that nesiritide may be associated with an increased risk of death after treatment for acutely decompensated heart failure when compared with noninotrope-based control therapy [27].

The lead author reviewed the paper and is not convinced about the methodology of the study outlined above (Sackner-Bernstein *et al.* 2005 [27]). It is a retrospective meta-analysis. Out of 12 trials, three were selected. Out of many thousands of patients in the 12 randomized trials, 485 patients were selected to represent the nesiritide group and 377 to represent the placebo patients. Just by these selective representations, there was a sense of data bias and manipulation. The selected patients represented a minority of patients of all the RCTs. The analyzed data were not clean data. This author is not convinced of the methodology and so the results of the meta-analysis. All the meta-analyses quoted in this book have more than 10,000 patients each and they are represented as "Emerging trend" boxes. Sackner-Bernstein *et al.* 2005 showed the trend but they are not considered as evidence-based medicine from rigorously controlled randomized trials. The management of acute myocardial infarction (AMI) or acute coronary syndrome (ACS) is not based on a single small trial or a retrospective meta-analysis. The data about AMI and ACS were so much convincing because the data came from both sides of the Atlantic, from both sides of the Pacific, from both north and south parts of the American continent, from small and large hospitals, from academic and community hospitals, from believers and their critics. This author does not believe on data from one source, one RCT and from small retrospective meta-analysis. This is why this author agrees with and congratulates the authors of the meta-analysis for their provocative idea (even I appreciate provocative ideas: however, we have to look at them or at any data, with a critical eye) that the possibility of an increased risk of death should be investigated in a large-scale, adequately powered, controlled trial. This author believes the data of the meta-analysis were not convincing to the authors themselves, (as to everybody who read any retrospective meta-analysis or subset analysis with small number of subjects), this is why the authors of the meta-analysis asked (and all of us too) for a new larger randomized trial.

Management in the First 24 Hours

Within a few hours of admission and after symptomatic improvement, ACEI or BB could be restarted, if the patient is barely congested and if the blood pressure is high enough (>100 mmHg). Other measures include bed rest on the day of admission and ambulation with the cardiac rehabilitation team on the following day, instruction on low sodium diet, fluid restriction and exercise, daily weight, daily check of electrolytes, BUN, creatinine, prevention of deep vein thrombosis and strict documentation of intake and output for a goal of negative fluid balance. After 24 hours of hospitalization, if the patient has symptomatic improvement, continuing excellent urine output and negative fluid balance, the IV diuretic is changed to oral form and the patient is prepared for long term chronic HF treatment with discharge planned in the next 48 hours. The average length of stay in 2005 for an American patient hospitalized with HF is 4.9 days (data from the Center of Medicare and Medicaid Services).

The benefits from BB, ACEI, ARB are evidenced from large RCTs. In a meta-analysis of ACEI for HF, mortality was lower with ACEI than with placebo (23.4% vs. 29.1%), as were the rates of readmission for HF (11.9% vs. 15.5%), reinfarction (10.8% vs. 13.2%). These benefits were observed early after the start of therapy and persisted long after. The benefits of treatment on all outcomes were independent of age, sex, and baseline use of diuretics, aspirin, and BBs [30]. On top of ACEI, BB was tried successfully in patients with NYHA FC 1 or 2, then BB was given again to patients with NYHA FC 3 and 4.

Evidence-based Medicine: The MERIT-HF trial

3391 patients with chronic HF, NYHA FC II to IV, and EF of 0.40 or less who were stabilized with optimal standard therapy. Then the patients were randomized to metoprolol CR/XL, 25 mg once per day (NYHA class II), or 12.5 mg once per day (NYHA class III or IV), titrated for 6–8 weeks up to a target dosage of 200 mg once per day (n = 1990); or matching placebo (n = 2001). After a mean follow up of one year, the incidence of all predefined end points was lower in the metoprolol CR/XL group than in the placebo group, including total mortality or all-cause hospitalizations (risk reduction, 19%; 95%CI 10–27%; P < 0.001); total mortality or hospitalizations due to worsening HF (risk reduction, 31%; 95%CI, 20–40%; P < 0.001), number of hospitalizations due to worsening HF (317 vs. 451; P < 0.001); and number of days in hospital due to worsening HF (3401 vs. 5303 days; P < 0.001). NYHA functional class, improved in the metoprolol CR/XL group compared with the placebo group (P = 0.003) [8].

In this study of patients with symptomatic HF, metoprolol CR/XL improved survival, reduced the need for hospitalizations due to worsening HF, improved NYHA functional class, and had beneficial effects on patient well-being [8]. These patients were at optimal medical therapy which includes ACEI. It is recommended that BB therapy be continued in most patients experiencing a symptomatic exacerbation of HF during chronic maintenance treatment [24].

However, a substantial proportion of patients experienced intolerance or side-effect with ACE inhibitors. The most common causes were cough (72%), symptomatic hypotension (13%) and renal dysfunction (12%), so ARB were tried on these patients with side-effect on ACEI.

So candesartan was generally well tolerated and reduced cardiovascular mortality and morbidity in patients with symptomatic chronic HF and intolerance to ACE inhibitors [29].

Evidence-based Medicine: The CHARM-alternative trial

In the Candesartan in Heart Failure-Assessment of Reduction in Mortality and Morbidity-Alternative trial, 2028 patients with symptomatic HF and LVEF 40% or less who were not receiving ACEI because of previous intolerance, were randomly assigned candesartan (target dose 32 mg once daily) or matching placebo. After 2 years, the results showed that 33% patients in the candesartan group and 40% in the placebo group had cardiovascular death or hospital admission for HF (unadjusted hazard ratio 0.77 [95% CI, 0.67–0.89], P = 0.0004). Each component of the primary outcome was reduced, as was the total number of hospital admissions for HF. Study-drug discontinuation rates were similar in the candesartan (30%) and placebo (29%) groups [29].

The Second Day of Hospitalization

On the second day of hospitalization for HF, the management is focused on titration of oral medications to its optimal dose while the patient is being watched for side effects of medications and monitored for anticipated recovery.

> **CLINICAL PEARLS**
> **Maximize or optimize medical treatment**
>
> - ACEIs are started at low dose and titrated upwards in order to avoid hypotension, especially in patient with hyponatremia. ARBs can be used if patients can not tolerate ACEI.
> - BBs should be started slowly, (e.g. metoprolol 12.5 mg BID) while watching for short term possible worsening of HF, fatigue, hypotension or bradycardia.
> - Diuretic is used to remove excess fluid, relieve the symptoms of congestion and is monitored for continuing excellent negative fluid balance on optimal oral dosage. Low dose aldosterone antagonist (aldactone 25 mg QD) is indicated for remodeling reversal in severe HF while high dose of aldosterone antagonist (Aldactone 25 mg TID) is used to remove ascitic fluid due to excessive aldosterone production by the liver.
> - Digitalis is best when patient has atrial arrhythmia, fibrillation or flutter with rapid ventricular response.
> - African-American patients could benefit from a combination of hydralazine and nitrates for symptom improvement and mortality reduction.

However, some patients with maximal dose of medical therapy do not improve maximally or revert to NYHA FC 2. Is there any other way to improve the symptoms of these patients so they can have a normal life? If they have EF <35%, bundle branch block then there is another option as described below.

Device Therapy for Symptom Improvement and Reduction of Mortality

LV failure can occur when the right and left ventricles fail to contract in a timely physiologic concordance due to conduction delays in the electrical activation of the ventricle (ventricular dyssynchrony). It happens in 15–30% of HF patients with dilated cardiomyopathy and bundle branch block [30].

In order to correct the dyssynchrony between the two ventricles, CRT by biventricular pacing was tried in these patients. At first, the COMPANION study randomized the HF patients for a CRT device with a defibrillator (CRT-D) or a device with CRT pacing capabilities only (CRT-P). The results showed that CRT-D reduced risk of mortality by 36% ($P = 0.003$), while CRT-P reduced risk of death from any cause by 24% ($P = 0.059$) which was not statistically significant [31]. However, the CARE-HF trial proved that CRT reduced mortality and improved morbidities by reducing the interventricular mechanical delay, the end-systolic volume index, the area of the mitral regurgitant jet; increased the LVEF; and improved symptoms and the quality of life [32].

Evidence-based Medicine: The CARE-HF trial

813 patients with NYHA class III or IV HF due to LV systolic dysfunction and cardiac dyssynchrony who were receiving standard pharmacologic therapy were randomly assigned to receive medical therapy alone or with cardiac resynchronization. The primary end point was the time to death from any cause or an unplanned hospitalization for a major cardiovascular event. The principal secondary end point was death from any cause. The patients were followed for a mean of 29.4 months. The primary end point was reached by 39% of patients in the cardiac-resynchronization group, as compared with 55% of patients in the medical-therapy group (HR: 0.63; 95% CI, 0.51–0.77; $P < 0.001$). There were 20% deaths in the CRT group, as compared with 30% in the medical-therapy group (HR: 0.64; 95% CI, 0.48–0.85; $P < 0.002$). Moreover, there was a dramatic improvement at 18 months in plasma levels of N-terminal pro-brain natriuretic peptide (NT pro-BNP), a marker of HF disease severity in the CRT group [32].

Since then, the recommendations of the ACC/AHA guidelines for device therapy are listed in Table 8.14. ICD placement is not recommended in chronic, severe refractory HF when there is no reasonable expectation for improvement. Biventricular pacing therapy is not recommended in patients who are asymptomatic or have mild HF symptoms [24].

Table 8.14 Indications for cardiac resynchronisation and implanted cardioverter defibrillators.

1. CRT is for patients with LVEF of 35% or less, sinus rhythm, and NYHA functional class III or ambulatory class IV symptoms despite OMT and who have cardiac dyssynchrony, which is currently defined as a QRS duration >120 ms (Class I recommendation; level of evidence: A) [1]
2. ICD is indicated in patients with reduced EF who had a history of cardiac arrest, ventricular fibrillation, or hemodynamically destabilizing VT (Class I recommendation; level of evidence: A). It is a secondary prevention
3. ICD is also indicated in patients with ischemic cardiomyopathy, at least 40 days post-MI, with EF of 30% or less, NYHA FC class II or III on chronic OMT (Class I recommendation; level of evidence: A). ICD is also indicated in patients who have non-ischemic cardiomyopathy and an EF of 30% or less, in NYHA FC II or III with OMT (Class I recommendation; level of evidence: B) These indications are for primary prevention [1]

CRT, cardiac resynchronisation therapy; EF, ejection fraction; ICD, implanted cardioverter defibrillators; LVEF, left ventricular ejection fraction; MI, myocardial infarction; OMT, optimal medical therapy.

The Third Day of Hospitalization

The preparations for discharge require thorough review of the chart with emphasis on all the laboratory results, medications and level of exercise. Then the patient, patient's caregivers and family members should be prepared and instructed on medications, diet, exercise, symptoms and signs of deterioration of HF and preventive measure for relapse.

The Day of Discharge

On this important day, the HF patients are checked for the last time before discharge (Table 8.15).

Table 8.15 Checklist before discharge.

1. All exacerbating factors have been addressed
2. Near optimal volume status
3. Oral medication regimen stable for 24 hours
4. Ambulation acceptable for NYHA FC 2
5. Patient and family instruction completed
6. Follow-up office visit scheduled
7. Home health set up and ready (scale at home, visiting nurse follow-up arranged)

Performance Assessment

In order to ensure that the patient received comprehensive therapy for HF, the American College of Cardiology issued a checklist of performance indicators for HF before being discharged. These local results are compared with the national level which serves as benchmark set by the Center of Medicare and Medicaid Service (Table 8.16). The complete instructions in item **5** of Table 8.16 include activity level, diet, discharge medications, follow-up appointment, weight monitoring, and what to do if symptoms worsen [1].

Table 8.16 Performance indicators for hospitalized heart failure patients.

Indicator	*Benchmark for 2005*
1. EF documented in chart	55.42%
2. ACEI and BB given at discharge	81.81%
3. Smoking cessation teaching	79.19%
4. Anticoagulant if the patient has AF	80.00%
5. Comprehensive discharge instruction	55.42%

ACEI, ACE inhibitors, AF, atrial fibrillation; BB, β-blockers; EF, ejection fraction.

Management of Stage C Heart Failure With Recurrent Hospitalization

In this stage C, patients had or are having frequent relapses of HF requiring hospitalization. The typical patient at this stage is an elderly patient with severe low EF, with multiple co-morbidities (chronic obstructed pulmonary disease (COPD), chronic kidney disease (CKD), diabetes type 2, HTN, hypercholesterolemia); or a middle-aged (frequently female) patient with severely low EF, limited education, and limited emotional or social support at home. The common causes of relapse are listed in Table 8.17.

Table 8.17 Causes of recurrent heart failure and hospitalization.

1. Non compliance of fluid restriction and insufficient dose of diuretics
2. Sub-optimal dose of BB and ACEI
3. Intolerance to medications
4. Severity of co-morbidities
5. Progression to end stage disease

ACEI, ACE inhibitors; BB, β-blockers.

Lifestyle Change

The patient at this stage C HF used to live alone or with an equally elderly and sick partner (spouse, roommate, friend). Despites many health problems, the patient has to stay mentally sharp and fit in order to balance the budget (on fixed income from a social security check), pay the bills on time at the end of the month (if not the basic services: telephone, electricity, heating etc. could be cut), buy the groceries (so the patient needs to be able to drive a car to the supermarket), prepare the meals for one or two people, and do the house chores (including cleaning, dusting, cutting grass, or shoveling the snow during winter). If the patient relies on meal prepared by others (meal-on-wheel program) then it is difficult to maintain a low salt low cholesterol diet. The patient eats what is delivered. Some patients cannot tolerate or do not purposely maintain a low salt diet or fluid restriction, so the diet and fluid restriction becomes a major problem (what else an elderly patient enjoys in this stage of life? Is it a favorite meal with egg, bacon and Polish sausage? or a puff of a cigarette?). As the patients become older, many become forgetful, do not take medication at all or on time, do not follow a diet. Slowly, the patients could not do all of the housework or chores which can make the HF worse. The patients could move to live with a son or daughter if they have one, or at least the patient could move into a supervised independent adult environment. However, these ideal solutions are the exceptions rather then the rules. So a nursing home becomes the last station of many elderly patients with HF.

Physical Examination

During these hospitalizations, the patient is examined daily to assess the extent of fluid retention and the disappearance of these fluids upon treatment. How to evaluate the extent of fluid retention is discussed below.

CLINICAL PEARLS

Search for fluid retention In patients with severely low EF, the physical examination could show no leg edema. Where is the fluid?

1 Ascite: the patient retains 5 L of fluid before having leg edema.
2 Abdominal wall: with fluid retention, the abdominal wall is thickened with fluid. It can shift with position. With treatment, it disappears slowly.

3 Presacral area: it is a major source of fluid retention especially after a long night sleep.
4 Thigh: it is a major area of fluid retention.
5 Ankle: this is the last and latest part of fluid retention.
6 Genital area: scrotal edema in men and labial edema in women.
7 Pleural effusion.
8 Arm: the backs of both arms can be filled with fluid especially in patients who are in bed for a long time.

Pharmacologic Treatment

As the patients live longer with BB, ACEI and CRT, many patients come with severe progressing end stage HF. The first treatment in this stage is removal of fluid excess with IV diuretic and fluid restriction. Frequent checks of K level, BUN and creatinine are needed. IV vasodilators (nitroprusside, nitroglycerin, or nesiritide) may be considered in patients with ADHF and advanced HF who have persistent severe HF despite aggressive treatment with diuretics and standard oral therapies (Strength of evidence = C) [24].

Digoxin is indicated especially if there is atrial arrhythmia, however, these patients carry higher risk for toxicity. The complete inpatient management of these patients is listed in Table 8.18.

As patients are older and sicker, they need more medications and at higher dose. They need new medications including the aldosterone antagonists or vasodilators (isosorbide and hydralazine). Then they are subjected to more complications or side effects, such as orthostatic hypotention, elevation of BUN or creatinine. So the two strategies in this phase are to give more medications or to optimize the dose of existing ones while at the same time ward off more frequent and severe side-effects.

During the daily visit, besides the daily weight, edema should be looked for diligently in the ankle, calf, thigh, presacral area, abdominal cavity (ascites), abdominal wall and back of arms. The other signs of fluid overload are liver

Table 8.18 Management of severe and recurrent heart failure.

1. Elimination of all medications which can aggravate HF (with emphasis on NSAID, thiazolidinediones, etc)
2. IV diuretics with daily electrolytes, BUN, creatinine level
3. IV vasodilator including nitroglycerin or nesiritide
4. Exercise (restart slowly)
5. New medications on top of BB, ACEI, CRT: hydralazine-ISDN, aldosterone antagonists
6. Enrollment in a HF clinic for daily follow-up after discharge
7. Nursing home care
8. Referral to cardiac transplant program
9. Ultrafiltration (investigational)

ACEI, ACE inhibitors; BB, β-blockers; BUN, blood urea nitrogen; CRT, cardiac resynchronisation therapy; HF, heart failure; ISDN, isosorbide dinitrate; IV, intravenous; NSAID, nonsteroidal anti inflammatory drug.

CLINICAL PEARLS

Diuretic efficacy At first, in the urgent setting of inpatient care, IV diuretic should be given. If the effect is not optimal, with less than maximal diuresis, IV diuretics can be increased to twice or three times per day for more diuresis and less physiologic perturbation than larger single doses. Changing the usual furosemide to torsemide may be considered in patients in whom poor absorption of oral medication or erratic diuretic effect may be present, particularly those with right-sided HF and refractory fluid retention despite high doses of other loop diuretics. Addition of chlorothiazides or metolazone, once or twice daily, should be considered in patients with persistent fluid retention. Metolazone is more potent and lasts much longer in patients with renal insufficiency; therefore, the dosage and the interval between doses should be adjusted accordingly [24].

If the patient can rest supine for a few hours after ingestion of diuretics, the urine output will increase. If there is slow response from diuretics, this author's experience with nesiritide IV would improve the diuresis without causing too much elevation of BUN and creatinine, while clearly improve the congestion symptoms of patients.

and spleen enlargement, hepato-jugular refux, jugular vein distention, and rale in the lungs.

Aldosterone Antagonist

Plasma aldosterone levels may be elevated 20-fold in patients with HF. This effect is due to increased production by the adrenal glands, which are stimulated by high plasma angiotensin concentrations, and to decreased hepatic aldosterone clearance secondary to hepatic hypoperfusion.

Evidence-based Medicine: The RALES trial

1663 patients with severe HF and a LVEF <35% and who were being treated with an ACEI, a loop diuretic, and in most cases digoxin were randomly assigned to receive 25 mg of spironolactone daily, or to receive placebo. After a mean follow-up period of 24 months, there were 46% deaths in the placebo group and 35% in the spironolactone group (relative risk of death, 0.70; 95% CI, 0.60–0.82; $P < 0.001$). This 30% reduction in the risk of death among patients in the spironolactone group was attributed to a lower risk of both death from progressive HF and sudden death from cardiac causes. The frequency of hospitalization for worsening HF was 35% lower in the spironolactone group than in the placebo group ($P < 0.001$). In addition, patients who received spironolactone had a significant improvement in the symptoms of heart failure, as assessed on the basis of the NYHA FC ($P < 0.001$) [12].

Blockade of aldosterone receptors by spironolactone, in addition to standard therapy, substantially reduces the risk of both morbidity and death among patients with severe HF. The dosage for HF is low: 25 mg/daily, while the diuretic dosage in patients with ascites is higher at 25–50 mg TID. According to the HFSA, aldosterone antagonist is recommended for patients with NYHA class IV or class III, previously class IV, HF from LV systolic dysfunction (LVEF = 35%) while receiving standard therapy, including diuretics. It should be considered in patients after acute MI, with clinical HF signs and symptoms and an LVEF <40%. Patients should be on standard therapy, including an ACEI (or ARB) and a β-blocker. It is not recommended when creatinine is >2.5 mg/dL (or creatinine clearance is <30 mL/min), or serum potassium is >5.0 mmol/L or in conjunction with other potassium-sparing diuretics. Serum potassium concentration should be monitored frequently following initiation or change in an aldosterone antagonist [24]. For African-Americans, there is another option: they may benefit from a combination of venous and arterial dilators.

Evidence-based Medicine: The A-HeFT trial

The African-American Heart Failure Trial evaluated the effects of isosorbide dinitrate (ISDN) plus hydralazine at a total daily dose of up to 120 mg ISDN and 225 mg hydralazine compared with placebo in 1050 African-American patients with NYHA functional class II–IV HF (mean age ~57 years; mean LVEF ~24%). Diuretics were given in ~90% of patients, ACE inhibitors in ~70%, BBs in ~74%, carvedilol in ~55%, and digoxin in ~59%. The results showed a significantly lower mortality rate in patients randomized to ISDN-hydralazine (6.2%) compared with placebo (10.2%; $P = 0.02$), ($P < 0.001$), and a statistically significant improvement of quality of life in response to the Minnesota Living with Heart Failure questionnaire [13].

With the results of the A-HeFT trial, the ACC and AHA guidelines suggested to use ISDN plus hydralazine in African-Americans patients and non-African-American who remain symptomatic despites maximal therapy with BB and ACEI.

Complications in the Treatment of Patients With Severe Heart Failure

At this stage, a patient with HF takes an average of nine medications a day: BB, ACEI, diuretic, digoxin, ASA, nitroglycerin, statin, aldosterone antagonist, and for African-American patients, hydralazine-ISDN, etc. (besides K, medication of diabetes, COPD etc.). The occurrence of side effects or the non-compliance are due to multiple medications, complex multiple daily dosing, and need of frequent adjustment with titration or holding one drug at a time. What the problems are and how to handle them is discussed in Table 8.19.

Table 8.19 Complication of treatment in patients with heart failure Stage C.

1. Increased BUN and creatinine
2. Hypotension
3. Dizziness
4. Polypharmacy
5. Destabilizing co-morbidities

BUN, blood urea nitrogen.

Increased BUN and Creatinine

As more patients survive into advanced stages of HF, it is increasingly difficult to maintain optimal fluid balance with high dose of diuretics while preserving renal function. Usually creatinine increased 0.3 mg/dL or proportional rises of 25% following diuresis in more than 20% of HF hospitalisations [33]. Worsening renal function limits symptomatic and neuro-hormonal therapy, lead to longer hospital stay, and predict higher rate of early rehospitalization and death. At this late stage of HF, the problem is multiple hospitalizations for congestion, with diuresis interrupted each time because of increasing levels of creatinine. The present treatment of increased BUN and creatinine continues to be decreasing dose or discontinuation of diuretics on top of more liberal fluid intake.

CLINICAL PEARLS

How to manage elevation of BUN and creatinine? In many instances, the HF patients can stay asymptomatic with a baseline level of BUN and creatinine in the high-normal or a little higher level. This is also the way to be sure the patient is dry enough or the patient benefits the most from optimal dosage of diuretics: the BUN and creatinine level is at its high-normal or a little above that level. Once the BUN and creatinine increases higher, the first therapeutic strategy is to hold diuretics, if the ratio of BUN/creatinine increases <50% and the patient is not congested. Cut the dose of ACEI in half if the BUN/creatinine ratio increases more than 50%. Stop ACEI if the ratio increases more than 100%. If the problem persists, change ACEI to ARB. In the experience of this author, the patient could have good diuresis without increasing BUN and creatinine when the patient is receiving diuretics under coverage of nesitiride.

It is very comforting to see the patients improving symptomatically and clinically. The increased BUN and creatinine, which requires discontinuation of diuretics and liberal fluid intake, is a contradiction in the treatment of patient with fluid retention. It also prolongs the length of stay. So with nesiritide coverage, diuresis can be better. Without the headache of increasing BUN and creatinine, is there another way to remove fluid quickly without causing problems?

CRITICAL THINKING

Ultrafiltration for higher urine output without Increasing BUN and creatinine. Some patients with ADHF manifested by volume overload, with clinical evidence of renal insufficiency or somewhat loosely defined diuretic resistance, underwent ultrafiltration (UF) and improved with euvolemia and early discharge (≤3 days) without adverse effects. UF was continued until the patients achieved relief of their presenting symptoms of congestion. The removal of fluid was aggressive, with an average fluid removal of 8.6 ± 4.2 L and a mean decrease in weight of approximately 6 kg at discharge. As expected with the removal of fluid and solute, clinical signs and symptoms and laboratory indices of hypervolemia improved by discharge. Another important effect of UF is a decrease in neurohormonal activity, manifested by declining levels of renin, norepinephrine, and aldosterone, as opposed to the effects seen with diuretic therapy [34].

Destabilizing Co-morbidities

As a patient lives longer, other co-morbidities can appear or become more severe or prominent. The list of co-morbidities and their problems is shown in Table 8.20. Once the co-morbidities are under control, then the HF symptoms can also be kept under control. However, if the problems with co-morbidities are not resolved, a stable HF can become decompensated.

Table 8.20 Co-morbidities and differential diagnoses in patients with heart failure.

Myocardial ischemia	Depression
Venous stasis	Hypoalbuminemia
Malnutrition	Renal failure
Obesity	Deconditioning
Hepatic failure	Anemia
Anxiety and hyperventilation syndromes	
Pulmonary disease (pneumonia, asthma, chronic obstructive pulmonary disease, pulmonary embolus, primary pulmonary hypertension, sleep-disordered breathing).	

CLINICAL PEARLS

Controlling co-morbidities In patients with DM, DM should be well controlled: HbA1c should be less than 7%, no thiazolidinediones if there is sign of congestion, body weight within 15% of ideal, no hypo- or hyperthyroidism.

- In patients with HF and COPD, the patient should stop smoking, live in a smoke-free environment, have influenza/pneumonia vaccine, aggressive prevention of flu and early treatment of upper respiratory infection, have any sleep apnea checked and treated, bronchodilator and 24-hour oxygen use if needed.
- For patients with arthritis, the patients should avoid use of NSAIDs, keep weight 15% of ideal and exercise regularly. Control BP well. Uncontrolled BP could aggravate the HF symptoms.
- Some patients came because of new onset of AF or recurrent PAF, then the ventricular response of AF has to be controlled. In other way, AF should be converted to regular sinus rhythm, if it can be done.

CLINICAL PEARLS

How to differentiate SOB from severe COPD and SOB from HF? At this stage, many HF patients also have severe COPD. The patient arrives to the hospital with increased SOB, even on oxygen 24 hours a day. The questions to ask are about fatigue and SOB (Table 8.21).

Table 8.21 Differential diagnosis of SOB from heart failure
or cronic obstructed pulmonary disease.

Symptom	HF	COPD
Fatigue at low level of activity	++	(−)
Fatigue at rest	(+++)	(−)
Fatigue first with activity	(+)	(−)
Shortness of breath first with activity	(−)	(+)

Maximize Medical Therapy

Once the patient is given BB or ACEI/ARB, the question is how much medication is enough. For the purist, the way is to use the same dosage as in the CRT; however, for others, if the BP is decreased to a little above 100 mmHg or the heart rate to the 60 bpm, then the patient has enough BB or ACEI. At this BP, some patients complain of feeling dizzy. How should one handle the problem?

CLINICAL PEARLS

Titration of medication in patients with hypotension The first thing to do is to confirm orthostatic hypotension (decrease of >15 mmHg) after standing for 2 minutes. Then diuretics can be discontinued if congestion is under control. The time of taking BB or ACEI should be at least 2 hours from each other; or long-acting BB (Toprol XL) can be given before going to sleep while ACEI is given in the morning. Every effort has to be made so that BB and ACEI should not be discontinued. ACEI can cause significant hypotension in patients with low sodium.

There are other options including: CRT, treatment of anemia, or statins, and avoidance of any situation or drug which can aggravate HF.

CRITICAL THINKING

Statin for Heart Failure. 54960 Medicare beneficiaries who were hospitalized with a primary discharge diagnosis of HF were evaluated. 16.7% of these patients received statins on discharge. In a Cox proportional-hazards model that took into account demographic, clinical characteristics, treatments, physician specialty, and hospital characteristics; discharge statin therapy was associated with significant improvements in 1- and 3-year mortality (hazard ratio 0.80; 95% CI, 0.76–0.84; and hazard ratio, 0.82; 95% CI, 0.79–0.85, respectively). Regardless of total cholesterol level or coronary artery disease status, statin therapy was associated with significant differences in mortality [35].

Discharge Planning

In the treatment of severe HF, the main strategy during follow-up for patients stable enough to be discharged and followed-up closely at home is to keep this status quo condition, by having daily monitoring and earliest prevention of any precipitating factor. The patient is to be kept on maximal dose of BB,

ACEI/ARB if tolerated. The patient is followed-up daily at a HF clinic run by a nurse. Every day, the patient should be monitored by telephone with questions shown in Table 8.22.

Table 8.22 Telemedicine: how to detect at earliest worsening heart failure?

Reminder questions
Did you weigh yourself today?
What is your current daily weight?
Have you taken your medications?

Evaluation questions
Do you have any chest discomfort?
Are you more short of breath?
Does your abdomen feel bloated?
Are you urinating less than usual? Or the same amount?
Are you more tired than usual?
Do you feel dizzy or light-headed?
If there are many "Yes" in the evaluation question set then the patient has signs of possible early deterioration. Prompt intervention is needed with pre-emptive measures:
    Withhold diuretics if vomiting or diarrhea
    Relax fluid restriction regimen when patient has vomiting or diarrhea
    Hold ACEI or BB if dizziness or low BP. Call again from the office in the afternoon if worse
    Take extra dose of diuretic if gain more than 2 lbs. Call again from the office if urine output no higher

ACEI, ACE inhibitors; BB, β-blockers; BP, blood pressure.

Life at Home Alone

Once the patient is stable, if the patient is mentally capable of understanding and be compliant with medical treatment, diet, fluid restriction, exercise (activity restriction), then the chance for being asymptomatic for a long time is high. Once the patient arrives home, the patient needs a lot of social and physical support to recuperate at home. The social support from the family is critical to set up the routine program for medication, exercise, meals, bowel movement, personal hygiene, etc. The problem with depression should be addressed because it can cause non-compliance with medication and diet. Anxiety attacks in patients living alone is also a common reason for decompensation and hospitalization. Without support of a family, the patient will return to the hospital and end up in a nursing home, which could be a blessing because now the patient is forced to be on a low sodium diet with fluid restriction and no heavy house-chores.

REAL WORLD QUESTION: What To Do When the Patient Does Not Do Well Even with Optimal Medical Treatment?

In the US and throughout the world, millions of patients suffer from myocardial infarction and many succumb to the morbidity and mortality of the ensuing cardiac failure, a protracted condition in need of healing. Despite improvements in the understanding and therapy of many stages of cardiovascular disease, there has been little progress in treating HF. While pharmacological agents have been the mainstay intervention that ameliorates cardiac failure through increased contractility or reduction of cardiac workload, these agents do not inherently heal the wounds inflicted by poor perfusion of the affected cardiac tissue. The ischemically injured failing heart lacks contractile myocardium, functional vasculature, and electrical integrity, which has made treatment of the underlying injury untenable in the past. Restoring all of these components at once seems to be an overwhelming challenge. Current options are cell therapy, cardiac transplantation and long term mechanical support. Cell therapy, however, holds the promise of repleting the damaged heart with new contractile cells that can be engineered to secrete concoctions that promote healing by recruiting new blood vessel development or angiogenesis.

Human Myoblast Genome Therapy

Human Myoblast Genome Therapy (HMGT) is a platform technology of cell transplantation, nuclear transfer, and tissue engineering. Unlike stem cells, myoblasts are differentiated, immature cells destined to become muscles. Myoblasts cultured from satellite cells of adult muscle biopsies survive, develop, and function to revitalize degenerative muscles upon transplantation. Injection injury activates regeneration of host myofibers that fuse with the engrafted myoblasts, sharing their nuclei in a common gene pool of the syncytium. Thus, through nuclear transfer and complementation, the normal human genome can be transferred into muscles of genetically ill patients to achieve phenotype repair or disease prevention. Myoblasts are safe and efficient gene transfer vehicles endogenous to muscles that constitute 50% of body weight.

The results of the phase II, first randomized, placebo-controlled trial Myoblast Autologous Grafting in Ischemic Cardiomyopathy (MAGIC) presented at the 2006 American Heart Association Scientific Sessions in Chicago, showed that partly reversed remodeling (heart enlargement) happened in the high-dose treatment group, (about 800 million myoblasts via 30 injections in and around the infarct area). The results failed to show a significant increase in ejection fraction or regional wall motion, however a significant decrease (by 12%–13% from baseline preoperative values) of LV volumes in patients receiving the high dose of cells was documented whereas there were no significant changes in the placebo group. Because LV volumes are predictors of outcomes, this finding might be clinically relevant. Furthermore, ejection fraction was also measured by nuclear angiography in a subgroup of 48 patients and was then found to be significantly increased in those that had received the high dose of myoblasts compared with the placebo group.

Left Ventricular Assist Device Destination Therapy

As the HF patients journey to their end, it is difficult for the cardiologists to reverse, correct the endstage pathological changes of HF. It is also a struggle just to keep the patient comfortable and functionally independent. In this hopeless situation, the Left Ventricular Assist Device (LVAD) Destination Therapy (DT) becomes a viable option since the complication rate decreases significantly compared with the REMATCH study. The rate of sepsis was 8%, and the mechanical failure from the device (LVAD) was only 15%. It is a big jump compared with the REMATCH data thank to many changes in the design of the LVAD and guidelines for infection prevention and treatment [39–41].

These are very exciting times in the development of mechanical circulatory support for patients with advanced or end-stage HF. As there continue to be improvements indevice design, patient selection, and patient management, new devices, and increased awareness of LVADs as treatment option, it is apparent that many patients with advanced HF will have improved survival and quality of life [42].

Take Home Message

For the stage A HF patient: the main message is to change lifestyle and treatment of risk factors in order to prevent ventricular remodeling.

For the asymptomatic stage B HF patient: the main treatments of stage B asymptomatic HF patients with abnormal structural changes emphasize primarily on prevention with healthy lifestyle change (low salt, low cholesterol diet, fluid restriction, exercise and medications (BB and ACEI). Revascularization is indicated if there is reversible ischemia. Avoidance of all precipitating or aggravating factors is very important to prevent any clinical deterioration. ICD implantation is indicated if the EF is still <35% after a few months of optimal medical treatment (including BB and ACEI). CRT is not indicated because the patient is asymptomatic. Medications or any treatment to reverse the structural abnormality (LVH or dilation) are to be pursued aggressively.

For the stage C HF patient after being symptomatic: because the patient is symptomatic for the first time, mainly due to fluid retention, so the shot term treatment is focused on effective diuresis. The patient should have oral diuretic with potassium replacement. Frequent blood tests to check the sodium and K level with BUN and creatinine is suggested. Fluid restriction has to be enforced, because diuretics will not work if the patient does not decrease oral intake. BB and ACEI/ARB are the main pharmacologic treatment for long term stabilization, and delay of disease progression. Eventually as fluid retention is controlled, diuretics can be discontinued or given intermittently or as needed. ICD is indicated if the EF is still <35% after a few months of optimal medical treatment (including BB and ACEI).

For the severe HF patients with multiple relapses: the two criteria for success in the treatment of HF with multiple relapse are: maximal medical therapy especially diuretics; and prevention of complications. During hospitalization while receiving intensive treatment, the patient needs to have the medications maximized (BB, ACEI/ARB, aldosterone blockers, IDSN/hydralazine, CRT and ICD, as needed). The complications need to be addressed include hypotension, dizziness, increasing BUN and creatinine. On the second day of hospitalization, the patient is encouraged to exercise with help. Then on the third or fourth day, instructions are given to patients and family on low salt diet, fluid restriction, exercise, (including avoidance of heavy activities), compliance with medications and office visit. Ideally, the patient is arranged to be follow up daily with a nurse through a dedicated HF clinic.

References

1 Hunt SA, Abraham WT, Chin MH *et al.* The ACC/AHA Guideline Update for the Diagnosis and Management of Chronic Heart Failure in the Adult. JACC 2005;46: 1116–1143.
2 Gersh B. Revascularization Decisions in Heart Failure: Who Needs Viability Assessment? www.cardiosource.com/ExpertOpinions/accel/interviewdetail.asp?interviewID=116 (Cardiosource accessed 5/14/06).
3 The SOLVD Investigators. Effect of enalapril on mortality and the development of heart failure in asymptomatic patients with reduced left ventricular ejection fractions. N Engl J Med 1992;3:327.
4 Packer M, Bristow MR, Cohn JN *et al.*, for the US Carvedilol Heart Failure Study Group. The effect of carvedilol on morbidity and mortality in patients with chronic heart failure. N Engl J Med 1996;334:1349–1355.
5 Packer M, Coats AJ, Fowler MB *et al.* Effect of carvedilol on survival in severe chronic heart failure. N Engl J Med 2001;344:1651–1658.
6 Ramipril. The Acute Infarction Ramipril Efficacy (AIRE) Study Investigators. Effect of ramipril on mortality and morbidity of survivors of acute myocardial infarction with clinical evidence of heart failure. Lancet 1993;342:821–828.
7 Kober L, Torp-Pedersen C, Carlsen JE *et al.* A clinical trial of the angiotensin-converting-enzyme inhibitor trandolapril in patients with left ventricular dysfunction after myocardial infarction. Trandolapril Cardiac Evaluation (TRACE) Study Group. N Engl J Med 1995;333(25):1670–1676.
8 Tepper D. Frontiers in congestive heart failure: Effect of Metoprolol CR/XL in chronic heart failure: Metoprolol CR/XL Randomised Intervention Trial in Congestive Heart Failure (MERIT–HF). MERIT–HF Study Group. Congest Heart Fail 1999;5:184–185.
9 Hjalmarson A, Goldstein S, Fagerberg B *et al.* Effects of controlled-release metoprolol on total mortality, hospitalizations, and well-being in patients with heart failure: The Metoprolol CR/XL Randomized Intervention Trial in congestive heart failure (MERIT–HF). MERIT–HF Study Group. JAMA 2000;283(10):1295–1302.
10 Pitt B, Poole-Wilson PA, Segal R *et al.* Effect of losartan compared with captopril on mortality in patients with symptomatic heart failure: Randomised trial – the losartan heart failure survival study ELITE II. Lancet 2000;355:1582–1587.
11 Cohn JN, Tognoni G. A randomized trial of the angiotensin-receptor blocker valsartan in chronic heart failure. The Valsartan Heart Failure Trial Investigators. N Engl J Med 2001;345:1667–1675.
12 Pitt B, Zannad F, Remme WJ, Cody R, Castaigne A, Perez A *et al.* The effect of spironolactone on morbidity and mortality in patients with severe heart failure. Randomized Aldactone Evaluation Study Investigators. N Engl J Med 1999;341:709–717.
13 Taylor AL, Ziesche S, Yancy C *et al.* for the African-American Heart Failure Trial Investigators. Combination of Isosorbide Dinitrate and Hydralazine in Blacks with Heart Failure. N Engl J Med 2004;351:2049–2057.
14 Shimoni S, Frangogiannis NG, Aggeli CJ *et al.* Identification of hibernating myocardium with quantitative intravenous myocardial contrast echocardiography: comparison with dobutamine echocardiography and thallium-201 scintigraphy. Circulation 2003;107:538–544.
15 La Canna G, Rahimtoola SH, Visioli O *et al.* Sensitivity, specificity, and predictive accuracies of non-invasive tests, singly and in combination, for diagnosis of hibernating myocardium. Eur Heart J 2000;21:1358–1367.

16 Wajg JM, Cwajg E, Nagueh SF *et al.* End-diastolic wall thickness as a predictor of recovery of function in myocardial hibernation:relation to reST-redistribution T1-201 tomography and dobutamine stress echocardiography. J Am Coll Cardiol 2000;35:1152–1161.

17 Allman KC, Shaw LJ, Hachamovitch R, Udelson JE. Myocardial viability testing and impact of revascularization on prognosis in patients with coronary artery disease and left ventricular dysfunction: A meta-analysis. J Am Coll Cardiol 2002;39:1151–1158.

18 Tarakji KJ, Brunken R, McCarthy PM *et al.* Myocardial Viability Testing and the Effect of Early Intervention in Patients With Advanced Left Ventricular Systolic Dysfunction. Circulation 2006;113:230–237.

19 Hohnloser SH, Kuck KH, Dorian P *et al.*, for the DINAMIT Investigators. Prophylactic use of an implantable cardioverter-defibrillator after acute myocardial infarction. N Engl J Med 2004;351:2481–2488.

20 CABG-Patch Trial Investigators. Bigger JT Jr. Prophylactic use of implanted cardiac defibrillators in patients at high risk for ventricular arrhythmias after coronary-artery bypass surgery. N Enl J Med 1997;337:1569–1575.

21 Moss AJ, Zareba W, Hall WJ *et al.*, for the Multicenter Automatic Defibrillator Implantation Trial II Investigators Prophylactic Implantation of a Defibrillator in Patients with Myocardial Infarction and Reduced Ejection Fraction. Circulation 346:877–883.

22 Bardy GH, Lee KL, Mark DB *et al.* Amiodarone or an implantable cardioverter-defibrillator for congestive heart failure. N Engl J Med 2005;352:225–237.

23 Colucci WAS, Kolias TJ, Adams KR *et al.* Metoprolol reverses LV remodeling in patients with asymptomatic systolic dysfunction: The REVERT trial. Recent and late breaking clinical trials. Program and abstracts from the 9th Annual Scientific Meeting of the Heart Failure Society of America, September 18–21, 2005, Boca Raton, Florida.

24 Adams KF, Lindenfeld J, Arnaold JMO *et al.* Executive Summary: HFSA 2006 Comprehensive Heart Failure Practice Guideline. J Cardiac Failure 2006;12:10–38.

25 Fonarow GC, Adams KF Jr, Abraham WT *et al.* for the ADHERE Scientific Advisory Committee, Study Group, and Investigators Risk Stratification for In–Hospital Mortality in Acutely Decompensated Heart Failure Classification and Regression Tree Analysis. JAMA 2005;293:572–580.

26 Publication Committee for the VMAC Investigators Intravenous Nesiritide vs. Nitroglycerin for Treatment of Decompensated Congestive Heart Failure A Randomized Controlled Trial. JAMA 2002;287:1531–1540.

27 Sackner-Bernstein JD, Kowalski M, Fox M *et al.* short-term Risk of Death After Treatment With Nesiritide for Decompensated Heart Failure A Pooled Analysis of Randomized Controlled Trials. JAMA 2005;293:1900–1905.

28 Norman K. Hollenberg. Angiotensin Receptor Blockers: What Is Their Current Status? Medscape Cardiology www.medscape.com/viewarticle/511795 (accessed 5/14/06).

29 Granger CB, McMurray JJ, Yusuf S, and the CHARM Investigators and Committees. Effects of candesartan in patients with chronic heart failure and reduced left-ventricular systolic function intolerant to angiotensin-converting-enzyme inhibitors: The CHARM-Alternative trial. Lancet 2003;362:772–776.

30 Nelson GS, Berger RD, Fetics BJ *et al.* Left ventricular or biventricular pacing improves cardiac function at diminished energy cost in patients with dilated cardiomyopathy and left bundle–branch block. Circulation 2000;102:3053–3059. [Erratum, Circulation 2001;103:476.]

31 Bristow MR, Saxon LA, Boehmer J for the Comparison of Medical Therapy, Pacing, and Defibrillation in Heart Failure for the COMPANION Investigators. Cardiacresynchronization therapy with or without an implantable defibrillator in advanced chronic heart failure N Engl J Med 2004;350:2140–2150.

32 Cleland JG, Daubert JC, Erdmann E *et al.*, for the Cardiac Resynchronization – Heart Failure (CARE–HF) Study Investigators The Effect of Cardiac Resynchronization on Morbidity and Mortality in Heart Failure. Circulation 352:1539–1549.

33 Weinfeld MS, Chertow GM, Warner Stevenson L. Aggravated renal dysfunction during intensive therapy for advanced chronic heart failure. Am Heart J 1999;138(2 Pt 1):285–290.

34 Costanzo MR, Saltzberg M, O'Sullivan J, Sobotka P. Early ultrafiltration in patients with decompensated heart failure and diuretic resistance. J Am Coll Cardiol 2005;46:2047–2051.

35 Foody JM, Shah R, Galusha D *et al.* Statins and Mortality Among Elderly Patients Hospitalized With Heart Failure. Circulation 2006;113:1086–1092.

36 Rigatelli G, Zanon F. Stem cell Therapy for Failing Hearts: There is Something Else Beyond the Cells The Journal of Geriatric Cardiology, 9/2006 (in press).

37 Law PK, Law DM, Lu P *et al.* Review: Human Myoblast Genome Therapy The Journal of Geriatric Cardiology, 9/2006 (in press).

38 Chat Dang. Muscling Up Damaged Hearts through Cell Therapy The Journal of Geriatric Cardiology, 9/2006 (in press).

39 Long J, Kfoury, Slaughter M *et al.* Long term "Destination Therapy" with the Hearmat® XVE Left ventricular Assist Device: Improved outcomes since the Rematch Study (in press).

40 Slaughter M, Deng M. Permanent Mechanical Circulatory support in Frazier OH, Kirklin JK editors Mechanical Circulatory Support. Elsevier 2006.

41 Rose E, Gelinjns AC, Moskowitz AJ *et al.* Long term use of a LVAD for end stage HF. NEJM 2001;345:1453–43.

42 Slaughter M. Destination therapy: A future is arriving. Congestive Heart Fail (in press).

CHAPTER 9

Ventricular Tachycardia

Thomas Bump, Pham Quoc Khanh, Pham Nhu Hung, Ta Tien Phuoc, Abdul Wase and Vuong Duthinh

Introduction

Ventricular tachycardia (VT) is an arrhythmia that originates in the ventricles and presents with wide QRS complexes and a rate greater than 120 bpm. The rhythm may be regular or irregular. The QRS complexes during tachycardia are identical to each other in the case of *monomorphic VT*, and are varying in the case of *polymorphic VT*. Episodes of VT that terminate spontaneously within 30 seconds of their onset are said to be *non-sustained* (NSVT), and the term *sustained* is applied to episodes that last longer than 30 seconds or require therapy for termination. Ventricular fibrillation (VF) is an arrhythmia in which distinct beats are not discernible in the surface electrocardiogram (ECG).

VT can be lethal in one patient and benign in another. The consultant must seek to prevent death from lethal forms of VT without over-treating patients who have relatively benign forms of ventricular arrhythmias. To this end the consultant must assess the present and likely future impact of VT on the patient and weigh the therapeutic options with their risks and benefits (Table 9.1).

Table 9.1 Management strategies for patients with ventricular tachycardia.

1. Make a diagnosis of VT or supraventricular tachycardia on the basis of a 12 lead ECG. If in doubt, treat as VT until proven otherwise
2. Treat VT and its causes on an emergency basis
3. Once VT is controlled, plan for long term treatment and prevention of recurrences

VT, ventricular tachycardia.

However, not all wide complex tachycardias are VT and some can occur at a rate slower then described, particularly in patients who are on anti-arrhythmic therapies. Supraventricular tachycardia (SVT) can mimic VT whenever either bundle branch block or ventricular pre-excitation is also present. It is especially important for the consultant to differentiate SVT from VT because SVT usually carries a more benign prognosis than VT, and because therapeutic options are different for SVT and VT. Table 9.2 lists criteria that have been identified as supporting the diagnosis of VT in a 12 lead ECG of wide complex tachycardia.

Table 9.2 Electrocardiographic criteria suggestive of ventricular tachycardia.

1. Atrioventricular dissociation
2. Absence of RS complex in any precordial lead
3. If there is an RS complex in at least one precordial lead, the interval from the onset of the R-wave to the nadir of the S-wave is >100 msec
4. If bundle branch block is present during sinus rhythm, the QRS morphology during tachycardia is different from the QRS morphology during sinus rhythm

Etiologies

VTs are caused by a variety of mechanisms. Monomorphic VT in a patient with a healed myocardial infarction (MI) is usually due to re-entry near the border of the scar [1]. The VT arising in the setting of digitalis toxicity is probably due to triggered automaticity arising from late afterdepolarizations [2]. Patients with dilated cardiomyopathy are subject to a type of monomorphic VT, usually with a left bundle branch block (LBBB) morphology, that is due to macroreentry with a wavefront that travels down the right bundle branch (RBB), across the interventricular septum, up the left bundle branch, and into the His bundle before starting another circuit [3]. Torsades de pointes (TdP), a polymorphic VT that arises in various settings, may be initiated by triggered automatically due to early afterdepolarizations [4]. The early afterdepolarizations are in turn caused by disorders of potassium or sodium channels. A catecholamine-dependent VT, which typically originates from the right ventricular (RV) outflow tract of patients with structurally normal hearts, may be due to cyclic adenosine monophosphate (cAMP)-mediated triggered activity [5]. The same mechanism may underlie repetitive monomorphic VT, which occurs at rest and usually originates from the right or left ventricular (LV) outflow tract [6]. A verapamil-sensitive VT, which typically originates in the region of the left posterior fascicle in patients with structurally normal hearts, may be caused by re-entry [7]. VF is probably caused by multiple simultaneous re-entrant wavefronts, which might migrate through the ventricles.

Evaluation

All patients with heart disease should be evaluated for the presence of characteristics that reveal a significant risk for lethal ventricular arrhythmias (Table 9.3).

Table 9.3 Characteristics that indicate increased risk of lethal ventricular tachyarrhythmias.

1. LV dysfunction (EF <30 or 35%)
2. Symptomatic congestive heart failure
3. Unrevascularized CAD with myocardial ischemia
4. Hypertrophic cardiomyopathy with any of the following:
   (a) History of syncope
   (b) History of non-sustained or sustained VT
   (c) Markedly thickened septum, greater than 25 mm
   (d) Genetic markers of mutations that are high risk for VT
   (e) Family history of SCD
5. Familial disorders of VT
   (a) Long QT syndrome
   (b) Arrhythmogenic RV dysplasia
   (c) Brugada syndrome

CAD, coronary artery disease; EF, ejection fraction; LV, left ventricular; RV, right ventricular; SCD, sudden cardiac death; VT, ventricular tachycardia.

History

Special attention is paid to eliciting information about the frequency and severity of symptoms, as more aggressive therapy is indicated when the symptoms are more severe. On the other hand, an implantable cardioverter-defibrillator

(ICD) might not be indicated as the only therapy for a patient with frequent episodes of VT, because patients tolerate frequent shocks poorly. Other important historical information includes any clues as to the possible presence of previous MI, ongoing ischemia, LV dysfunction, valvular abnormalities, and family history of VT, syncope, or premature sudden cardiac death (SCD). One must identify any causative factors such as ischemia, drug use (illicit or prescribed), electrolyte disturbances, or excessive catecholaminergic tone imbalance. The consultant must identify what therapies might have already been used for the patient, and with what degree of success they were met.

Other diagnostic measures in patients known to have VT include physical examination, 12-lead ECGs during tachycardia and during sinus rhythm, echocardiogram, stress testing, and cardiac catheterization. Depending on the type of presentation of VT or VF, acute MI might have to be ruled out by serial cardiac enzymes and ECGs.

ECG

The 12-lead ECG during VT is invaluable. It heightens the ability of the consultant to differentiate between VT and SVT with aberrant conduction. It also aids the consultant in determining if a type of VT might be present, such as idiopathic VT arising from the RV or LV outflow tracts, idiopathic VT arising from the inferoseptal left ventricle, or bundle branch re-entry, which might be treated with ablation. Furthermore, the 12-lead ECG during VT can be compared with ECGs obtained during electrophysiologic (EP) studies to determine if VT that is induced during the study is the same as what that the patient had outside the laboratory. In a patient who has had wide QRS tachycardia, the ECG obtained during sinus rhythm should be examined for evidence of bundle-branch block or ventricular pre-excitation (i.e. presence of a delta wave) that would indicate a susceptibility to SVT with aberrant conduction. In a patient with VT, the ECG during sinus rhythm might provide clues of the cause of VT, such as evidence of an acute old myocardial infarction, long QT syndrome, arrhythmogenic right ventricular dysplasia, or Brugada syndrome. Echocardiograms, stress tests, and cardiac catheterization may permit the identification of correctable causes of VT in the particular patient.

Ejection Fraction

Measurement of LV function is particularly important. Good LV function is associated with good prognosis even in patients with non-sustained VT, as long as there are no other markers of high risk. The presence of severe LV dysfunction alone is evidence of high risk for developing lethal VT and can be an indication for placement of an ICD. The Multicenter Automatic Defibrillator Implantation Trial (MADIT)-II and the Sudden Cardiac Death-Heart Failure trial (SCD-HeFT) studies showed that ICDs improve the chances for survival in patients with persistent severe LV dysfunction (LVEF <0.30 or 0.35, respectively) [8,9]. The Comparison of Medical Therapy, Pacing, and Defibrillation in Heart Failure (COMPANION) trial revealed that biventricular pacing defibrillators improve the chances for survival in patients with persistent severe left dysfunction and LBBB [10].

CRITICAL THINKING

Why did the outcomes not improve after implantable cardioverter defibrillator? There have been two studies in which ICDs were not found to help survival of patients with LV dysfunction. In trial CABG-Patch, the patients with LV dysfunction who were undergoing coronary artery bypass were randomized to receive or to not receive an ICD at the time of surgery [11]. In DINAMIT, patients who had LV dysfunction in the setting of recent acute myocardial infarction (AMI) were randomized to receive or to not receive an ICD [12]. ICDs did not improve survival in either of these studies. It is thought that LV function improved sufficiently in enough subjects in these trials to reduce the benefit that ICDs might provide in patients with persistent LV dysfunction.

ECG Monitoring

Patients with unexplained palpitations, near-syncope or syncope should be evaluated to find out if VT is the cause of any of their symptoms. Evaluation of these patients includes electrocardiographic monitoring and provocative testing. Monitoring can be performed in the hospital, or on an outpatient basis with ambulatory electrocardiographic recording, transtelephonic arrhythmia monitor, implantable event recorder, or continuous outpatient telemetry.

Patients with regular tachycardia with wide QRS complex are evaluated in order to determine whether the tachycardia is caused by supraventricular tachycardia with aberrant conduction or by VT. The ECGs obtained during sinus rhythm and during tachycardia are inspected and compared. The diagnosis of VT is made with certainty if atrioventricular dissociation is present during tachycardia, but this finding is apparent in only 21% of ECGs obtained during ventricular tachycardia. Other electrocardiographic criteria have also been found to be very helpful.

Provocative testing might include exercise stress testing, epinephrine infusion to test for long QT syndrome, procainamide infusion to test for the Brugada syndrome, and EP testing.

Genetic testing is available to be used in highly selected patients for the purpose of detecting the presence of a mutation that causes the long QT syndrome or another of the inherited arrhythmia syndromes. When a diagnosis cannot be reached with certainty using the ECGs, EP testing can be definitive, as long as the clinical tachycardia can be induced in the laboratory.

Electrophysiological Studies

An EP study is performed in a specialized cardiac catheterization laboratory that is equipped with a programmable stimulator, EP amplifiers, and recording equipment. These devices are connected to multipolar electrode catheters that are advanced to various intracardiac positions such as the high right atrium, the His bundle position, and the RV apex. The timing of local activation during different cardiac rhythms can be measured from bipolar recordings that are made through closely spaced electrodes on the catheters. Different rhythms may be induced in susceptible patients by provocative stimulation protocols that are delivered through the catheters from the programmable stimulator. The electrophysiologist can then determine if a particular rhythm is VT or SVT with aberrant conduction. Another reason to perform an EP study is to see if a patient has inducible VT. In certain situations, the presence of inducible VT indicates that the patient has an increased risk of developing spontaneous VT, and the absence of inducible VT implies a more benign prognosis.

Strength and Weakness

The predictive accuracy of EP testing varies greatly according to the type of VT that is being investigated and the nature of the heart disease that is present. For example, polymorphic VT can be induced by aggressive provocative stimulation protocols even in patients who are known to be at minimal risk for developing spontaneous VT or VF. Thus, induced polymorphic VT is a non-specific finding of EP studies, particularly when closely spaced triple premature beats are required for induction. The induction of monomorphic VT is usually taken to be a meaningful finding, but induction of very rapid monomorphic VT (in the range of 300 or more bpm) has less specificity than induction of slower monomorphic VTs. The sensitivity of EP for detecting susceptibility to VT is high in patients with LV dysfunction due to coronary disease, and relatively low in patients with non-ischemic cardiomyopathy.

Indications

EP studies can be helpful in defining the level of risk for lethal VT in patients, especially when there might be uncertainty concerning whether an implantable defibrillator might be helpful. In a patient with persistent severe LV dysfunction with EF of less than 35%, an EP study isn't necessary to determine if an ICD is indicated. However, a study of patients with history of MI, non-sustained VT, and EF less than 40%, found that patients with inducible VT have improved survival with ICDs. This suggests that EP testing should be considered in patients with non-sustained VT, history of MI, and EF of 35–40%. On the other hand, EP studies have such a low sensitivity in the presence of nonischemic cardiomyopathy that they are generally not performed in these patients unless syncope, near syncope, or a sustained wide complex tachycardia have occurred. Patients with non-ischemic cardiomyopathy might be better screened for the presence or absence of T wave alternant [13].

Another indication for EP testing is to evaluate the patient for possible cure of the arrhythmia by catheter ablation (discussed below). Candidates for catheter ablation first undergo EP evaluation to determine if VT can be induced in the laboratory and to see if the induced VT is similar or identical to the VT that the patient has had in the past. The hemodynamic status of the patient during the induced VT is evaluated to determine if the patient is stable enough during VT to undergo possibly prolonged efforts to locate the site in the ventricles where a small lesion might eradicate the VT. Testing is performed to see if the patient has multiple forms of VT, which, if present, might render attempts at catheter ablation futile.

EP testing is relatively safe. The chief risks are vessel damage, thrombophlebitis, and perforation of a vessel or the heart. The patient may require electrical defibrillation during the study. The risk of death as a complication of an EP study is approximately one in 10,000. If the EP study leads to catheter ablation, then other risks may be encountered. These risks are discussed below.

CLINICAL PEARLS

Work-up for patients with ventricular tachycardia A systematic approach to the evaluation of patients presenting with VT includes a 2D echocardiography for evaluation of the EF and an evaluation for ischemia, either with a form of stress test, or cardiac catheterization.

1 After revascularization is performed, if indicated, measurement of the post revascularization EF (which hopefully improves) is taken to see whether the patient still needs an ICD.

2 For patients who need an EP study, the results are most reliable in the setting of ischemic cardiomyopathy. They have less sensitivity and specificity, or prognostic value for patients with non-ischemic dilated cardiomyopathy who might be better screened for the presence or absence of T wave alternans.

Therapy

General Principle

Ventricular tachyarrhythmias do not respond uniformly well to a single kind of therapy. Therefore, the consultant must be acquainted with indications for different therapies including anti-arrhythmic drugs, anti-tachycardia pacing, electrical cardioversion and defibrillation, catheter ablation, anti-arrhythmic surgery, and implantation of anti-tachycardia devices.

If the patient is hemodynamically stable, a 12-lead ECG and rhythm strip should be obtained and the diagnosis of VT confirmed from among the other causes of a wide QRS complex tachycardia. The conscious patient with VT does not need to be electrically cardioverted on an emergent basis, but preparations can be made for elective synchronized cardioversion. Intravenous (IV) amiodarone, lidocaine, or procainamide can be administered. Rarely, the consultant may have the option of pace-terminating the episode of VT (e.g., in patients who have temporary ventricular pacing leads in place).

Once an episode of VT has been terminated, the consultant must turn his or her attention to preventing recurrences. Efforts should be made to identify and treat any of the causes of VT. Careful attention should be paid to the most common precipitants of ventricular ectopy, including electrolyte disturbances, hypoxemia, cardiac ischemia, intracardiac catheters, and drugs such as digoxin, aminophylline, and adrenergic agents. To prevent recurrences of

VT, an infusion of an anti-arrhythmic drug can be administered. Typically, the selected drug is the one which successfully terminated the initial episode of VT. The infusion may be necessary for up to 24–48 hours until the cause of the VT has been fully evaluated and managed. Lidocaine is the most commonly used agent in this setting, although it may be replaced by amiodarone or procainamide [14].

CLINICAL PEARLS

What to do when ventricular tachycardia recurs despite standard IV anti-arrhythmic drugs? Occasionally, VT immediately recurs despite the administration of standard anti-arrhythmic agents. In these situations, several options exist.

- High-dose IV magnesium sulfate (eg, 5 g over 4 hours) has been effective in both hypomagnesemic and normomagnesemic patients with intractable VT, in patients with TdP, and in patients with digitalis intoxication [15].
- In patients without digitalis intoxication, this regimen of magnesium administration may produce hypokalemia, necessitating concomitant potassium administration. Contraindications to continued administration include renal failure, a loss of deep tendon reflexes, rise in serum magnesium above 5 mEq/L, fall in systolic blood pressure below 80 mmHg, or pulse below 60 bpm.
- If the underlying cause is ischemia, then coronary angiogram with intervention if indicated would control the ventricular arrhythmias. Intra-aortic balloon pumping can provide dramatic improvement in arrhythmia control, especially in cases where cardiac ischemia underlies refractory VT.
- VT in the setting of slow intrinsic heart rates (sinus bradycardia or AV block) may respond to measures to increase the heart rate such as atropine, isoproterenol, or pacing.

Many patients with VT do not have an easily identifiable or correctable cause of their arrhythmia. Effective anti-arrhythmic therapy for each patient must be identified prior to discharge from a monitored setting. The consultant should not take false encouragement from an absence of VT during monitoring after conversion of an episode of sustained VT; it is the nature of some cases of sustained VT to recur after long periods of remission. As described previously in this chapter, EP testing is often used at this point to confirm that the patient is susceptible to VT and not SVT with aberrant conduction. EP testing is more useful for patients who have had VT or a sustained wide complex tachycardia than it is for patients who have had VF [16]. In the former group of patients, EP testing can identify which patients are suitable candidates for catheter ablation. These include patients with bundle branch re-entry and patients with a single inducible VT that is hemodynamically stable enough to permit careful mapping. Also, ablation therapy is a very reasonable option for patients with idiopathic monomorphic VT.

For patients who are not candidates for ablation therapy, treatment options include chronic oral anti-arrhythmic drug therapy or implantation of an ICD. ICDs have been found to improve survival rates compared to anti-arrhythmic drug therapy in patients with a history of sustained VT or VF [17]. Anti-arrhythmic drugs may be used in combination with ICD therapy in patients with frequent recurrences of VT or VF, to reduce the frequency of shocks from the device [18]. Also, anti-arrhythmic drugs (usually β-blockers, amiodarone, or sotalol) are used as solo therapy in patients with symptomatic non-sustained VT if the patient does not appear to be susceptible to sustained VT.

Anti-arrhythmic Drugs

Anti-arrhythmic drugs are often classified according to their presumed mechanism of action. The chief merit of this classification scheme is to provide a framework for discussing anti-arrhythmic drugs. This scheme, however, has important limitations [19]. For example, a patient may respond well to one anti-arrhythmic drug but not to other drugs from the same class or subclass [20,21]. Also, some drugs do not fit neatly into one class: for instance, amiodarone has characteristics that could place it in Classes IA, II, III, and IV. Quinidine, procainamide, and disopyramide have Class III properties as well as Class IA properties.

CLINICAL PEARLS

Myths and realities of anti-arrhythmic drugs Even when a drug is said to be effective against an arrhythmia, it does not mean that the drug will always suppress the arrhythmia. For example, lidocaine is often said to be effective against ventricular arrhythmias, but in fact it is effective at terminating episodes of sustained VT less than 50% of the time.

For most arrhythmias there is no way to predict if a drug will be effective in a particular patient. Ultimately, an element of trial and error always comes into play.

Anti-arrhythmic drugs all have the potential to cause considerable toxicity. It is not surprising that drugs that can suppress tachycardias can also suppress normal cardiac rhythm, especially in patients with intrinsic dysfunction of the cardiac conduction system. Thus, virtually every anti-arrhythmic drug has been reported to cause sinus bradycardia or heart block. Furthermore, these drugs are notorious for their proarrhythmic effect (i.e., their capacity to cause a new tachycardia to appear in a patient or to exacerbate the pre-existing arrhythmia by causing it to occur more frequently, be more sustained, or be less well tolerated) [22,23].

Side Effects

Several different mechanisms for proarrhythmia are likely. Drugs that delay repolarization may contribute to the appearance of early afterpotentials, which may underlie rhythms ranging from ventricular extrasystoles to TdP, a rapid and dangerous form of VT [24]. Digitalis toxicity probably causes arrhythmias by producing late after potentials [25]. Drugs that slow conduction can stabilize re-entry and turn non-sustained tachycardia into sustained [26]. Drugs with negative inotropic effects might reduce a patient's ability to tolerate an arrhythmia, and increase the likelihood that the tachycardia will degenerate into a more dangerous form. Amiodarone can lead indirectly to sudden worsening of arrhythmia by causing hyperthyroidism.

Some anti-arrhythmic drugs have negative inotropic effects [27,28]. These effects usually are not manifested in patients with normal LV function, but can be devastating in patients with LV dysfunction, particularly those with a LVEF less than 30%. Disopyramide, Class Ic agents, β-blockers, and calcium channel blockers are the most notorious anti-arrhythmic drugs for precipitating heart failure in patients with underlying LV dysfunction. Finally, anti-arrhythmic drugs may have non-cardiac side effects. These range from those that are a nuisance to those that are lethal. Sodium channel blocking drugs (the drugs in Class I and amiodarone) can produce dose-related neurologic effects such as headache, visual disturbances, tremor, and even confusion, seizures, or coma. They also can cause gastrointestinal side effects such as epigastric pain and nausea. β-blocking drugs can exacerbate asthma or can prevent diabetic patients from recognizing hypoglycemia when it occurs. Calcium channel blocking drugs can cause edema, constipation, and headache. Certain individual drugs can cause particular side effects. The side effects of amiodarone are particularly troublesome because the half-life of elimination of amiodarone is as much as several months and therefore side effects persist for a long time and often progress even after the drug has been discontinued.

Pharmacokinetics

The side effects caused by anti-arrhythmic drugs often occur at serum concentrations only a little higher than their minimum therapeutic concentration. These drugs must be administered in such a way as to produce serum concentrations within a narrow therapeutic window. During long-term maintenance therapy, this is usually accomplished by administering enough drug to offset elimination, at intervals equal to the elimination half-life. When anti-arrhythmic therapy is not emergently required, treatment can begin at a low dose, with gradual dose escalation until the desired effect is produced. However, it is common for ventricular arrhythmias to require urgent therapy. Here the goal is to quickly produce a therapeutic serum concentration and, subsequently, to keep the concentration in the therapeutic range. Typically, a loading dose is given to raise the serum concentration into the therapeutic range. At the same time, a maintenance dose is started in order to offset drug elimination. But if only these steps are taken, the patient may be transiently unprotected following the bolus. This is because most anti-arrhythmic drugs follow two-compartment pharmacokinetics, i.e., following a bolus, drugs disappear from the circulation (the central compartment) by two routes: (1) elimination; and (2) distribution into adipose tissue and other sites (the peripheral compartment). A drug leaves the central circulation by the latter route until its concentrate in the peripheral compartment equals the concentration in the central compartment. To keep the serum concentration of a drug within the therapeutic range following a bolus, the consultant should supplement the maintenance dose with additional boluses to offset distribution.

Dosing schedules have been developed for each anti-arrhythmic drug. Use of these schedules should be tempered by an appreciation of how pharmacokinetics might be altered in the particular patient. The dose of an anti-arrhythmic drug should be adjusted with a view to potential interactions with other drugs that the patient might be taking. Also, various disease states can affect the pharmacokinetic characteristics of drugs. The absorption of oral drugs (i.e., their bioavailability) can be reduced by bowel resection, mesenteric ischemia, or congested intestinal mucosa. On the other hand, bioavailability can be increased by hepatic dysfunction, which reduces the extent to which the liver removes orally administered drugs from the portal circulation (i.e., the first-pass effect). Drug elimination can be reduced or even abolished by hepatic or renal dysfunction, depending on the site of metabolism or elimination of the drug. Disease states have a variable effect on the size of the central and peripheral compartments, which are critical determinants of the appropriate size of a loading dose. The usual way to compensate for variability in pharmacokinetics is to monitor for efficacy and side effects and to monitor serum concentrations of drugs. Serum concentration measurements are useful, although the concentrations of active metabolites may not be measured (eg, 3-hydroxyquinidine and 2-oxoquinidinone). Also, serum concentrations of drugs do not reflect the free or protein-bound fractions. α-1 acid glycoprotein, the serum protein which binds most anti-arrhythmic drugs, is an acute-phase reactant, and its serum concentration rises during acute MI, during renal transplant, with malignancy, in the postoperative period, in old age, and in general as a response to any physical stress [29]. As a consequence, in these situations the percentage of drug available to act on the cardiac membrane can be reduced.

CLINICAL PEARLS

How to avoid lidocaine toxicity? Lidocaine deserves special consideration as an example of the importance of pharmacokinetics in anti-arrhythmic therapy. Lidocaine is almost entirely metabolized in the liver, and its rate of clearance approaches the rate of hepatic blood flow. Impaired clearance can be anticipated in the presence of liver disease, as well as during hypotension, low output states, and in the setting of congestive heart failure – conditions in which hepatic blood flow is reduced.

In addition to reducing clearance, congestive heart failure has been found to reduce the central compartment of the volume of distribution by as much as 50% [30,31], and may necessitate reductions in both the loading dose and the maintenance dose.

Lidocaine clearance has also been shown to be reduced in the elderly, during prolonged infusions lasting over 24 hours, and by the concomitant administration of β-blockers (propranolol, metoprolol) and cimetidine.

Signs and symptoms of lidocaine toxicity (confusion) should be watched for carefully in all patients receiving lidocaine infusion, but in particular in those who are receiving high infusion rates (>2 mg/min), or who have any of the aforementioned factors predisposing toward lidocaine accumulation.

Because the half-life of lidocaine is short, when lidocaine toxicity with confusion is suspected, discontinuation of the drug will correct the confusion episode in a matter of minutes.

Amiodarone

Among the anti-arrhythmic drugs, amiodarone, a leading drug for treatment of ventricular and supraventricular tachyarrhythmias, is notable for its relative freedom from causing proarrhythmia. It is metabolized by the cytochrome P-450 subfamily of enzymes to N-desethylamiodarone, which has anti-arrhythmic activity. Amiodarone inhibits the P-450 enzymes, causing increased levels of digoxin, quinidine, procainamide, warfarin, dextromethorphan, cyclosporine, simvastatin, and many other drugs. When amiodarone is administered intravenously, hypotension is the most common side effect, occurring in about 16% of patients. Fatal hepatocellular necrosis has occurred in two patients who received high doses of IV amiodarone. Oral amiodarone can cause pulmonary fibrosis, cirrhosis, hypothyroidism or hyperthyroidism, skin discoloration, visual disturbances, peripheral neuropathy, and ataxia.

Flecainide and Propafenone

Flecainide and propafenone are Class IC drugs that are very potent against ventricular and supraventricular extrasystoles. Since extrasystoles can trigger re-entrant tachycardias, marked reduction of extrasystoles can lead to a significant reduction in the frequency of episodes of tachycardia. On the other hand, these drugs produce slowed conduction in re-entrant circuits, and thereby stabilize re-entry because slower conduction causes the re-entering impulse to be less likely to encounter refractoriness. So, with flecainide and propafenone, episodes of tachycardia might be less frequent but more likely to be sustained. Data from the CAST study suggested that the use of flecainide for the treatment of VT should be best avoided in the setting of coronary disease and decreased EF [32].

Sotalol

Sotalol is an interesting drug in that its levo-isomer has β-blocking effects while its dextro-isomer has Class III anti-arrhythmic effects. Racemic sotalol is used in the treatment of both ventricular and supraventricular arrhythmias. In the Electrophysiologic Study vs. Electrocardiographic Monitoring trial (ESVEM), sotalol was found to have a significantly more favorable effect on survival than any of the other drugs [33]. Sotalol should be used with extreme caution in patients with renal insufficiency or renal failure, as the drug can accumulate rapidly to toxic level in this setting.

Anti-arrhythmic drugs are an important therapeutic option in patients with ventricular arrhythmias. But, these drugs have not been found to improve survival in patients with VT or other forms of ventricular ectopy in the setting of ischemic or non-ischemic cardiomyopathy, compared to best medical therapy (e.g., with no anti-arrhythmic drugs). In these patients, ICD therapy has been found to help survival more than anti-arrhythmic drug therapy. The main roles for anti-arrhythmic drug therapy in these patients are in the acute management of VT in a monitored setting, and in the reduction in frequency of episodes of VT in patients who have ICDs.

CLINICAL PEARLS

Which tachycardia is refractory to anti-arrhythmic drugs? Several types of VT are refractory to direct-current shock or to the usual anti-arrhythmic drugs.

Extreme hyperkalemia (with serum potassium concentration >8 mEq/L) can cause an incessant VT with a sinusoidal morphology. It should be treated with IV calcium (10–30 mL 10% calcium gluconate given over 1–5 minutes), hypertonic glucose plus insulin, and sodium bicarbonate (44–132 mEq, or 1–3 ampules).

Class Ic anti-arrhythmic drugs (flecainide, encainide, and propafenone) cause a similar VT, which occasionally responds to lidocaine but can be highly refractory. Theoretically, this arrhythmia might respond best to hypertonic sodium, which would counteract the sodium channel blocking effects of the Class Ic agent [34,35].

Refractory VT or VF can be the terminal event in patients with truly end-stage heart disease in which mechanical cardiac function is so severely diminished that the patient would not survive even if the VT could be terminated. In this situation the arrhythmia is called secondary VF or VT.

Statins

A few studies have suggested that lipid-lowering drugs may have anti-arrhythmic effects in patients with CAD. The question of whether statins have anti-arrhythmic effects may be answered by exploring the association of statin use with appropriate ICD therapy for VT/VF in the Multicenter Automatic Defibrillator Implantation Trial (MADIT)-II.

EMERGING TREND

Statins in the treatment of ventricular tachycardia in the MADIT-II study

Patients receiving an ICD ($n = 654$; US centers only) in the MADIT-II study were categorized by the percentage of days each patient received statins during follow-up (90–100%, $n = 386$; 11–89%, $n = 116$; and 0–10%, $n = 152$). The results showed that the cumulative rate of ICD therapy for VT/VF or cardiac death was significantly reduced in those with ≥90% statin usage compared to those with lower statin usage ($P = 0.01$). The time-dependent statin: no statin therapy hazard ratio was 0.65 ($P < 0.01$) for the end point of VT/VF or cardiac death and 0.72 ($P = 0.046$) for VT/VF after adjusting for relevant covariates. Statin use in patients with an ICD was associated with a reduction in the risk of cardiac death or VT/VF, and was associated with a reduction in VT/VF episodes. These findings suggest that statins have anti-arrhythmic properties [36].

Non-pharmacologic Therapy

In the management of VT as indicated above, non-pharmacologic therapies are important options. Antitachycardia pacing (ATP) or direct-current shock can be used to terminate episodes of tachycardia, and in some cases pacing can be used to prevent recurrences of tachycardia. These therapies can be delivered by either external devices or by ICDs. Other treatments, which are potentially curative, include catheter ablation and cardiac surgery.

Antitachycardia Pacing

Re-entrant tachycardias are vulnerable to ATP when the re-entry circuit is anatomically defined and there is an excitable gap between a circulating wavefront and its wake of refractoriness. Given these conditions, it is possible for a stimulated impulse to invade the circuit and create a bidirectional block. This will occur if the invading impulse proceeds in both directions in the circuit, clockwise and counter-clockwise. In one direction, the invading impulse collides with and extinguishes the re-entering wavefront; in the other direction, it is itself extinguished when it runs into the wake of refractoriness of the re-entering impulse. ATP cannot terminate VF or polymorphic VT.

The usual technique of ATP is to deliver a train of stimuli at a somewhat faster rate than that of the tachycardia. A train of stimuli is more likely than a single stimulus to produce an impulse that penetrates the re-entrant circuit. With trains of stimuli, however, there is a risk that one stimulus will terminate a tachycardia and a subsequent one will restart the tachycardia. It may be necessary for the consultant to deliver literally dozens of trains of stimuli of different rates and durations, until finally a train is delivered that fortuitously ends with a pulse that extinguishes the tachycardia rather than re-inducing it. As this process may take from ten seconds to a minute or more, ATP is usually used for VTs that do not cause immediate hemodynamic compromise. Also, ATP often causes VT to accelerate or even degenerate into VF. For this reason, ATP must be used only when back-up electrical defibrillation is available. The typical indication for ATP is for treatment of a recurrent re-entrant sustained VT which is refractory to drugs and which does not cause immediate hemodynamic compromise. ATP would be used in preference to electrical cardioversion, since patients much better tolerate the former. Most ICDs have the capacity to deliver ATP as first-line therapy for VT, thereby reducing the frequency of shocks.

Direct-current Cardioversion

Direct-current cardioversion has the broadest spectrum of anti-arrhythmic activity of any therapy. If properly applied, it is nearly always effective against those arrhythmias that are thought to result from re-entry, including atrio-ventricular (AV) nodal re-entrant tachycardia, AV re-entrant tachycardia using a bypass tract, atrial flutter, and most cases of paroxysmal atrial tachycardia and paroxysmal VT. In addition, high doses of electricity can defibrillate the heart, which is not surprising since atrial and ventricular fibrillation probably often arise from a re-entrant mechanism. Finally, direct-current cardioversion (DCC) can terminate TdP, which may result from a non-reentrant mechanism – namely, triggered activity.

CLINICAL PEARLS

Which tachycardia is resistant to electrical shock? DCC is ineffective against tachycardias that arise from enhanced automaticity. Arrhythmias in this category include sinus tachycardia, some forms of ectopic atrial tachycardia, multifocal atrial tachycardia, accelerated junctional rhythm, and even some cases of VT.

Any rhythm that occurs in the setting of digitalis intoxication can be exacerbated by direct-current shock, probably because shocks depolarize sympathetic nerve terminals in the heart, causing them to release norepinephrine, which then accelerates the tachycardia or even causes a more malignant arrhythmia to appear.

Electrical shock can fail to terminate incessant VT that is caused by Class IC anti-arrhythmic drugs (i.e., flecainide, encainide, and possibly propafenone), even though this rhythm is probably caused by re-entry [37]. Arrhythmias that cannot be terminated by cardioversion are often referred to as incessant.

Another VT that is refractory to direct-current shock and to Class I drugs is a rare form of verapamil-responsive VT, which occurs in young patients with no identifiable heart disease [38]. The QRS morphology of this VT resembles right bundle branch block with left axis deviation. This VT provides an exception to the rule that verapamil has no role in the management of VT.

In order to terminate fibrillation, a shock must produce a sufficient voltage gradient throughout the fibrillating chamber to bring all myocardial cells to the same electrical state. When all of the cells within a re-entrant circuit are depolarized, a condition of electrical homogeneity is established that is inimical to re-entry. This is because ongoing re-entry requires that at all times some part of the chamber not be depolarized, so that this part can be next in line to be activated. In order to be successful, a shock must produce a period of electrical homogeneity that persists for a sufficient period of time. In an elegant series of animal experiments, fibrillation was demonstrated to reappear immediately if the period of homogeneity lasted for less than 130 milliseconds [39]. Re-entrant arrhythmias that are more organized, such as atrial flutter or VT, may require depolarization only of the excitable portion of the re-entry circuit. This may explain the clinical observation that less energy and current are necessary to terminate these arrhythmias than is the case with atrial or ventricular fibrillation.

The minimum amount of energy required to defibrillate the heart is called the defibrillation threshold. Even in a single individual, the defibrillation threshold is not a single value but rather is described by a sigmoidal dose – response relationship: the greater the energy in a shock, the more likely it is to defibrillate a given heart [40]. Typical energy thresholds for external defibrillation of the atria or ventricles are between 50–100 J. Defibrillation thresholds for intracardiac electrodes, such as are used in ICD systems, are in the neighborhood of 10 J. Biphasic shocks have lower thresholds than monophasic shocks.

CLINICAL PEARLS

Factors which change the defibrillation threshold There is marked variability from patient to patient in the energy threshold for external defibrillation, mainly because of interpatient differences in transthoracic impedance. The latter has several determinants: interelectrode distance (chest size), electrode size, electrode – chest wall contact pressure, couplant ("electrode paste"), and respiratory phase.

Increases in transthoracic impedance during lung expansion have implications for patients receiving mechanical ventilation and positive end-expiratory pressure.

Impedance declines after repeated shocks, partly because of hyperemia and edema in the current pathway [41]. Since current, not energy, is the determinant of successful defibrillation, an external defibrillator has been developed that automatically delivers more energy when the impedance has been found to be high [42].

Other factors besides transthoracic impedance can influence the defibrillation threshold. Lidocaine, flecainide, and amiodarone have been found to raise defibrillation thresholds significantly [43–46]. Sotalol lowers defibrillation thresholds [47]. Most other anti-arrhythmic drugs have neutral or else very mild effects on defibrillation thresholds. β-agonists and aminophylline lower defibrillation thresholds [48,49]. The duration of VF prior to attempted defibrillation affects the defibrillation threshold in a biphasic manner. The energy requirement may actually decrease after 2 minutes of VF, perhaps because of a favorable increase in extracellular potassium [50]. When VF has persisted for more than 10 minutes, it becomes increasingly difficult and ultimately impossible to defibrillate the heart.

Implantable Cardioverter Defibrillator

ICDs are invaluable for treating patients with VT. These devices can be programmed to deliver different types of therapy for different types of VT, such as anti-tachycardia pacing or direct current shocks ranging from 1–40 J. When a milder treatment fails to convert a tachycardia, the device can proceed to deliver a stronger therapy. The ICD systems include an ICD pulse generator plus one or more leads which have electrodes for sensing cardiac rhythm and for delivery of pacing stimuli or shocks of up to 40J to the heart. The usual current pathway for a shock from the device is between an electrode coil in the RV apex and the can of the pulse generator. Other electrodes may also be employed in the high voltage shocking circuit, such as a proximal electrode coil situated in the superior vena cava, and less frequently electrodes that are located either on the epicardium or subcutaneously. ICDs can deliver anti-tachycardia pacing even while charging internal capacitors in preparation for automatically shocking the heart. After charging, and before shocking, the ICD re-examines the heart rate to see if VT is still present. If VT is recon-firmed, a shock is delivered to the heart. Even ICDs with single leads have algorithms that are able to differentiate SVT from VT, based on the morphol-ogy of the intracardiac signal, suddenness of onset, and regularity of the ven-tricular rhythm. Some ICDs have both an atrial lead and a ventricular lead, which greatly enhances their capacity to distinguish VT from other rhythms such as atrial fibrillation with rapid response, sinus tachycardia, and other forms of SVT. This greatly diminishes the incidence of inappropriate shocks or therapies when the heart rate increases because of SVT rather than VT. Some ICDs offer atrial therapies for treating SVT, atrial flutter, and atrial fib-rillation, in addition to shocking and pacing therapies for VT.

CLINICAL PEARLS

Myths and realities of implantable cardioverter defibrillator ICDs are very effective in preventing sudden death [51]. They have drawbacks, however. ICDs are expensive and require surgery for implantation. The surgical technique is similar to that employed during pacemaker implantation. Surgical risks include bleeding complications, infection, lead dislodgement, and pneumothorax.

ICDs do not always prevent syncope, because it can take 10–20 seconds for the device to complete a cycle of arrhythmia detection, capacitor charging, and shock delivery.

Also, shocks delivered to conscious patients are not well tolerated. Defibrillators, unfortunately, may deliver inappropriate shocks when the patient is not in VT. For example, a rapid ventricular rate during atrial fibrillation or sinus tachycardia can cause the rate threshold for detection of VT to be exceeded, triggering a shock. In fact, the first shock or two may cause the patient enough distress to cause the heart rate during atrial fibrillation or sinus tachycardia to remain elevated so that multiple shocks are triggered.

ICDs can malfunction as a result of lead dislodgement, poor connection between the lead and the pulse generator, lead fracture, or breakdown of insulation of the lead. Rarely, the ICD itself may malfunction because of a flaw in manufacturing. Occasionally, manufacturers have issued recalls or techni-cal warnings and physicians and their patients have had to weigh whether to explant and replace a possibly defective device.

Indications of Implantable Cardioverter Defibrillator

The basis for indications of ICDs is based on the results of clinical trials listed in Table 9.4.

Table 9.4 Implantable Cardioverter Defibrillator indications according to patients' subsets and supported trials.

	Clinical trials
Primary prevention	
Ischemic cardiomyopathy EF <35%	MADIT II and SCD-HFT
Non-ischemic cardiomyopathy EF <35%	SCD-HeFT, DEFINITE
NSVT, EF = 35–40% needs EPS	MUSTT and MADIT I
Secondary prevention	
Ischemic cardiomyopathy	AVID and CIDS
Non ischemic cardiomyopathy	AVID and CIDS

EF, ejection fraction; EPS, electrophysiology test; NSVT, non-sustained VT.

Evidence-based Medicine: The MADIT trial

The Multicenter Automatic Defibrillator Implantation Trial [52] is the first prospective, randomized trial to compare the efficacy of defibrillators with that of conventional medical therapy in patients with non-sustained VT after a previous MI and an EF < 35%. If sustained VT was inducible at the EP study, and was not suppressible by procainamide, then the patients were randomized for ICDs or conventional anti-arrhythmic medical therapy. The 2-year mortality in the medical treatment group (mostly with amiodarone) was high at 32%. ICD therapy reduced the risk of death by 54%. However, further analysis showed that survival with ICD therapy was significantly greater only in the subgroup of patients with LVEF < 26%.

Evidence-based Medicine: The MUSTT trial

In the Multicenter Unsustained Tachycardia Trial Investigators [53] the patients with CAD, an LVEF of 40% or less, and asymptomatic NSVT were evaluated for electrophysiologically-guided anti-arrhythmic therapy. The patients with induced sustained VT were randomized for either ICDs, anti-arrhythmic therapy, or no anti-arrhythmic therapy. The results showed the incidence of the primary end points of cardiac arrest or death from arrhythmia were 25% among patients receiving electrophysiologically guided anti-arrhythmic therapy compared to 32% in patients without anti-arrhythmic therapy (*P* = 0.04). The five-year estimates of overall mortality were 42% and 48%, respectively. The risk of cardiac arrest or death from arrhythmia among the patients with ICDs was significantly lower than that among patients discharged without ICDs. However, there was no difference in the rate of cardiac arrest, death from arrhythmia or overall mortality, between the patients on medical therapy or no therapy [53]. This trial showed that the benefit was totally due to ICDs, rather due to anti-arrhythmic drugs. In fact, the event rate trend was slightly higher with in patients receiving anti-arrhythmic drugs, even the trend was not statistically significant.

Primary Prevention for Patients with Ischemic Cardiomyopathy

A series of randomized trials have investigated the role of ICDs for primary prevention of SCD. First, MADIT and MUSTT found that survival was increased by ICD therapy in patients with history of MI, EF <35% (MADIT) or <40% (MUSTT), NSVT on monitor, and inducible VT at electrophysiologic (EP) study. The MADIT trial found that patients with EF <35%, history of MI, and NSVT on monitor, had an unacceptably high risk for SCD even if they did not have inducible VT at EP testing. So, subsequent trials, including MADIT II, SCD-HeFT, and COMPANION, have not required EP testing to identify high-risk patients. These studies still found that ICDs improve survival in previously asymptomatic patients with severe left ventricular systolic dysfunction. SCD-HeFT and COMPANION found that ICDs significantly improve survival in patients with either nonischemic or ischemic left ventricular systolic dysfunction.

Secondary Prevention for Ventricular Tachycardia or Fibrillation in Patients with Ischemic Cardiomyopathy

In order to study the effects of SCD in patients with witnessed VT or VF, the Anti-arrhythmic vs. Implantable Defibrillators (AVID) trial was conducted. These VT or VF were not secondary to a reversible cause such as an acute MI, proarrhythmia from drugs, or electrolyte disturbance.

Evidence-based Medicine: The AVID trial

This is a randomized comparison of these two treatment strategies in patients who had been resuscitated from near-fatal VF or who had undergone cardioversion from sustained VT. Patients with VT also had either syncope or other serious cardiac symptoms, along with a LVEF of 0.40 or less. One group of patients was treated with ICD; the other received Class III anti-arrhythmic drugs, primarily amiodarone at empirically determined doses. 1016 patients (45% of whom had ventricular fibrillation, and 55% VT), 507 were randomly assigned to treatment with ICDs and 509 to anti-arrhythmic-drug therapy. The results showed that the overall survival was greater with the implantable defibrillator, with unadjusted estimates of 89.3%, as compared with 82.3% in the anti-arrhythmic-drug group at one year, 81.6% vs. 74.7% at two years, and 75.4% vs. 64.1% at three years ($P < 0.02$) [17].

In the Canadian Implantable Defibrillators Study (CIDS), patients with VT, VF or syncope that was deemed to be secondary to arrhythmia, were randomized to ICD or amiodarone [55]. However, after a five-year follow-up, the total mortality with ICD was not significantly reduced compared to amiodarone (8.3% vs. 10.2% per year, $P = 0.142$). There was no difference in arrhythmic death, (3% vs. 4.5% per year, $P = 0.094$). Then the outcome of the high-risk patients in the two above trials was analyzed retrospectively. When separating patients according to ventricular function, the AVID data indicate that patients with a relatively well-preserved EF ($\geq$35%) do not have better survival when treated with the ICD compared with anti-arrhythmic drugs (mostly amiodarone). On the contrary, the patients with lower EF benefit the most from ICD therapy and were associated with better survival [56]. These findings were evidenced again in the CIDS trial, where the patients were classified in four risk quartiles based on reduced EF, advanced age, and NYHA functional class. In the highest risk quartile, a 50% relative risk reduction in death occurred with ICD therapy, when compared with amiodarone. There was no benefit from ICD over amiodarone in the three lower risk quartiles [57]. In all these four trials, is the sickest patients who benefit the most from ICD therapy [58]. In patients with advanced heart disease or severe LV dysfunction, (EF < 20%), the role of heart failure on survival must be considered before recommending ICD [59].

The results of the AVID, CIDS trials provide compelling data to support Class I status of implantation of an ICD as therapy of first choice in patients who have experienced VF or hemodynamically unstable sustained VT [59].

Primary Prevention in Patients Without Dilated Cardiomyopathy

Implantation of ICDs is recommended as a Class II indication for patients who are felt to be at high risk of experiencing life-threatening ventricular tachyarrhythmias, who had experienced no spontaneous episodes, and/or in whom invasive electrophysiology testing is not expected to provide additional prognostic information. This category includes specific inherited conditions associated with a high risk of SCD such the long QT syndrome [60] and arrhythmogenic RV dysphasia [61] under certain circumstances, as well as the Brugada syndrome [62] and high risk individuals with hypertrophic cardiomyopathy [59,63].

Class III indications emphasize on inappropriate use of ICD. They include patients with incessant VT unless controlled with drugs, catheter ablation, or endocardial resection. Similarly, tachyarrhythmias associated with Wolff – Parkinson – White syndrome or VT in the absence of structural heart disease should be treated with antiarrhythmias, catheter ablation, or surgical techniques. Sustained VT or VF in the setting of acute myocardial ischemia or infarction, profound electrolyte imbalance, proarrhythmic drug effects, or other remedial causes does not qualify as indications for ICD therapy [59] (see Table 9.4).

Evidence-based Medicine: The SCD-HeFT trial

RCT

In the Sudden Cardiac Death-Heart Failure trial (SCD-HeFT), 2521 patients with NYHA Class II or III and a LVEF of 35% or less were randomized to conventional therapy for CHF plus placebo (847 patients), conventional therapy plus amiodarone (845 patients), or conventional therapy plus a conservatively programmed, shock-only, single-lead ICD (829 patients) (no pacing for bradycardia). The primary end point was death from any cause. The cause of was ischemic in 52% and non-ischemic in 48%. The median follow-up was 45.5 months. The results showed that there were 29% mortality in the placebo group, 28% in the amiodarone group, and 22% in the ICD group. The number needed to treat (NNT) to prevent one death was 14.

The results did not vary according to either ischemic or non-ischemic causes, however, the benefits of ICD were more marked (and significant only) among patients in NYHA FC II, with an absolute reduction in mortality of 11.9% (NNT = 8). Over 5 years of follow-up, the average appropriate shocks for rapid sustained VF or VT were 5.1% [64].

This indication would greatly simplify the implantation protocol. The results of DEFibrillators In Non-Ischemic Cardiomyopathy Treatment Evaluation (DEFINITE) [65] and SCD-HeFT argue strongly for implantation of an ICD in patients with non-ischemic dilated cardiomyopathy with reduced LVEF and moderate heart failure (NYHA functional Class II and III) for mortality benefits.

Evidence-based Medicine: The DEFINITE trial

458 patients with non-ischemic dilated cardiomyopathy, a LVEF of less than 36%, and premature ventricular complexes or non-sustained VT were enrolled. 229 patients were randomly assigned to receive standard medical therapy, and 229 to receive standard medical therapy plus a single-chamber ICD. Patients were followed for a mean (±SD) of 29.0 ± 14.4 months. The mean LVEF was 21%. The vast majority of patients were treated with angiotensin converting enzyme inhibitors (ACEI) (86%) and β-blockers (85%). There were 68 deaths: 28 in the ICD group, as compared with 40 in the standard-therapy group (hazard ratio, 0.65; 95% CI, 0.40–1.06; P = 0.08). The mortality rate at two years was 14.1% in the standard-therapy group (annual mortality rate, 7%) and 7.9% in the ICD group. There were 17 sudden deaths from arrhythmia: three in the ICD group, as compared with 14 in the standard-therapy group (hazard ratio, 0.20; 95% CI, 0.06–0.71; P = 0.006) [65].

In patients with severe, non-ischemic dilated cardiomyopathy who were treated with ACEI and β-blockers, the implantation of a cardioverter – defibrillator significantly reduced the risk of sudden death from arrhythmia and was associated with a non-significant reduction in the risk of death from any cause [65].

As a result of these studies, the Centers for Medicare & Medicaid Services (CMS) broadened the coverage for ICD implantation. Other data suggest that only subsets of this patient population would truly benefit from such an aggressive intervention, notably the use of T wave alternans to further identify that subset of patients with a depressed EF and CAD that are truly at risk for SCD. The issue becomes more complex as some critics suggest that patients in this category who received prophylactic ICD will not succumb to arrhythmic deaths, but still may die from pump failure, so that overall mortality may not change. In this regard, ICD implantation with devices capable of resynchronization (bi-ventricular ICD) may change the outcome. Clearly, more data are needed to clarify the issue.

Table 9.5 Recommendations for implantable cardioverter defibrillator.

Class I

1. Cardiac arrest due to VF or VT not due to a transient or reversible cause (A)
2. Spontaneous sustained VT (B)
3. Syncope of undetermined origin with clinically relevant, hemodynamically significant sustained VT or VF, induced at electrophysiological study when drug therapy is ineffective, not tolerated, or not preferred (B)
4. Non-sustained VT with coronary disease, prior MI, LV dysfunction, and inducible VF or sustained VT at electrophysiological study that is not suppressible by a Class I anti-arrhythmic drug (B)

Class IIb

1. Cardiac arrest presumed to be due to VF when electrophysiological testing is precluded by other medical conditions (C)
2. Severe symptoms attributable to sustained ventricular tachyarrhythmias while awaiting cardiac transplantation (C)
3. Familial or inherited conditions with a high risk for life-threatening ventricular tachyarrhythmias such as long QT syndrome or hypertrophic cardiomyopathy (B)
4. Non-sustained VT with CAD, prior MI, and LV dysfunction, and inducible sustained VT or VF at electrophysiological study (B)
5. Recurrent syncope of undetermined etiology in the presence of ventricular dysfunction and inducible ventricular arrhythmias at electrophysiological study when other causes of syncope have been excluded (C)

Class III

1. Syncope of undetermined cause in a patient without inducible ventricular tachyarrhythmias (C)
2. Incessant VT or VF (C)
3. VF or VT resulting from arrhythmias amenable to surgical or catheter ablation; for example, atrial arrhythmias associated with the Wolff – Parkinson – White syndrome, RV outflow tract VT, idiopathic LV tachycardia, or fascicular VT (C)
4. Ventricular tachyarrhythmias due to a transient or reversible disorder (e.g., AMI, electrolyte imbalance, drugs, trauma) (C)
5. Significant psychiatric illnesses that may be aggravated by device implantation or may preclude systematic follow-up (C)
6. Terminal illnesses with projected life expectancy <6 months. (level of evidence: C)
7. Patients with coronary artery disease with LV dysfunction and prolonged QRS duration in the absence of spontaneous or inducible sustained or non-sustained VT who are undergoing coronary bypass surgery (level of evidence: B)
8. NYHA Class IV drug-refractory congestive heart failure in patients who are not candidates for cardiac transplantation (level of evidence: C)

AMI, acute MI; CAD, coronary artery disease; MI, myocardial infarction; RV, right ventricular; VF, ventricular fibrillation; VT, ventricular tachycardia. A. Level of evidence A: Data derived from multiple randomized clinical trials. B. Level of evidence B: Data derived from a single randomized trial or non-randomized studies. C. Level of evidence C: Only consensus opinion of experts, case studies.

Catheter Ablation

Catheter ablation is an excellent non-pharmacologic option for some types of VT. The goal of catheter ablation is to destroy the substrate of the tachycardia with as small a lesion as possible. The first step in catheter ablation is to position an electrode catheter so that its ablating electrode is adjacent to the arrhythmogenic substrate, through a process called mapping. The ablating electrode is almost always at the distal end of the catheter and is usually larger than the other electrodes on the catheter. For example, the ablating electrode is usually 4–10 mm in length instead of the 1 or 2 mm length of pacing or stimulating electrodes.

Once it is determined that the ablating electrode is in a suitable location, adjacent either to the focus of a tachycardia or to a vulnerable point of a re-entrant circuit, up to 100 W of radiofrequency electrical energy (150 kHz to 1 MHz) is then delivered through the electrode to a reference electrode patch on the patient's chest wall. The purpose is to heat the myocardium adjacent to the ablating electrode and to destroy the arrhythmogenic substrate. Ablation creates injury by heating the myocardium at the electrode – tissue interface to a temperature of up to 70°C. The residuum of radiofrequency ablation is a well-demarcated spherical or oval zone of coagulation necrosis. Other catheter-based approaches are undergoing evaluation, including microwave energy, ultrasound, and cryotherapy.

Different mapping techniques are used for different types of VT. For VTs that arise from a small focus, such as the idiopathic VT that arises from the RV outflow tract, the electrophysiologist uses activation mapping and pace mapping. In activation mapping the ablating electrode is positioned at the site in the ventricle that is activated earliest during each beat of tachycardia. This is the site from which the VT arises. Local activation of this site is usually 20–40 milliseconds earlier than the onset of the QRS in the 12 lead surface ECG during VT. In pace mapping, the concept is that pacing at the exact focus where the VT originates should duplicate the QRS morphology of the clinical VT. The chance for a successful ablation at such a site will be high [66]. Success rates of at least 90% have been reported for ablation of these VTs [66].

In the case of idiopathic VTs arising from the inferoseptal wall of the left ventricle, the ablating catheter is also positioned at the site of earliest activation during VT. The electrical signal at this site usually has a distinct high-frequency potential, similar to a His bundle potential, which appears before the onset of the QRS on the surface ECG. This has led to speculation that this VT may be caused by re-entry involving the left posterior fascicle. Again, success rates of 90% can be expected for ablation of this kind of VT.

In the case of bundle branch re-entrant VT, the ablating electrode is positioned near the distal right bundle branch, which can be easily found by first locating the His bundle and then moving the tip of the catheter more distally until the distal electrode records the electrical signal of the distal right bundle branch. This potential looks like a His bundle potential, but its timing is much closer to the onset of the surface QRS during sinus rhythm than is the His bundle potential. The re-entry circuit of bundle branch re-entrant VT is vulnerable at this point, and often this VT can be eliminated by an application of energy here without producing complete heart block (although permanent right bundle branch block will be produced) [67]. Success rates of close to 100% may be expected for this kind of VT. Unfortunately, many patients with bundle branch re-entrant VT have severe LV dysfunction and are subject to other forms of VT that are not eliminated by ablation of the right bundle branch.

Mapping techniques are different in the case of VTs that originate from the region of a previous infarction. These VTs are usually caused by re-entry circuits that include a zone of slow conduction that passes through the scar. During VT this zone produces an activation signal that occurs after one surface QRS complex and before the next (that is, when the bulk of normal ventricular myocardium is in diastole – therefore, this signal is called a "diastolic potential"). Usually there are other areas in the scar that also conduct slowly and exhibit diastolic potentials during VT, even though they do not participate in the re-entry circuit. Therefore, diastolic potentials are not a specific finding. In order to determine if a site with diastolic potentials is part of the re-entry circuit, pacing stimuli are delivered through the mapping/ablating catheter at a rate slightly faster than the tachycardia. If the site is within the re-entry circuit, the pacing stimuli should produce paced QRS complexes with similar morphology as the QRS complexes during VT; and, during pacing, the interval from stimulus to the onset of the paced QRS should be identical to the interval from the diastolic potential to the QRS during VT. If the site is in a zone of slow conduction that is not part of the re-entry circuit, then the interval of pacing stimulus to the onset of paced QRS is much longer than the interval of diastolic potential to onset of QRS during VT [68,69]. The success rate of ablation for treatment of postinfarction VT is highly dependent on patient selection. Higher success rates (perhaps 80% to 90%) are achieved in patients who have one slow, hemodynamically stable VT. Lower success rates are achieved in patients with multiple different types of VT (that is, a history of VTs with different rates and morphologies), severe LV dysfunction, and rapid, hemodynamically unstable VT.

Newer mapping technologies for ablation may negate the complicated traditional techniques employed for VT ablation. Whereas conventional techniques required mapping for the site of origin of the tachycardia while the patient is in VT, with the inherent limitations dictated by hemodynamic stability, newer imaging capabilities allow for VT ablation either in sinus rhythm (using substrate voltage mapping as reported by Marchlinski *et al.* [70]) or mapping of hundreds of points simultaneously during only a few beats of tachycardia, thus obviating the need to have the patient be in VT for prolonged periods of time. However, despite these advances, ablation for VT in the setting of coronary disease and the existence of prior scars in the ventricles are still at best a palliative approach to minimize the chance of repetitive and recurrent shocks from ICDs, because of the complex morphology and histology of the substrate to be altered by ablation. Ablation for VT as a primary therapeutic approach has the best result (+90% success rate) in the setting of normal ventricles, such as in repetitive monomorphic VT (also known as exercise induced VT or RV outflow tract VT), or in bundle branch re-entry VT in idiopathic dilated VT, as the target for ablation is well described and circumscribed.

Catheter ablation carries a small risk. Complete heart block can be produced by inadvertent destruction of the normal AV conduction system. Other complications can include vascular damage (eg, hematoma, arteriovenous fistula, or pseudoaneurysm), cardiac perforation with tamponade, thromboembolism, valvular damage (particularly when mapping or ablating catheters are advanced retrogradely across the aortic valve), infection, and adverse reactions to drugs used during the procedure. The risk of a serious complication is less than 5%. Catheter ablation procedures can last many hours unless an arbitrary limit is placed on the permissible duration of the procedure. Exposure to fluoroscopic radiation can be considerable and is a concern for patient and staff.

Cardiac Surgery

Cardiac surgery can be used to treat VT. The site from which the VT emerges can be identified through EP mapping. Once it is localized, it can be surgically excised, ablated with radiofrequency energy, or frozen by cryosurgery [71]. An alternative approach is to use visual guidance and remove scarred endocardium, for the re-entrant loop seems to pass through endocardial scar in most cases [72]. With either approach the efficacy rate is approximately 75%, with a perioperative mortality rate of 10–15%. This is an attractive therapeutic option for patients with discrete anterior or apical aneurysms, especially if the patient might benefit hemodynamically from aneurysmectomy or if the patient needs coronary bypass surgery. Inferior wall aneurysms are not as accessible to the surgeon, and inferior wall surgery is more likely to compromise the papillary muscles and mitral apparatus. Other therapeutic options, such as the implantable defibrillator, are more attractive than endocardial resection for patients with inferior aneurysms.

Difficult Situations and Suggested Solutions

Real World Question How to Manage Cardiac Arrest?

Cardiac arrest must be managed with cardiopulmonary resuscitation including airway management, mechanical ventilation, chest compressions, and immediate electrical defibrillation with 120–200 J biphasic shock or 360 J monophasic shock. In general, successful defibrillation is closely correlated to the time to delivery of countershock [63]. If the patient remains in pulseless VT despite these measures, 1.0 mg of 1 : 10,000 epinephrine or 40 units vasopressin should be given intravenously followed by another attempt at electrical defibrillation. This dose of epinephrine should be repeated every 5 minutes while the patient remains in pulseless VT or VF. When VT persists, either IV amiodarone (bolus of 300 mg followed if necessary by an additional 150 mg) or lidocaine (an initial IV bolus of 1 mg/kg followed by repeated boluses of 0.5 mg/kg every 8 minutes, to a total of 3 mg/kg) may be given. Throughout this process, the utmost attention must be paid to recognizing and correcting metabolic abnormalities. Once an adequate rhythm is restored, evidence for underlying myocardial ischemia or infarction should be sought; this may dictate the need for specific interventions such as intra-aortic balloon pumping or emergent coronary revisualization [73].

Real World Question How to Treat Ventricular Tachycardia Due to Digoxin Toxicity?

Certain types of VT are refractory to electrical shock and to the usual anti-arrhythmic drugs. VT from digitalis intoxication may require management with antidigoxin antigen binding fragments (Fab). The dose of antidigoxin Fab to be delivered can be calculated by calculating the total body load of digoxin as the serum concentration of digoxin (in ng/L) multiplied by the volume of distribution (equal to the patient's weight in kilograms multiplied by 5.6 L/kg). The total body load of digoxin is then divided by 600 (the number of nanograms of digoxin bound by each vial) to determine the number of vials that should be administered to the patient. Antidigoxin Fab also binds digitoxin, and the same calculations can be used to determine the number of vials to be given, except that the volume of distribution of digitoxin is 0.56 L/kg. Patients usually respond clinically to the antibody fragments within 30 minutes of administration. The serum concentration of digoxin climbs after administration of the antibody fragments, because they remove digoxin from extravascular binding sites. The Fab – digitalis complexes are excreted by the kidneys, and have a half-life of 16–20 hours in patients with normal renal function. It is not clear how the complexes are eliminated in patients with renal insufficiency; however, such patients have responded well to antidigoxin Fab.

Real World Question How to Treat Polymorphic Ventricular Tachycardia?

Polymorphic VT arises in different clinical settings. It appears in various genetic syndromes such as the long QT syndrome, the Brugada syndrome, the catecholaminergic polymorphic VT syndrome, and the short QT syndrome. It can appear in patients with acquired long QT syndromes such as are caused by Class IA and Class III drugs, hypomagnesemia, and hypokalemia. It also can appear in acute ischemia, so patients with polymorphic VT should be screened for ischemia unless another cause is apparent. The Brugada syndrome also produces episodes of polymorphic VT. It has not been found to reliably respond to anti-arrhythmic drugs, so symptomatic patients and high-risk asymptomatic patients are best treated with implantation of an ICD.

Real World Question How to Treat Torsades De Pointes?

Torsades de pointes (TdP) receives its name, which translates as "twisting of the points," from the manner in which the QRS complexes appear to rotate around the isoelectric baseline, with variability in axis and morphology. It often occurs in the setting of a prolonged QT interval. Other features of TdP include episodes that are often non-sustained. Some forms of TdP are catecholamine-dependant, while others are pause-dependant. Often there is T wave alternans prior to episodes, and occasionally the episodes degenerate into VF.

β-adrenergic blockade is the best therapy for adrenergic-dependent TdP, including the congenital abnormalities of the potassium channel (LQT1 and LQT2) and certain acquired forms caused by neurologic disorders (subarachnoid hemorrhage, stroke, or encephalitis). Pause-dependent TdP (including most of the commonly acquired forms) is chiefly treated by temporary or permanent pacing and by removal of any offending drugs (e.g., Class IA and Class III anti-arrhythmics) and correction of electrolyte abnormalities. Episodes of sustained TdP respond to electrical cardioversion. While waiting for the underlying disorder to be corrected, recurrent TdP can be prevented with use of interventions that shorten the QT interval, such as atrial or ventricular pacing at rates of 90–110 bpm or isoproterenol. Pacing is preferred in patients with concomitant coronary artery disease. Lidocaine is often ineffective in the treatment of TdP, and Class IA anti-arrhythmic agents should be avoided because they can further prolong the QT interval. Magnesium sulfate has been reported to abolish TdP with a high rate of success [74].

Real World Question Can We Prevent all Sudden Cardiac Deaths?

In both ischemic and non-ischemic heart disease the severity of LV dysfunction has emerged as the key determinant affecting the decision of which patient should receive an ICD for prophylaxis against a future risk of arrhythmic sudden death. A documented EF of ⩽35% in an otherwise suitably treated patient will commonly result in an electrophysiology referral and an ICD implant. Although such treatment has yielded mortality benefit in the qualifying patient, whether it can significantly impact on overall sudden death in the general population is less clear. A population-based study unfortunately showed that only a small proportion of sudden death victims could have benefited from the current primary prevention ICD guidelines.

CRITICAL THINKING

The Oregon Sudden Unexpected Death Study All cases of SCD in Multnomah County, Oregon (population 660,486; 2002–2004) were prospectively ascertained in the ongoing Oregon Sudden Unexpected Death Study. LVEFs were retrospectively assessed among subjects who underwent evaluation of LV function before SCD (normal: ⩾55%; mildly to moderately reduced: 36–54%; and severely reduced: ⩽35%). Of a total of 714 SCD cases (annual incidence 54 per 100,000), LV function was assessed in 121 (17%). The results showed that the LVEF was severely reduced in 36 patients (30%), mildly to moderately reduced in 27 (22%), and normal in 58 (48%). Patients with normal LVEF were distinguishable by younger age (66 ± 15 years vs. 74 ± 10 years; $P = 0.001$), higher proportion of females (47% vs. 27%; $P = 0.025$), higher prevalence of seizure disorder (14% vs. 0%; $P = 0.002$), and lower prevalence of established coronary artery disease (50% vs. 81%; $P < 0.001$). So in this community-wide study, only one-third of the evaluated SCD cases had severe LV dysfunction meeting current criteria for prophylactic cardioverter-defibrillator implantation. The SCD cases with normal LV function had several distinguishing clinical characteristics. These findings support the aggressive development of alternative screening methods to enhance identification of patients at risk [75].

Of 714 sudden deaths occurring over a two-year period, only 121 patients had a previous assessment of LV function and only 36 of these patients (5% of the total) had an EF of ≤35%. The concept that only a minority of sudden deaths occurs in patients previously identified as having significant LV dysfunction has been previously well documented in a number of studies. So far it remains far less than perfect at predicting at what time and for which patient the unfortunate substrates and triggers cross to result in sudden death. The second corollary is that not all SCDs are from arrhythmias. Clearly, these patients died of AMI, which could not be prevented by ICD [76].

References

1 Harris L, Downar E, Mickleborough L *et al.* Activation sequence of ventricular tachycardia:Endocardial and epicardial mapping studies in the human ventricle. J Am Coll Cardiol 1987;10:1040–1047.

2 Wieland JM, Marchlinski FE. Electrocardiographic response of digoxin-toxic fascicular tachycardia to Fab fragments: Implications for tachycardia mechanism. PACE 1986;9:727–738.

3 Caceres J, Jazayeri M, McKinnic J *et al.* Sustained bundle branch reentry as a mechanism of clinical tachycardia. Circulation 1989;79:256–270.

4 Benson DW, MacRae CA, Vesely MR *et al.* Missense mutation in the pore region of HERG causes familial long QT syndrome. Circulation 1996;93:1791–1795.

5 Lerman BB. Response of nonreentrant catecholamine-mediated VT to endogenous adenosine and acetylcholine: Evidence for myocardial receptor – mediated effects. Circulation 1993;87:382–390.

6 Lerman BB, Stein K, Engelstein ED *et al.* Mechanism of repetitive monomorphic ventricular tachycardia. Circulation 1995;92:421–429.

7 Okumura K, Matsuyama K, Miyagi H *et al.* Entrainment of idiopathic VT of left ventricular origin with evidence for reentry with an area of slow conduction and effect of verapamil. Am J Cardiol 1988;62:727–732.

8 Moss AJ, Zareba W, Hall WJ *et al.*, for the Multicenter Automatic Defibrillator Implantation Trial II Investigators Prophylactic Implantation of a Defibrillator in Patients with Myocardial Infarction and Reduced Ejection Fraction Circulation 346:877–883.

9 Bardy GH, Lee KL, Mark DB *et al.* Amiodarone or an implantable cardioverter-defibrillator for congestive heart failure. N Engl J Med 2005;352(3):225–237.

10 Bristow MR, Saxon LA, Boehmer J, for the Comparison of Medical Therapy, Pacing, and Defibrillation in Heart Failure for the COMPANION Investigators Cardiac-resynchronization therapy with or without an implantable defibrillator in advanced chronic heart failure N Engl J Med 2004;350:2140–2150.

11 CABG-Patch Trial Investigators. Bigger JT Jr. Prophylactic use of implanted cardiac defibrillators in patients at high risk for ventricular arrhythmias after coronary-artery bypass surgery. N Enl J Med 1997;337:1569–1575.

12 Hohnloser SH, Kuck KH, Dorian P *et al.*, for the DINAMIT Investigators. Prophylactic use of an implantable cardioverter-defibrillator after acute myocardial infarction. N Engl J Med 2004;351:2481–2488.

13 Bloomfield DM, Bigger JT Jr, Steinman RC *et al.* Microvolt T-wave alternans and the risk of death or sustained ventricular arrhythmias in patients with left ventricular dysfunction. J Am Coll Cardiol 2006;47:456–463.

14 Mostow ND, Vrobel TR, Noon D, Rakita L. Rapid suppression of complex ventricular arrhythmias with high-dose oral amiodarone. Circulation 1986;73:1231–1238.

15 Iseri LT, Brodsky MA. Magnesium therapy of cardiac arrhythmias in critical-care medicine. Magnes Res 1989;8:299–306.

16 Poole JE, Mathisen TL, Kudenchuk PJ et al. long-term outcome in patients who survive out of hospital ventricular fibrillation and undergo electrophysiologic studies: Evaluation by electrophysiologic subgroups. J Am Coll Cardiol 1990;16:657–665.

17 The Antiarrhythmics vs. Implantable Defibrillators (AVID) Investigators. A Comparison of antiarrhythmic-drug therapy with implantable defibrillators in patients resuscitated from near-fatal ventricular arrhythmias. N Engl J Med 1997;337:1576–1583.

18 Pacifico A, Hohnloser SH, Williams JH et al. Prevention of implantable-defibrillator shocks by treatment with sotalol. N Engl J Med 1999;340:1855–1862.

19 Task Force of the Working Group on Arrhythmias of the European Society of Cardiology. The Sicilian Gambit: A new approach to the classification of antiarrhythmic drugs based on their action on arrhythmogenic mechanisms. Circulation 1991;84:1831–1851.

20 Bauernfeind RA, Swiryn S, Petropoulos AT et al. Concordance and discordance of drug responses in atrioventricular reentrant tachycardia. J Am Coll Cardiol 1983;2: 345–350.

21 Hession M, Blum R, Podrid PJ et al. Mexiletine and tocainide:Does response to one predict response to the other? J Am Coll Cardiol 1986;7:338–343.

22 Selzer A, Wray HW. Quinidine syncope. Paroxysmal ventricular fibrillation occurring during treatment of chronic atrial arrhythmias. Circulation 1964;30:17–26.

23 Velebit V, Podrid PJ, Lown B, Raeder E. Aggravation and provocation of ventricular arrhythmias by antiarrhythmic drugs. Circulation 1982;65:886–894.

24 Brachmann J, Scherlag BJ, Rozenshtraukh LV, Lazzara R. Bradycardia-dependent triggered activity: Relevance to drug-induced multiform ventricular tachycardia. Circulation 1983;68:846–856.

25 Hoffman BF, Rosen MR. Cellular mechanisms for cardiac arrhythmias. Circulation Res 1981;49:1–15.

26 Rinkenberger RL, Prystowsky EN, Jackman WM et al. Drug conversion of nonsustained ventricular tachycardia to sustained ventricular tachycardia during serial electrophysiologic studies:Identification of drugs that exacerbate tachycardia and potential mechanisms. Am Heart J 1982;103:177–184.

27 Gottlieb SS, Weinberg M. Hemodynamic and neurohumoral effects of quinidine in patients with severe left ventricular dysfunction secondary to coronary artery disease or idiopathic dilated cardiomyopathy. Am J Cardiol 1991;67:728–731.

28 Ravid S, Podrid PJ, Lampert S, Lown B. Congestive heart failure induced by six of the newer antiarrhythmic drugs. J Am Coll Cardiol 1989;14:1326–1330.

29 Kupersmith J. Monitoring of antiarrhythmic drug levels:Values and pitfalls. Ann NY Acad Sci 1984;432:138–154.

30 Thomson PD, Melmon KL, Richardson JA et al. Lidocaine pharmacokinetics in advanced heart failure, liver disease, and renal failure in humans. Ann Intern Med 1973;78:499–508.

31 Kessler KM, Kayden DS, Estes DM et al. Procainamide pharmacokinetics in patients with acute myocardial infarction or congestive heart failure. J Am Coll Cardiol 1986;7: 1131–1139.

32 CAST Investigators. Preliminary report:effect of encainide and flecainide on mortality in a randomized trial of arrhythmia suppression after myocardial infarction. N Engl J Med 1989;32:406–412.

33 Olshansky B, Hahn E, Hartz V *et al.* and the ESVEM Investigators; Clinical Significance of Syncope in the Electrophysiologic Study vs. Electrocardiographic Monitoring (ESVEM) Trial Am Heart J 137(5):878–886.

34 Winkelmann BR, Leinberger H. Life-threatening flecainide toxicity. Ann Intern Med 1987;106:807–814.

35 Pentel PR, Goldsmith SR, Salerno DM *et al.* Effect of hypertonic sodium bicarbonate on encainide overdose. Am J Cardiol 1986;57:878–880.

36 Vyas AK, Guo HS, Moss AJ *et al.* for the MADIT-II Research Group Reduction in Ventricular Tachyarrhythmias With Statins in the Multicenter Automatic Defibrillator Implantation Trial (MADIT)-II J Am Coll Cardiol 2006;47:769–773.

37 Winkle RA, Mason J, Griffin JC, Ross D. Malignant ventricular tachyarrhythmias associated with the use of encainide. Am Heart J 1981;102:857–864.

38 German LD, Packer DL, Bardy GH, Gallagher JJ. Ventricular tachycardia induced by atrial stimulation in patients without symptomatic cardiac disease. Am J Cardiol 1983;52:1202–1507.

39 Chen PS, Shibata N, Dixon EG *et al.* Activation during ventricular defibrillation in open-chest dogs. Evidence of complete cessation and regeneration of ventricular fibrillation after unsuccessful shocks. J Clin Invest 1986;77:810–823.

40 Davy J-M, Fain ES, Dorian P, Winkle RA. The relationship between successful defibrillation and delivered energy in open-chest dogs: Reappraisal of the "defibrillation threshold" concept. Am Heart J 1987;113:77–84.

41 Sima SJ, Kieso RA, Fox-Eastham KJ *et al.* Mechanisms responsible for the decline in thoracic impedance after direct current shock. Am J Physiol 1989;257:H180.

42 Kerber RE, Martins JB, Kienzle MG *et al.* Energy, current, and success in defibrillation and cardioversion: Clinical studies using an automated impedance-based method of energy adjustment. Circulation 1988;77:1038–1046.

43 Ujhelyi MR, Schur M, Frede T *et al.* Differential effects of lidocaine on defibrillation threshold with monophasic vs. biphasic shock waveforms. Circulation 1995;92: 1644–1650.

44 Hernandez R, Mann DE, Breckinridge S *et al.* Effects of flecainide on defibrillation thresholds in the anesthetized dog. J Am Coll Cardiol 1989;14:777–781.

45 Guamieri T, Levine JH, Veltri EP *et al.* Success of chronic defibrillation and the role of antiarrhythmic drugs with the automatic implantable cardioverter/defibrillator. Am J Cardiol 1987;60:1061–1064.

46 Jung W, Manz M, Pizzulli L *et al.* Effects of chronic amiodarone therapy on defibrillation threshold. Am J Cardiol 1992;70:1023–1027.

47 Wang M, Dorian P. DL and D sotalol decrease defibrillation energy requirements. PACE 1989;12:1522–1529.

48 Ruffy R, Schechtman K, Monje E, Sandza J. Adrenergically mediated variations in the energy required to defibrillate the heart: Observations in closed-chest, nonanesthetized dogs. Circulation 1986;73:374–380.

49 Ruffy R, Monje E, Schechtman K. Facilitation of cardiac defibrillation by aminophylline in the conscious, closed-chest dog. J Electrophysiol 1988;2:450–454.

50 Babbs CF, Whistler SJ, Kim GKW *et al.* Dependence of defibrillation threshold upon extracellular/intracellular K + concentrations. J Electrocardiol 1980;13:73–78.

51 Echt DS, Armstrong K, Schmidt P *et al.* Clinical experience, complications, and survival in 70 patients with the automatic implantable cardioverter defibrillator. Circulation 1985;71:289–296.

52 Moss AJ, Hall WJ, Cannom DS *et al.* Improved survival with an implanted defibrillator in patients with coronary disease at high risk for ventricular arrhythmia. N Engl J Med 1996;335:1933–1940.

53 Buxton A, Lee K, Fisher J *et al.* A randomized study of the prevention of sudden cardiac death in patients with coronary artery disease. N Engl J Med 1999;341:1882–1890.

54 Link MS, Costeas XF, Griffith JL *et al.* High incidence of appropriate cardioverter-defibrillator therapy in patients with syncope of unknown etiology and inducible arrhythmias. J Am Coll Cardiol 1977;2:370–375.

55 Connolly SJ, Gent M, Roberts RS *et al.* for the CIDS investigators. Canadian Implantable Defibrillators Study (CIDS): A randomized trial of the implantable cardioverter against amiodarone. Circulation 2000;101:1297–1302.

56 Domanski MJ, Sakseena S, Epstein AE *et al.* for the AVID investigators. Relative effectiveness of the implantable cardioverter-defibrillator and antiarrhythmic drugs in patients with varying degrees of LV dysfunction who have survived malignant ventricular arrhythmias. J Am Coll Cardiol 1999;34:1090–1095.

57 Sheldon R, Connolly S, Krahn A *et al.* on behalf of the CIDS investigators. Identification of patients most likely to benefit from ICD therapy: The Canadian Implantable Defibrillators Study. Circulation 2000;101:1660–1664.

58 Moss A. Implantable cardioverter defibrillator therapy. The sickest patients benefit the most. Circulation 2000;101:202–230.

59 Committee Members, Gregoratos G, Abrams J, Epstein AE *et al.* ACC/AHA?NASPE 2002 Guideline update for implantation of cardiac pacemakers and antiarrhythmia devices-summary article: A report of the American College of Cardiology/American Heart Association Task Force on Practice Guidelines (ACC/AHA/NASPE Committee to update the 1998 pacemaker guidelines) J Am Coll Cardiol 2002;40:1703–1719.

60 Groh WJ, Silka MJ, Oliver RP *et al.* Use of ICD in the congenital long QT syndrome. Am J Cardiol 1990;78:703–705.

61 Breithardt G, Wichter T, Havorkamp W *et al.* ICD therapy in patients with arrhythmogenic right ventricular dysplasia, long QT syndrome, or no structural heart disease. Am Heart J 1994;127:1151–1158.

62 Brugada P, Brugada R, Brugada J *et al.* Use of the prophylactic ICD for patients with normal heart. Am J Cardiol 1999;83:98D–100D.

63 Maron BJ, Shen WK, Links MS *et al.* Efficacy of ICD for the prevention of SCD in patients with hypertrophic cardiomyopathy. N Engl J Med 2000;342:365–373.

64 Bardy GH ;Lee KL ;Mark DB *et al.* Amiodarone or an implantable cardioverter-defibrillator for congestive heart failure. N Engl J Med 2005;352(3):225–237.

65 Kadish A, Dyer A, Daubert JP *et al.*, for the Defibrillators in non-Ischemic Cardiomyopathy Treatment Evaluation (DEFINITE) Investigators Prophylactic Defibrillator Implantation in Patients with Nonischemic Dilated Cardiomyopathy NEJM 350: 2151–2158.

66 Klein LS, Shih HT, Hackett FK *et al.* Radiofrequency catheter ablation of ventricular tachycardia in patients without structural heart disease. Circulation 1992;85: 1666–1674.

67 Tchou P, Jazayeri M, Denker S *et al.* Transcatheter electrical ablation of right bundle branch. A method of treating macroreentrant ventricular tachycardia attributed to bundle branch reentry. Circulation 1988;78:246–257.

68 Stevenson WG, Weiss JN, Weiner I *et al.* Resetting of ventricular tachycardia: Implications for localizing the area of slow conduction. J Am Coll Cardiol 1988;11:522–529.

69 Fitzgerald DM, Friday KJ, Wah J *et al.* Electrogram patterns predicting successful catheter ablation of ventricular tachycardia. Circulation 1988;77:806–814.

70 Marchlinski FE, Callans DJ, Gottlieb CD *et al.* Linear ablation lesions for control of unmappable ventricular tachycardia in patients with ischemic or non-ischemic cardiomyopathy. Circulation 2000;101:1288–1296.

71 Horowitz LN, Harken AH, Kastor JA, Josephson ME. Ventricular resection guided by epicardial and endocardial mapping for treatment of recurrent ventricular tachycardia. N Engl J Med 1980;302:589–593.

72 Kehoe R, Zheutlin T, Finkelmeler B *et al.* Visually directed endocardial resection for ventricular arrhythmia: Long term outcome and functional status. J Am Coll Cardiol 1985; 5(suppl 2):497.

73 Hazinski MF, Chameides L, Elling B *et al.* 2005 American Heart Association guidelines for cardiopulmonary resuscitation and emergency cardiovascular care. Circulation 2005; 112:IV–1–IV–211.

74 Tzivoni D, Banal S, Schuger C *et al.* Treatment of torsade de pointes with magnesium sulfate. Circulation 1988;77:392–397.

75 Stecker EC, Vickers C, Waltz J *et al.* Population-Based Analysis of Sudden Cardiac Death With and Without Left Ventricular Systolic Dysfunction: Two-Year Findings from the Oregon Sudden Unexpected Death Study 2005.11.045 (Published online 21 February 2006).

76 Groh WJ Lessons From a Population The Limitations of Left Ventricular Ejection Fraction as the Major Determinant for Primary Prevention Implantable Cardioverter-Defibrillators. 2005.12.031 (Published online 21 February 2006).

CHAPTER 10

Atrial Fibrillation

Hung-Fat Tse and Chu-Pak Lau

Introduction

Atrial fibrillation (AF) is the most commonly occurring cardiac arrhythmia associated with increased cardiovascular morbidity and mortality. Epidemiological data from the Framingham Heart Study indicate the cumulative incidence of AF over a 22 year follow-up was 2.1% in men and 1.7% in women. The prevalence of AF increases with age, affecting over 1 in 25 persons aged 60 years or older, and 1 in 10 persons aged 80 years or older [1]. Even in an ethnic group with a low incidence of coronary artery disease (CAD), AF occurs in 1.3% of population with age >60 years [2]. Furthermore, recent data suggests that the prevalence of AF is increasing even after adjusting for age and other risk factors. In conjunction with congestive heart failure (CHF), AF has been described as one of the two emerging epidemics of cardiovascular disease due to the aging population [3]. AF is associated with a 3- to 5-fold increase risk of stroke, a 3-fold increase risk of CHF and a significant 1.5–3-fold increase in risk of death [1]. In contrast to other risk factors for stroke which decrease with increasing age, risk of AF-related stroke remains high at all ages. Although AF is often associated with heart diseases or other risk factors (Table 10.1), it can also occur in about 30% of patients without underlying etiological cause (lone AF) [4].

During AF, the atria activates at >350 bpm, resulting in no effective atrial contraction. These chaotic atrial impulses in turn activate the atrio-ventricular (AV) node at random intervals. As the AV node has a limited capacity in transmitting atrial activations, in most cases the ventricles are beating irregularly at rates between 80–120 bpm at rest. Ineffective atrial contraction leads to a reduction in left ventricular (LV) filling (hence decrease stroke volume), a higher left atrial (LA) pressure and stasis of blood that lead to clot formation. The ventricles are bystanders during AF. When the ventricular rate (VR) is inappropriately fast, adequate LV filling does not occur, and the depressed stroke volume results in a reduction in forward cardiac output despite the increase in rate. Very often, closely coupled cardiac cycles do not generate a detectable pulse because of small stroke volume, and pulse deficit is a feature

Table 10.1 Risk factors for atrial fibrillation.

1. Age
2. Male sex
3. Alcohol
4. Thyroid dysfunction
5. Chronic obstructive lung disease
6. Diabetes mellitus
7. Cardiovascular diseases
8. Hypertension
9. Valvular heart disease
10. Ischaemic heart disease
11. Cardiomyopathies
12. Heart failure
13. Congenital heart disease
14. Wolff–Parkinson–White syndrome
15. LV hypertrophy
16. Recent cardiac or non-cardiac surgery

LV, left ventricular.

of AF. Another adverse change is irregularity of the ventricular contraction, and it has been shown that it can further reduce the overall cardiac output compared to a regular rhythm. These ventricular responses are critically dependent on the AV node. For example, heightened conduction during stress or exercise can worsen the hemodynamic response. On the other hand, appropriate rate control by an AV nodal blocker can ameliorate much of the changes and improve symptomatology. Chronic inappropriately fast VR can lead to impair LV contraction, a condition known as tachycardiomyopathy.

Recent experimental and clinical studies have provided new insights into the mechanisms of AF. The mechanisms of AF are heterogeneous and are likely to differ in different clinical circumstances. However, three basic components are required for the occurrence of AF: (1) a specific trigger; (2) a suitable substrate; and (3) modifying factors. Experimental AF could be induced by a single source of very rapid impulses or by multiple re-entering wavelets that continuously travel randomly through the available myocardium [5,6]. If the cycle length of the firing focus is shorter than the refractory period in other parts of atria, rate-dependent functional conduction block occurs and non-uniform excitation will result. This type of AF is actually represented as "fibrillatory conduction". One of the important observation from Haissagurere *et al.* [7] was that a single source of rapid ectopic foci of automaticity, mainly originating from the pulmonary veins, can be the trigger for the initiation and maintenance of AF in patients with paroxysmal AF (PAF). Other ectopic foci are in the superior vena cava, coronary sinus, LA posterior wall, vein of Marshall, and interatrial septum have also been shown to trigger AF. Furthermore, atrial flutter or any supraventricular tachycardia may also serve to trigger AF.

In contrast, established AF often consists of multiple wavelets and was thought to be caused by multiple re-entries. Allessie *et al.* [8] provided the first experimental evidence to support the presence of multiple re-entering wavelet during AF by using a mapping technique, and postulated that perpetuation of AF depends on a critical number (i.e. 4–6) of simultaneously circulating wavelets. Subsequently, Cox *et al.* [9] documented the presence of multiple wave fronts, non-uniform conduction, bi-directional block and complete re-entrant circuits during AF in human atria using intra-operative electrophysiologic mapping. This type of AF requires the presence of appropriate atrial substrates which include an adequate atrial mass and the occurrence of short wavelength. Wavelength is a product of atrial refractory period and atrial conduction velocity. Therefore, any atrial structural and electrophysiological changes that resulted in a shortening of atrial refractoriness or slowing of conduction can facilitate the maintenance of AF [6]. Both animal and human studies have shown that the occurrence of AF leads to changes in the atrial refractory period, which favor the maintenance of AF [10,11]. Furthermore, heterogeneous changes of regional dispersion in atrial effective periods in the right and left atria further contribute to the chronicity of AF. These changes occurred in parallel with progressive increase in P wave duration, sinus node dysfunction and LA dilatation from paroxysmal to persistent AF, suggesting a progressive electromechanical remodeling process [12]. In addition, dispersion of conduction velocities when atrial dilatation occurred in HF may also be an alternative mechanism for persistence of AF [13]. These electromechanical remodelings are associated with cellular hypertrophy, atrial fibrosis and calcium overloading, which increase the propensity to AF [14,15]. Thus, a vicious cycle of progression to long standing AF occurs once the process begins. Therefore, aggressive treatment of AF if initiated early may potentially prevent these progressive atrial electromechanical remodeling.

A variety of modifying factors appears to be of importance in the initiation and maintenance of AF. In experimental models for AF, stimulation of the parasympathetic system or applying acetylcholine directly onto atrial tissue is required to produce sustained AF [16]. A change in autonomic tone with either parasympathetic or sympathetic stimulation directly affects atrial refractoriness to contribute to both multiple wavelets of re-entry and focal mechanisms with fibrillatory conduction [17]. Other modifying factors appear to be of importance in the initiation and maintenance of AF, including effects of drugs, inflammation, and metabolic and electrolyte changes may affect the onset of the atrial trigger and the atrial susceptibility for AF.

Clinical Manifestations and Evaluation of Atrial Fibrillation

Symptoms due to AF are highly variable and depend on several factors including VR, cardiac function, concomitant medical problems and individual patient perception. The rapid and irregular rhythm and the loss of synchronized atrial activity both contribute to impaired cardiac performance and symptomatology. While palpitation is the commonest presenting symptoms in over half (54%) of patients with AF [4], a significant proportion of patients may present with other symptoms, including dyspnea (44%), fatigue (14%) and dizziness (10%). Importantly, 11% of patients with AF are asymptomatic. Furthermore, the first clinical presentation of AF may be an embolic complication or aggravation of CHF. A history of alcohol use and athletic predisposition should be sought. On examination, signs of hyperthyroidism and evidence of peripheral embolisation should be evaluated. Underlying valvular disease, hypertension (HTN) and HF should also be assessed (Table 10.2).

There is no single widely accepted classification of AF. However, a clinical classification of AF, based on the temporal pattern of AF occurrence is useful to help the physician in selecting a therapeutic approach (Figure 10.1). In this classification, the main categories of are new, onset, and chronic AF. When AF is documented in a patient for the first time it is termed new onset of AF. This can be a transient event due to a reversible cause or may move to another category with further observation. For chronic AF, it can be paroxysmal (terminate spontaneously, usually within 48 hours and recurrent), persistent

Table 10.2 Assessment of patients with atrial fibrillation.

History	Frequency and severity of AF symptoms
	Exercise capacity
	Symptoms of concomitant cardiovascular diseases and thyroid dysfunction
	Risk factors of AF and thromboembolic complications (see Tables 10.1 and 10.6)
	Drugs including adverse effects
Physical examination	Heart rate – pulse and apex
	Signs of thyrotoxicosis
	Heart size and murmur
	Sign of pulmonary diseases
12-Lead ECG	Confirm diagnosis
	Rate and look for other arrhythmias, including pre-excitation syndromes
	Evidence of left ventricular hypertrophy or CAD
Chest X-ray	Heart size and evidence of cardiac diseases, such as mitral stenosis
	Pulmonary diseases
Blood biochemistry	Full blood count
	Liver and renal function tests
	Thyroid function
Echocardiogram	To diagnose underlying structural heart diseases, such as valvular diseases, LV hypertrophy, CAD and cardiomyopathies
	To assess left atrial size, LV size and function
Holter monitoring	To diagnosis paroxysmal AF
	To assess ambulatory ventricular rate during AF
Treadmill test	Diagnosis CAD and exercise-induced AF
	Assess ventricular rate during exercise

AF, atrial fibrillation; ECG, electrocardiogram; CAD, coronary artery disease; LV, left ventricular.

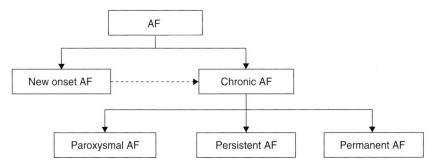

Figure 10.1 Classification of atrial fibrillation.

Table 10.3 Management strategies for atrial fibrillation.

1. Control the heart rate
2. Correct underlying disease and convert AF to regular rhythm
3. Prophylactic anticoagulation and prevention of embolism if indicated

AF, atrial fibrillation.

(sinus rhythm is restored by chemical or electrical cardioversion) or permanent (either failed conversion or a low success rate considered by the physician).

Routine blood tests that include thyroid and renal function and diabetic screening are essential. Other acute and reversible causes of AF, such as pulmonary diseases and infection, should be ruled out. If the patient is in AF, a 12-lead ECG should be recorded. This not only documents the rhythm, but also gives an idea of the rate and irregularity, and for possible LV hypertrophy or underlying myocardial infarction. If the symptoms are suggestive and the patient is in sinus rhythm, either a 24 hour ECG or event recording can be used to identify the arrhythmia. A 24 hours recording can also identify associated sinus node disease in bradycardia-tachycardia syndrome, and to assess the rate of AF over the 24 hour period. An echocardiogram should be performed in most patients with AF. This not only enable valvular diseases to be detected and quantified, but also will enable LV function and the size of the LA to be measured, and to assess clots in the LA. A transoesophagcal echocardiogram (TEE) may be needed when the transthoracic window is inadequate, or when a LA clot is suspected or needs to be excluded prior to defibrillation. An exercise test may be useful to evaluate underlying CAD (if suspected) and to assess rate control. The management strategies of AF are listed in Table 10.3.

New Onset Acute Atrial Fibrillation

In about 50% of patients, AF of recent onset converts spontaneously to sinus rhythm at presentation. Patients who remain in AF and hemodynamic unstable due to rapid VRs should undergo emergency cardioversion. These patients usually have pre-excitation syndrome with extremely rapid VR or significant structural heart disease, such as significant valvular heart disease, CHF or acute myocardial ischemia. Treatment for acute AF is summarized in Figure 10.2.

Acute Ventricular Rate Control

The majority of patients who present acutely in AF have rapid VR. Therefore, acute VR control is required to improve hemodynamic status and relieve

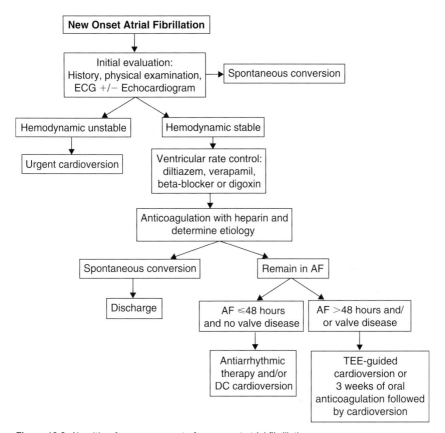

Figure 10.2 Algorithm for management of new onset atrial fibrillation.

symptoms. The goal of therapy should be a reduction of resting heart rate to less than 80–90 bpm by using AV nodal blocking agents (verapamil and dilti-azem, β-blocker, and digoxin) administrated intravenously (IV) or orally. The dosage, side-effects and indications for different AV nodal blocking agents are summarized in Table 10.4. For rapid and effective acute VR control, IV drugs are often required.

In patients with HF and AF, relief of pulmonary congestion by diuretics and vasodilators may aid in decreasing the heart rate. Digoxin has both negative chronotropic and positive inotropic effects and therefore is an appro-priate first-line drug in patients with HF and AF. Furthermore, in patients with borderline blood pressure, IV digoxin is useful alternative to β-blocker or calcium channel blockers that may cause further decrease in blood pressure.

Table 10.4 Drugs for control of the ventricular rate in patients with atrial fibrillation.

Drug	Acute intravenous therapy (loading dose)	Chronic oral therapy	Efficacy	Comments
Calcium channel blockers				
Diltiazem	IV bolus 20 mg or 0.25 mg/kg over 2 min followed if necessary by IV 25 mg or 0.35 mg/kg 15 min later. Maintenance infusion of 5–15 mg/h	90–360 mg daily as slow release form	Good	*Acute* Side effects: heart block, worsening of HF and hypotension (3%). Usually well tolerated and no effect on digoxin levels. *Chronic* Side effects: constipation and bradycardia. Useful in HTN and CAD
Verapamil	IV 5–10 mg over 2–3 min. Repeat 5–10 mg 30 min later if required. Maintenance infusion rate is not well documented	120–360 mg/day in divided doses or in slow release form	Good	*Acute* Side effects: heart block, worsening of HF and hypotension (5–10%). Synergistic with digoxin but also increases digoxin levels. *Chronic* Side effects: constipation and bradycardia. Useful in HTN and CAD
Beta-blockers				
Metoprolol	IV 5 mg every 5 min; total 15 mg	50–100 mg twice daily or in slow release form	Good	*Acute* Side effects: heart block, worsening of HF and bronchospasm and hypotension. Useful in post-operative setting. *Long term* Side effects: fatigue and depression. Useful in HTN, HF and CAD
Propranolol	IV 1–5 mg (1 mg every 2 min)	10–120 mg three times daily or in slow release form	Good	Acute and chronic side effects as above. Useful in HTN thyrotoxicosis and CAD

Atenolol	IV 5 mg over 5 mins, repeat in 10 mins	80–320 mg in slow release form	Good	Acute and chronic side effects as above Useful in HTN and CAD
Esmolol	IV 0.5 mg/kg over 1 min. Repeat if necessary Maintenance infusion 0.05 mg/kg/min	25–100 mg once daily	Short-acting	Acute and chronic side effects as above Useful in post-operative setting; hypotension (20–50%) is common
Pindolol		2.5–20 mg/twice to three times daily	Fair	Chronic side effects as above, but can avoid excessive bradycardia
Carvedilol		3.125–25 mg twice daily	Good	Chronic side effects as above bradycardia Useful in HTN, CAD and HF
Cardiac glycoside				
Digoxin	IV 0.25–0.5 mg (total 1 mg/24 hr)	0.125–0.5 mg daily	Moderate to low	Delayed onset of AV node slowing (hours) Caution for digoxin toxicity in patients with electrolytes imbalance and renal failure Useful in patients with HF
Amiodarone	IV 5–7 mg/kg up to 1500 mg/24 hours	PO loading 600–800 mg daily, maintenance 100–200 mg QD	Good	*Acute* Side effects: bradycardia, hypotension and thrombophlebitis. Useful in critically ill patients and hypotension *Chronic* Side effects: (see Table 10.3). Useful in refractory patients and HF

AV, atrio-ventricular; CAD, coronary artery disease; HF, heart failure; HTN, hypertension; IV, intravenous.

CLINICAL PEARLS

β-blockers or calcium channel blockers for control of ventricular response In many acute situations, either a β-blocker or calcium channel blocker is the preferred agent for slowing VR. The non-dihydropyridine (or rate-limiting) calcium channel blockers – verapamil and diltiazem – prolong AV nodal refractory period to slow AV nodal conduction, and are effective agents for VR control during AF.

Since IV verapamil has more potent negative inotropic and peripheral vasodilator effect, IV diltiazem has became a more popular drug for acute VR control during AF, especially in patients with LV dysfunction and hypotension.

IV β-blockers are also effective AV nodal blocking agent through their sympatholytic properties. They are more effective in conditions in which the rapid VR is due to heightened adrenergic tone, such as in the postoperative periods. Except for esmolol, all the β-blockers have a slower onset of action than diltiazem. However, IV esmolol has a very short half-life which requires careful monitoring and titration of dosage.

Both β-blockers and calcium channel blockers should be used with caution in patients with hypotension or HF and should be started with a smaller dose and administered slowly.

CLINICAL PEARLS

Digoxin or amiodarone for control of heart rate As the effect of digoxin on VR is mediated by its vagotonic effect on the AV node, the onset of action may take several hours. For the same reason, digoxin is usually ineffective in the acute setting with high catecholamines status, such as post-operative status, acute sepsis, myocardial ischemia and pulmonary diseases [18].

Both digoxin and verapamil are contraindicated for AF associated with the Wolff–Parkinson–White syndrome.

In critically ill patients with severe HF or hypotension for whom other agents are ineffective or contraindicated for VR control, IV amiodarone is an effective alternative (preferable administrated via central IV line). The most common side effects of IV amiodarone include hypotension, bradycardias, and thrombophlebitis.

Cardioversion

Within the first 24 hours, up to 70–80% of patients with new onset AF convert back to sinus rhythm [18]. If the patient does not convert spontaneously, pharmacological or electrical cardioversion should be attempted. In general, patients with non-valvular AF >48 hours, cardioversion can be safety performed with a low risk of thromboembolism after anticoagulation with heparin. However, in patients with AF >48 hours or in those with higher risk of thromboembolism due to underlying valvular heart disease, 3 weeks of adequate oral anticoagulation prior to cardioversion is recommended. Alternatively, a TEE to exclude atrial thrombi allows immediate cardioversion with IV heparin cover [19]. When LA appendage cannot be adequately visualized, cardioversion should be performed after 3 weeks of

CLINICAL PEARLS

Pharmacological and external electrical cardioversion For recent onset of AF in patients without mitral valve disease and CHF, pharmacological cardioversion should be tried first. It requires no anesthesia and can prevents early recurrence of AF. The disadvantage is that the efficacy is low, and proarrhythmia during cardioversion may occur.

External cardioversion is more effective, with an acute success rate of 90%, but will require heavy sedation or anesthesia.

A number of antiarrhythmic drugs (AADs) may be used for pharmacological cardioversion with variable success rate (Table 10.5). For AF < 48 hours, oral or IV administration of Class I or III AADs can achieve conversion in 60–90% of patients. However, for AF of longer duration, only 15–30% of patients convert to sinus rhythm with pharmacological cardio version [18,19].

The choice of AAD is based on the presence or absence of underlying structural heart diseases in the patient (Figure 10.3). In patients with structural heart diseases, such as CAD and LV dysfunction, Class I AADs are contraindicated as they have been shown to increase the risk of proarrhythmias. Careful monitoring of the patients is required during cardioversion for proarrhythmic events.

If pharmacological cardioversion failed, external electrical cardioversion can still be performed safely to restore sinus rhythm after administration of a either Class I or III AADs. In fact, it is not uncommon to combine the two approaches: an initial trial of AADs, followed by external cardioversion if drugs failed [19].

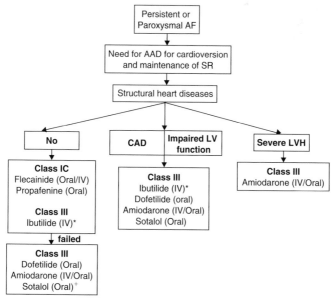

* For acute chemical cardioversion only
+ For maintenance of sinus rhythm in patients with normal LV function

Figure 10.3 Algorithm for choice of anti-arrhythmic agents for cardioversion of atrial fibrillation and maintenance of sinus rhythm.

Table 10.5 Antiarrhythmic drug therapy in atrial fibrillation.

Drug	IV dose	Oral dose	CV efficacy	Relapse rate	Useful in:	Comments
Class IA						
Quinidine gluconate		PO 1.2–1.6 g/day in divided dose	40–84%	46–89%	Renal failure	Vagolytic; many side effects including diarrhea, nausea, TdP and hypotension Avoid in patients with CHF
Procainamide	IV 100 mg bolus over 2 min up to 25 mg/min to 1 g, then 2–6 mg/min	PO 1 g, then up to 500 mg three-hourly	43–65%	NA	Men, short-term therapy	TdP rare; hypotension with IV dose Limit oral use to 6 months to reduce the risk of drug-induced lupus
Disopyramide		PO 100–200 mg six-hourly. Loading dose 300 mg	NA	46–56%	Women Vagally mediated AF	Vagolytic (urinary retention, dry mouth) and negative inotropic effects; hypotension and TdP Avoid in patients with CHF/renal failure
Class IC						
Flecainide	IV 1–2 mg/kg	PO 50–150 mg BD	67–95%	19–51%	Patients without heart disease Failure of Class IA drugs	Proarrhythmia; negative isotropic; central nervous system effects; increased incidence of sudden death postinfarct Avoid in patients with heart failure and CAD
Propafenone		PO 150–300 mg TDS	45–87%	54–70%	Patients without heart disease Failure of Class IA drugs	Proarrhythmia; modest negative inotropic effect; gastrointestinal side-effects; unknown effects postinfarct

Class III

Drug	IV dose	PO dose			Indication / Contraindication	Side effects
Sotalol	IV 1–2 mg/kg	PO 80–240 mg BD	8–54%	51–63%	CADs Failure of Class IA or IC drugs	Sinus bradycardia; AV block; negative inotropic, TdP if hyperaemic. Avoid in patients with congestive heart failure
Ibutilide	1–2 mg or 0.01–0.025 mg/kg		33–63%	NA	Acute therapy with short half-time (4 hrs)	Proarrhythmia. Avoid in patients with low EF and hypokalemia
Amiodarone	IV 5–7 mg/kg up to 1500 mg/24 hours	PO loading 600–800 mg daily, maintenance 100–400 mg QD	37–73%	17–47%	CHF Failure of other drugs Renal failure	Many side effects including pulmonary fibrosis, gastrointestinal upset, thyroid dysfunction, eye and skin changes. TdP uncommon

AF, atrial fibrillation; CAD, coronary artery disease; CHF, congestive heart failure; CV, cardiovascular; EF, ejection fraction; IV, intravenous; TdP, Torsades de pointes.

oral anticoagulation. Nevertheless, in both approaches, anticoagulation with warfarin should be continued for 3–4 weeks after cardioversion to prevent thrombi from forming in the postcardioversion period. Such method of anticoagulation before cardioversion decreases the overall risk of stroke from 6% to less than 1%. If the episode of AF lasts for more than 7 days, the chances of spontaneous cardioversion are greatly diminished. In those cases, restoration of sinus rhythm can be achieved by electrical or pharmacological cardioversion.

Chronic atrial fibrillation

After identifying and treating any underlying causes, there are three strategies to be considered for all patients with persistent AF: restore and/or maintain sinus rhythm, control VR and prevent thromboembolism.

Treatment Strategy

The perceived beneficial effects of restoration and maintenance of sinus rhythm in patients with AF have not been confirmed in clinical trial. Currently, several clinical trials comparing the two strategies of rhythm control versus rate control have been published: the Pharmacological Intervention in Atrial Fibrillation (PIAF) [20], Atrial Fibrillation Follow-up Investigation of Rhythm Management (AFFIRM) [21], Rate Control Versus Electrical Cardioversion for Persistent Atrial Fibrillation (RACE) [22], Strategies of Treatment of Atrial Fibrillation (STAF) [23], How to Treat Chronic Atrial Fibrillation (HOT CAFÉ) [24].

Evidence-based Medicine: Meta-analysis from PIAF, AFFIRM, RACE and STAF

A pooled analysis [25] of 4975 patients from PIAF, AFFIRM, RACE and STAF was performed. Overall, these four trials included elderly patients (mean age from 60–70 years old), greater than 60% were men and 75% patients had persistent and recurrent AF. In the rhythm control arm, amiodarone was the most common AAD used (followed by sotalol and propafenone) and only a small minority of patients had non-pharmacological therapies. In the rate control arm, AV nodal blocking agents were used in the majority of patients and <5% of patients with AV nodal ablation and pacemaker implant. In the pooled results of these trials, there was a non-significant trend for excess mortality in the rhythm control strategy (hazard ratio 1.12, 95% CI 0.98–1.28, $P = 0.09$), as seen in AFFIRM. There were no differences between rate control vs. rhythm control strategies with respect to the risks for thromboembolic stroke (hazard ratio 1.63, 95% CI 0.81–3.28, $P = 0.20$, favoring rate control).

Therefore, there is no particular advantage in major clinical outcome endpoints for rhythm control over the rate control. For functional endpoint, PIAF, AFFIRM and HOT CAFÉ; have demonstrated some improvement in exercise capacity in the rhythm control arm [20,24,26]. However, the costs, need for hospitalization and adverse drug effects, were also greater with rhythm control strategy [27]. These studies highlighted the low clinical efficacy of current AADs to maintain sinus rhythm, and this probably contributes to the stroke risk associated with rhythm control. Indeed, the presence of sinus rhythm (with or without AADs) was associated with a significant reduction in the risk for death, but the use of AADs is associated with increased mortality [28]. In AFFIRM, the risk of ischemic stroke was strongly related to the lack of or suboptimal anticoagulation therapy [21]. Therefore, independent of the use of rate control or rhythm control strategies, anticoagulation should be considered in patients with stroke risk factors (see below).

CRITICAL THINKING

When rhythm control is better than rate control? The equivalent status of the two therapeutic strategies (rate and rhythm control) may not be applicable to all patients with AF. In the PIAF AFFIRM, RACE and STAF studies [21–24], the majority of patients were elderly with persistent AF (>75%) and mild symptoms, had multiple risk factors for stroke, but with only a small proportion with valvular heart diseases, HF and symptomatic PAF. Indeed, recent studies in younger patients with valvular heart diseases and AF have demonstrated a possible benefit of rhythm control in term of reduction in mortality and improvement in functional class, quality of life and exercise time [29]. Therefore, there are different subsets of AF patients, both young and old, who are potential candidates for benefits from maintenance of sinus rhythm (Table 10.6).

Table 10.6 Choice of rate control vs. rhythm control strategy.

Favor rate control strategy	*Favor rhythm control strategy*
Persistent AF	Paroxysmal AF
No symptoms of AF	Severe and frequent symptoms of AF
Age >65 years old	Age <65 years old
Presence of HTN and CADs	Absence of HTN and CAD
Failure or contraindications to AADs	No previous failure of AADs
Patient preferences	Patient preferences
Failure or contraindication to	Valvular heart diseases
electrical cardioversion	CHF

AF, atrial fibrillation; AADs, antiarrhythmic drugs; CAD, coronary artery disease; CHF, congestive heart failure; HTN, hypertension.

Chronic Ventricular Rate Control

The aims of chronic VR controls during AF are to relieve symptoms and to prevent tachycardia-associated cardiomyopathy. However, there is very limited data to guide the optimal VR control in AF patients at rest and during exercise [25]. The rate is generally considered controlled when the ventricular response ranges between 60–80 bpm at rest and between 90–115 bpm during moderate exercise [19,30]. As a result, the patient's heart rate profile at rest and during moderate exercise are required for optimal rate control.

CLINICAL PEARLS

When is the heart rate considered controlled? The heart rate response on treadmill test and/or the heart rate trend during ambulatory Holter monitoring are valuable in assessing rate control in AF patients. In certain conditions, such as mitral stenosis and diastolic heart failure, an even lower resting heart rate may be desirable. However, excessive blunting of the heart rate response during exercise during AF can actually lead to a decrease in exercise capacity [31]. Furthermore, regularization of the VR during AF can further improve hemodynamic status. Unfortunately, current pharmacological agents have very limited efficacious in controlling rhythm irregularity during AF [32].

Either β-blockers or rate-limiting calcium antagonists are preferable initial choice of monotherapy for VR control in AF patients (see Table 10.4). Both class of agents are effective for controlling heart rate during exercise. In AF patients with concomitant CAD, HTN and systolic heart failure, the use of β-blockers (e.g. carvedilol and metoprolol) may provide additional benefit. The non-dihydropyridine (or rate-limiting) calcium channel blockers (diltiazem, vera-pamil) are also effective in reducing VR. These agents are also useful in AF patients with concomitant HTN and CAD, or with contraindication with β-blockers, such as asthma. Digoxin should only be considered for use as monotherapy in sedentary and elderly patients, as it is less effective for VR control during exercise. If monotherapy is inadequate to control the VR, combination therapy should be considered. Indeed, β-blockers or rate-limiting calcium channel blockers could be co-administered with digoxin to provide better over-all control of VR in chronic AF especially during exercise [33]. Furthermore, in patients with systolic HF and AF, a combination of digoxin and β-blockers can provide additional beneficial effect on rate control, symptoms and LV function. In refractory patients, long-term low dose amiodarone may be required for additional rate control. Alternatively, AV nodal ablation and permanent pacing (see below) are useful for rate control when other agents failed or contraindi-cated, especially in the setting of LV systolic dysfunction.

Restoration and Maintenance of Sinus Rhythm

Restoration of sinus rhythm can be achieved by either pharmacological or elec-trical cardioversion. As discussed above, if AF persists for more than 48 hours, the efficacy of pharmacological cardioversion is low and electrical cardioversion is usually required for restoration of sinus rhythm. Electrical cardioversion via external transthoracic synchronized electrical shock, especially with the recently available biphasic defibrillator, is a very effective method (success rate >90%) of restoring sinus rhythm [34]. However, all patients with persistent AF should receive appropriate anticoagulation therapy before and after cardioversion.

A more difficult task is to maintain sinus rhythm after successful cardioversion. Some patients may not have recurrence after a single episode of AF, especially in those with clear reversible causes of AF and no chronic form of drug therapy is needed after cardioversion. However, in most patients cardioverted from chronic AF, the early and late recurrence rate of AF without AAD therapy is high [19]. The efficacy of different AADs is comparable and only about 50% of patients remain in sinus rhythm, with the possible exception of amiodarone (see Table 10.5). The use of sequential AADs and repeated cardioversion has been suggested to increase the proportion of patients successfully treated and maintain in sinus rhythm [19]. However, it is unclear whether sinus rhythm was maintained by repeated defibrillation or because of the different drug efficacy. Because of the limited efficacy of all forms of drug therapy, a drug that maintains sinus rhythm for months or years should probably be given at least one more trial after a repeat cardioversion. Furthermore, caution should be taken for potential adverse effects when using AADs for suppression of AF. The choice of long-term AADs depends on the underlying co-morbidities (see Figure 10.2).

 CLINICAL PEARLS

Side effects of anti-arrhythmic drugs In addition to the general principle on the choice of AADs (as for chemical cardioversion, i.e., Class I agents should be avoided in patients with structural heart diseases) the long-term adverse effects of AADs should be considered (see Table 10.5).

The risk for drug-induced Torsades de pointes (TdP) is enhanced by metabolic disturbances, LV dysfunction, history of ventricular tachycardia, prolongation of QT interval and relative bradycardia.

Amiodarone appears to have a lower risk of proarrhythmia (<1%) as compared to other AADs. However, amiodarone has considerable extracardiac adverse effects-pulmonary fibrosis, hepatic and thyroid dysfunction, and neurologic and dermatologic effects, especially at higher dose and after long-term use. Furthermore, it increases the plasma levels of warfarin, digoxin and numerous other drugs, in which their dosage should be reduced after initiation of amiodarone [35]. Due to the unfavorable long term side effect profile, amiodarone should be used in patients with significant heart disease and as a last resort when other drugs have failed [19].

Newer AADs, such as azimilide, tedisamil, dronaderone, RSD-1235, with potentially better clinical efficacy and safety profiles are under development, and may ultimately be used for treatment of AF in the future.

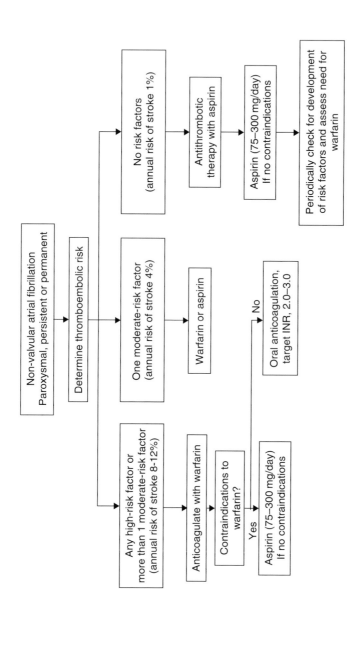

Figure 10.4 Algorithm for decision of the use of anti-thrombotic therapy in patients with non-valvular AF. (Adapted from Fuster V, Ryden LE, Cannon DS et al. ACC/HAH/ESC 2006 Guidelines for the management of patients with atrial fibrillation. J Am Coll of Cardiol 2006;48:854–906)

Paroxysmal Atrial Fibrillation

Patients with self-terminating recurrent AF often pose a management problem. In most of the major clinical trials [20–24] comparing rate control and rhythm control strategy, only ~25% of patients had PAF and highly symptomatic patients were excluded. Therefore, limited data is available in guiding the treatment in such patients.

CLINICAL PEARLS
How to treat PAF and assess its results? In patients with infrequent PAF and without structural heart diseases, a "pill-in-the-pocket" strategy with Class IC agents (single oral dose of propafenone 600 mg or flecainide 300 mg) could be considered [19].

In patients with symptomatic PAF, AV nodal blocking agents with digoxin or β-blockers should be the initial treatment option. Where rate control alone is ineffective, treatment with AADs, as discussed above, may be successful in reducing the frequency of paroxysms, a significant number of treated patients will continue to have symptomatic arrhythmia.

However, suppression of patient's symptomatic AF episodes may not abolish the arrhythmia. A lot of these patients still have asymptomatic episodes that are associated with an increase risk of thromboembolism.

Prevention of Thromboembolism

As discussed above, independent of the use of either rate control or rhythm control strategies, all patients with risk factor for AF-related stroke (Figure 10.4) should be considered for thromboembolism prophylaxis. Patients with different types of AF (paroxysmal, persistent and permanent AF) have a similar risk of stroke. The absence of AF symptoms does not confer a more favorable prognosis and anticoagulation should still be considered in patients with asymptomatic AF or PAF. Furthermore, patients with atrial flutter should be managed with antithrombotic therapy in a similar manner to those with AF, depending on the coexistence of stroke risk factors.

Evidence-based Medicine: Meta-analysis of effectiveness of thromboprophylaxis in patients with non-valvular atrial fibrillation
In a recent meta-analysis of 13 randomized controlled trials including 14,423 participants treated with adjusted-dose warfarin and aspirin, fixed low-dose (FLD) warfarin, ximelagatran or placebo. Outcome measures studied were ischemic stroke, systemic embolism, mortality and hemorrhage. The results showed the adjusted-dose warfarin significantly reduced the risk of ischemic stroke or systemic embolism compared with aspirin (relative risk [RR] 0.59; 95% CI, 0.40–0.86), FLD warfarin (RR 0.36; 95% CI, 0.23–0.58), or placebo (RR 0.33; 95% CI, 0.24–0.45). However, aspirin and

placebo had a lower risk of major bleeding compared to warfarin (RR 0.58; 95% CI, 0.35–0.97 and RR 0.45; 95% CI, 0.25–0.82, respectively), without statistically significant increase risk of intracranial hemorrhage (~0.3% per year) [36].

Furthermore, as compared with aspirin, warfarin was superior in reducing the risk of ischemic stroke or systemic embolism by 41%. Compared with placebo, aspirin alone reduced the risk of stroke by approximately 22%. This benefit is only similar to the effect of antiplatelet therapy on stroke prevention amongst high risk vascular disease patients, thus the protective effect of aspirin is mainly on vascular disease rather than on the AF *per se* [37,38].

All antithrombotic agents confer a risk of bleeding [39]. Therefore, the assessment of risk factors for bleeding complications (Table 10.7) is also an important part of evaluation before initiation of antithrombotic agents. The anticoagulation effect of warfarin is influenced by various food and drug–drug interactions, hepatic dysfunction, dietary vitamin K intake, and genetic variation in enzyme activity, and alcohol intake. The potential risks and benefits of antithrombotic therapy as well as the potential interaction of anticoagulation with food, herbs and drugs should always be explained to patients [40].

After initiation of antithrombotic therapy, continuous and frequent monitoring is essential to maintain safety and efficacy of treatment. Prior studies [41] have shown that the international normalized ratio (INR) should be

Table 10.7 Risk factors for thromboembolic and bleeding complications in patients with atrial fibrillation.

Risk factors for Thromboemoblism	Risk factors for bleeding complications
High-risk factors Previous CVA, TIA or embolism Mitral stenosis Prosthetic heart valve	Age >75 years old History of stroke History of gastrointestinal bleeding Uncontrolled HTN Renal dysfunction Concomitant drugs: aspirin and NSAIDs Underlying malignancy
Moderate-risk factors Age ≥ 75 Hypertension Heart failure LVEF < 35% Diabetes mellitus	
Less validated or weaker risk factors Female gender Age 65 to 74 Coronary artery disease Thyrotoxicosis	

AF, atrial fibrillation; HTN, hypertension; LV, left ventricular; NSAID, non-steroidal anti inflammatory drug. (Adapted from Fuster V, Ryden LE, Cannon DS *et al*. ACC/HAH/ESC 2006 Guidelines for the management of patients with atrial fibrillation. J Am Coll of Cardiol 2006;48:854–906)

maintained between 2.0–3.0 (target 2.5) when dose adjusted warfarin is used. At INRs >3.0, the risk of hemorrhage increases exponentially and at INRs <2.0 the risk of stroke increases.

Anti-thrombotic treatment of patients with AF presenting with acute stroke, after coronary intervention and during perioperative status presents a problem, as there are limited data on these aspects. After coronary stenting, the use of dual antiplatelet agents with aspirin plus clopidogrel, together with warfarin will significantly increase the risk of bleeding. Temporarily withdrawal of warfarin during the initial 2–4 weeks may be needed and then followed by warfarin plus clopidogrel [37].

The narrow therapeutic margin of warfarin in conjunction with numerous associated food and drug interactions requires frequent INR testing and dose adjustments. These liabilities of warfarin contribute to significant underutilization, even in high-risk patients. Therefore, alternative therapies that are easier to use are needed [42,43].

Currently, novel oral direct thrombin inhibitor, such as ximelagatran, combination antiplatelet with clopidogrel and aspirin, and long acting indirect factor Xa inhibitor, such as idraparinux are undergoing clinical evaluation, which may provide other viable alternatives to warfarin for prevention of thromboembolism in AF. Because ximelagatran does not need anticoagulation monitoring or dose adjustment, it was developed to be an easier drug to administer than adjusted-dose warfarin. However, ximelagatran has been recently withdrawn from the market due to the potential of liver toxicity. Currently, another oral direct thrombin inhibitor – dabigatran titillate – with potential low risk of liver dysfunction is undergoing phase III clinical study.

Finally, as the LA appendage appears to be the primary source of thrombus in AF, novel percutaneous mechanical devices have been developed to obliterate the LA appendage for stroke prevention in patients at high risk of stroke but not suitable for long-term anticoagulation [44]. Furthermore, surgical obliteration and/or removal of the LA appendage in those patients who undergo open heart surgery may be also a strategy for stroke prevention in high risk AF patients [45]. Both of these methods are currently undergoing clinical trials.

Non-pharmacological Approaches

The limited efficacy and proarrhythmic risks of AADs have led the exploration of a wide spectrum of alternative non-pharmacological therapies to treat AF. Furthermore, recent observations on the mechanisms of AF have resulted in the development of different non-pharmacological therapies that directed to eliminate the triggers and to modify the electrophysiological substrate for the prevention and treatment of AF. Indications and potential adverse effects of non-pharmacological treatments of AF include: surgical Maze procedure, device therapies, and catheter ablation are summarized in Table 10.8. In some patients, combined pharmacological and non-pharmacological therapies may be required for successful rhythm control.

Table 10.8 Non-pharmacological therapy for atrial fibrillation.

Non-pharmacological therapy	Current indications	Adverse effects
Surgical Maze procedures	Patients with AF undergoing concomitant open heart surgery such as mitral valve surgery or bypass surgery	Sinus node dysfunction necessitates permanent pacing (~6%) Postoperative bleeding (~5%) Stroke (~0.5%) Postoperative arrhythmias (~30%) Operative mortality (2–4%)
Device therapies Atrial pacing	In AF patients with conventional indications for pacemaker implantations	
Defibrillator	In AF patients with conventional indications for implantable cardioverter defibrillator	Shock discomfort Early reinitiation of AF
AV nodal ablation and permanent pacing	Symptomatic patients refractory to other rate and rhythm control therapies Patients who already have an implanted pacemaker or defibrillator	Pacemaker dependence Sudden death early after ablation (<0.1%)
Catheter ablation for AF	Symptomatic patients refractory to AADs Younger patients with lone AF Patients unable or unwilling to take long-term AADs	Vascular access complications (1%) Stroke and transient ischaemic attack (1%) Significant pulmonary vein stenosis (0.5–1%) Proarrhythmia (10–20%) Rare: valvular, phrenic nerve and oesophagus injury

AADs, antiarrhythmic drugs; AF, atrial fibrillation.

Surgical Maze Procedure

The surgical approach was designed to create conduction barriers at the critical area within the left and right atria to prevent the maintenance of AF. Based on the animal and human mapping studies, Cox *et al.* [46] described the surgical Maze procedure that involved encircling the pulmonary veins and multiple linear atrial incisions over both atria using either the classical "cut-and-sew" technique or different energy sources (radiofrequency, microwave, ultrasound and cryoablation) for curative ablation of AF [46]. The reported success rate of surgical Maze procedure ranged from 85–95%, and no significant difference was observed between different techniques [47]. Furthermore, with the removal or closure of the LA appendage together with maintenance of sinus rhythm, the long-term stroke rate after the surgical Maze procedure is rather low (<1%) [46,47]. The potential advantages of these alternative sources of energy over the "cut-and-sew" technique is less complex procedure, shorter procedure time and can be performed with minimally invasive procedure. Unfortunately, the surgical Maze operation is still very complex and technical demanding, the operator skills rather than tools are the critical determinant of the clinical outcome. Furthermore, because of the associated morbidity including sinus node dysfunction necessitates permanent pacing (~6%), postoperative bleeding (~5%), stroke (~0.5%), and arrhythmias (~30%) as well as the operative mortality (2–4%), surgical therapy for AF remains an unattractive option for patients without another indication for open heart surgery [46,47]. On the other hands, in patients with AF undergoing concomitant open heart surgery such as mitral valve surgery or bypass surgery, maze procedure is a viable option for treatment of drug-refractory AF [48].

Device Therapies – Atrial Pacing and Defibrillation

The utility of permanent atrial pacing as a treatment for PAF in patients without conventional indications for pacing has not been proven [49,50]. In patients with conventional indications for pacemaker implantations – such as sinus node disease, symptomatic bradycardia and chronotropic incompetence, the use of physiological pacemaker (dual chamber or atrial) rather than a single-chamber ventricular pacemaker have been shown to prevent AF [49]. Furthermore, in patients with intact AV conduction, efforts should be made to program the device to minimize the amount of ventricular pacing [51]. Although many of the latest pacemakers and implantable defibrillators have incorporated different features (overdrive pacing, antitachycardia atrial pacing and atrial defibrillation) designed to prevent and terminate AF, no consistent data from large randomized trials support their use. The uses of alternative single-site atrial pacing, multisite right atrial pacing and biatrial pacing have also been tested for treatment and prevention of AF, but no studies have convincingly show a significant benefit on long-term clinical outcome [49]. However, additional studies on these different pacing algorithms and sites are ongoing, which will help to clarify their role in the treatment of AF.

Currently, there is no role for stand alone atrial defibrillator for treatment of AF due to the issue of cost, patients' tolerability and early reinitiation of AF after shock. However, in AF patients implanted with an implantable cardioverter defibrillator for primary or secondary prevention of ventricular tachyarrhythmias, the appropriate use of physician- or patient-activated shock therapy device could effectively terminate AF and reduced AF burden in those patients [52].

Catheter Ablation

Ablation of AV node and permanent pacing is an effective strategy for symptomatic relief and/or rate control in patients with medically refractory AF. In a meta-analysis of 21 studies [53], there were significant improvements after ablation and pacing therapy in quality of life and clinical outcome measures (except fractional shortening), and the calculated 1-year total and sudden death mortality rates were 6.3% and 2.0%, respectively. In patients with symptomatic HF or impaired LV systolic function, biventricular pacing after AV nodal ablation for permanent AF appears to provide better improvement in functional capacity and LV function as compared with right ventricular pacing [54]. However, this approach is highly invasive and creates dependence in an implanted pacemaker. It is commonly considered in AF patients in whom other therapies failed to achieve either rate or rhythm control and in patients who already have an implanted pacemaker or defibrillator.

Based on the success of the surgical approach [46] and the recognition that the pulmonary veins are a common source of rapidly depolarizing arrhythmogenic foci that induce PAF [7], catheter ablation strategies for treatment of AF are primarily targeted to eliminate the triggers that initiate or perpetuate AF and to modify atrial substrate that sustain AF. In patients with PAF, arrhythmogenic foci from the pulmonary veins, or less commonly from other atrial sites (superior vena cava, coronary sinus, LA posterior wall, vein of Marshall, and interatrial septum) may play a more important role in the mechanism of AF. Therefore, elimination of these arrhythmogenic foci can achieve a relatively high successful rate (80–90%) in patients with PAF [55,56]. However, elimination of arrhythmogenic foci alone in patients with persistent AF has a lower success rate (~60%). In patients with persistent AF, the substrate for arrhythmia and changes in the substrate due to electrical remodeling induced by AF become more important. Therefore, as compared to PAF, curative ablation approach for persistent AF needs to target both additional triggers as well as linear or focal ablation over the atrial substrates outside the pulmonary veins [57]. Currently, different catheter ablation techniques to electrically isolate the pulmonary veins from the LA (segmental ostial isolation) and/or to modify the LA substrate around the pulmonary veins (circumferential ablation) are used by most investigators for curative ablation of AF. In specialized centers with extensive experience in performing AF ablation, the success rate achieved with different catheter ablation techniques appears to be comparable (~80%). Even in patients with HF and impaired LVEF, AF ablation restored sinus rhythm without AADs in 70% of patients and significantly improved LV function [58].

 EMERGING TREND

Catheter ablation vs. medication trial In order to determine whether pulmonary vein isolation (PVI) is feasible as first-line therapy for treating patients with symptomatic AF, a multicenter prospective study randomized 70 patients with symptomatic AF to receive either PVI using radiofrequency ablation ($n = 33$) or anti-arrhythmic drug treatment ($n = 37$), with a 1-year follow-up. At the end of 1-year follow-up, 22 (63%) of 35 patients who received anti-arrhythmic drugs had at least one recurrence of symptomatic AF compared with four (13%) of 32 patients who received PVI ($P < 0.001$). Hospitalization during 1-year follow-up occurred in 19 (54%) of 35 patients in the anti-arrhythmic drug group compared with three (9%) of 32 in the

PVI group ($P < 0.001$). In the anti-arrhythmic drug group, the mean (SD) number of AF episodes decreased from 12 (7) to 6 (4), after initiating therapy ($P = 0.01$). At 6-month follow-up, the improvement in quality of life of patients in the PVI group was significantly better than the improvement in the anti-arrhythmic drug group in five subclasses of the Short-Form 36 health survey. There were no thrombo-embolic events in either group. Asymptomatic, mild or moderate pulmonary vein stenosis was documented in two (6%) of 32 patients in the PVI group [59].

Despite the impressive reported success rates achieved with AF ablation [55–59], these procedures are associated with a significant risk of serious and life-threatening complications. Major complications from AF ablation include complications secondary to vascular access (1%), stroke and transient ischemic attack (1%), significant pulmonary vein stenosis (0.5–1%), proarrhythmia (10–20%), valvular, phrenic nerve and esophagus injury (rare) [54,55]. Furthermore, AF ablation procedures remain technically difficult and operator dependent, most centers have limited experience and a lower success rate than those reported series [60]. Recently, remote magnetic navigation for AF ablation is safe and feasible with a short learning curve. Although all procedures were performed by highly experienced operators, remote AF ablation can be performed even by less experienced operators [61].

In addition, repeat procedure is required in a significant proportion (10–40%) of patients to achieve the high reported success rate. Finally, limited data is available on the long-term clinical efficacy and risk of stroke after ablation. For now, AF ablation may perhaps be considered in symptomatic patients who were resistant to pharmacological treatment, especially those who are younger and have lone AF, and in patients unable or unwilling to take long-term AADs.

Recently, treatment with angiotension converting enzyme inhibitor (ACEI) and angiotensin receptor blockers (ARB) showed lower incidence of AF.

 EMERGING TREND

Angiotensin converting enzyme inhibition to prevent atrial fibrillation

A systematic review of the literature was performed to identify all reports of the effect of ACEIs or ARBs on the development of AF. The results showed that a total of 11 studies, which included 56,308 patients, were identified: four in heart failure, three in HTN, two in patients following cardioversion for AF, and two in patients following myocardial infarction. Overall, ACEIs and ARBs reduced the relative risk of AF by 28% (95% CI, 15–40%, $P = 0.0002$). Reduction in AF was similar between the two classes of drugs (ACEI: 28%, $P = 0.01$; ARB: 29%, $P = 0.00002$) and was greatest in patients with HF (relative risk reduction [RRR] = 44%, $P = 0.007$). Overall, there was no significant reduction in AF in patients with HTN (RRR = 12%, $P = 0.4$), although one trial found a significant 29% reduction in patients with LV hypertrophy. In patients following cardioversion, there appears to be a large effect (48% RRR), but the confidence limits are wide (95% CI, 21–65%). Both ACEIs and ARBs appear to be effective in the prevention of AF. This benefit appears to be limited to patients with systolic LV dysfunction or LV hypertrophy. The use of these drugs following cardioversion appears promising but requires further study [62].

Difficult Situations and Suggested Solutions

Real World Question Who are the Patients Who May Not Need Anticoagulant Therapy for Atrial Fibrillation?

Despite this clear evidence to support the use of antithrombotic therapy in AF, an individual's risk of stroke and hemorrhage needs to be considered when making the decision about the optimal antithrombotic therapy. In the new ACC/AHA/ESC 2006 guidelines for the management of patients with atrial fibrillation, multiple risk stratification models and guideline have been introduced based on the pooled analysis of the original anti-thrombotic treatment trials and expert consensus on the different clinical risk factors associated with AF (see Table 10.7) [63]. A simple risk score – the CHADS$_2$ scheme (CHF, HTN, Age >75, Diabetes mellitus, and prior Stroke or transient ischemic attack) has been validated in a national registry of elderly AF patients for stroke prediction [38].

Evidence-based Medicine: The CHADS$_2$ index

In order to assess the predictive value of classification schemes that estimate stroke risk in patients with AF, two existing classification schemes were combined into a new stroke-risk scheme, the CHADS$_2$ index, and all three classification schemes were validated. The CHADS$_2$ was formed by assigning one point each for the presence of CHF, HTN, age 75 years or older, and diabetes mellitus; and by assigning two points for history of stroke or transient ischemic attack. Data from peer review organizations representing seven states were used to assemble a National Registry of AF (NRAF) consisting of 1733 Medicare beneficiaries aged 65–95 years who had non-rheumatic AF and were not prescribed warfarin at hospital discharge. The main outcome measure is hospitalization for ischemic stroke. During 2121 patient-years of follow-up, 94 patients were readmitted to the hospital for ischemic stroke (stroke rate, 4.4 per 100 patient-years). As indicated by a c statistic greater than 0.5, the two existing classification schemes predicted stroke better than chance: c of 0.68 (95% CI, 0.65–0.71) for the scheme developed by the Atrial Fibrillation Investigators (AFI) and c of 0.74 (95% CI, 0.71–0.76) for the Stroke Prevention in Atrial Fibrillation (SPAF) III scheme. However, with a c statistic of 0.82 (95% CI, 0.80–0.84), the CHADS$_2$ index was the most accurate predictor of stroke. The stroke rate per 100 patient-years without antithrombotic therapy increased by a factor of 1.5 (95% CI, 1.3–1.7) for each one-point increase in the $CHADS_2$ score:

1.9 (95% CI, 1.2–3.0) for a score of 0
2.8 (95% CI, 2.0–3.8) for 1
4.0 (95% CI, 3.1–5.1) for 2
5.9 (95% CI, 4.6–7.3) for 3;
8.5 (95% CI, 6.3–11.1) for 4
12.5 (95% CI, 8.2–17.5) for 5
18.2 (95% CI, 10.5–27.4) for 6

The two existing classification schemes and especially the new stroke risk index, $CHADS_2$, can quantify risk of stroke for patients who have AF and may aid in selection of antithrombotic therapy [38]. However, this scheme did not provide a clear recommendation for antithrombotic therapy in patients with intermediate risk. A more practical treatment guideline for antithrombotic treatment in AF has been proposed in the guidelines of the ACC, AHA and ESC [63] (see Figure 10.4).

Anticoagulation with an oral VKA, such as warfarin, has far greater efficacy than aspirin in preventing stroke, and particularly in preventing severe ischemic stroke, in AF. Aspirin therapy was recommended for lower-risk groups, estimating that the absolute expected benefit of anticoagulant therapy may not be worth the increased hemorrhagic risk and burden of anticoagulation. Individual lower-risk patients may rationally choose anticoagulation over aspirin therapy to gain greater protection against ischemic stroke if they value protection against stroke much more highly than reducing risk of hemorrhage and burden of managing anticoagulation [63].

Besides ASA, another anti-platelet (clopidogrel) was tried in the Atrial Fibrillation Clopidogrel Trial with Irbesartan for Prevention of Vascular Events (ACTIVE-W) trial. It was stopped on the recommendation of the Data Safety and Monitoring Board before planned follow-up was completed because the combination of clopidogrel (75 mg daily) plus aspirin (75 to 100 mg daily) was proved to be inferior to warfarin (target INR 2.0 to 3.0) in patients with an average of 2 stroke risk factors in addition to AF [64].

Real World Question How to Anticoagulate the Atrial Fibrillation Patient Presenting with Acute Stroke?

In AF patients presenting with acute stroke, acute anti-thrombotic therapy with heparin reduces re-infarction, but the increased risk of hemorrhagic transformation may outweigh its benefit. The use of aspirin during the acute phase was associated with modest benefits for reduction of early recurrent stroke and functional outcome [42]. Therefore, aspirin followed by early initiation of warfarin for long-term secondary prevention is reasonable anti-thrombotic management. Before starting any anti-thrombotic agent, a CT scan of the brain be obtained to confirm the absence of intracranial hemorrhage. In patients with AF with no evidence of hemorrhage and small infarct size (or no evidence of infarction), anticoagulation (aiming for INR 2–3) can be started, provided the patient is normotensive. In patients with AF with a large cerebral infarction, the initiation of anticoagulation should be delayed for 2–4 weeks due to the potential risk of hemorrhagic transformation, which is an absolute contraindication to the immediate and future use of anticoagulation for stroke prevention in AF [37].

Real World Question How to Manage Anticoagulant Therapy in Atrial Fibrillation Patients with a Therapeutic INR Level Presenting with Acute Stroke?

An urgent imaging (CT scan or MRI) of the brain should be obtained to confirm the presence or absence of intracranial hemorrhage and to assess the size of any cerebral infarction, and INR level should be measured. In patient with no evidence of hemorrhage and small infarct, anticoagulation can be continued and maintained at therapeutic level providing that the patient is normotensive. In patients with hemorrhage, the INR should be corrected with vitamin K and fresh frozen plasma. In patients with no evidence of hemorrhage but large infarct, anticoagulation should be withheld until a repeated imaging at 2 weeks later shows no evidence of hemorrhage. The use of additional antiplatelet agents on top of warfarin with stroke is conflicting. Based on the potential vascular rather than cardiac source of stroke in AF patients, the combination therapy seems to be appropriate. However, the risk of bleeding will be higher especially during the first few weeks after acute stroke and currently, no data is available to support this approach. For patients with AF who suffer an ischemic stroke or TIA despite therapeutic anticoagulation, no data indicate that either increasing the intensity of anticoagulation or adding an antiplatelet agent provides additional protection against future ischemic events. If AF patients sustain cardioembolic events while receiving low intensity anticoagulation, then anticoagulation intensity should be increased to a maximum target INR of 3.0 to 3.5 rather than routinely adding antiplatelet agents [63]. In addition, both strategies are associated with an increase in bleeding risk.

Real World Question How to Interrupt Anticoagulation for Diagnostic or Therapeutic Procedures?

From time to time, it may be necessary to interrupt oral anticoagulant therapy in preparation for elective surgical procedures. In patients with AF who do not have mechanical valves, however, based on extrapolation from the annual rate of thromboembolism in patients with nonvalvular AF, anticoagulation may be interrupted for a period of up to 1 week for surgical or diagnostic procedures that carry a risk of bleeding without substituting heparin (UFH). In high-risk patients (particularly those with prior stroke, TIA, or systemic embolism) or when a series of procedures requires interruption of oral anticoagulant therapy for longer periods, UFH or low-molecular-weight heparin (LMWH) may be administered intravenously or subcutaneously. Laboratory monitoring is not required when LMWH is used except in patient with obesity, renal insufficiency, or pregnancy [63].

Take Home Message

AF is a common and growing problem due to an aging population, and is associated with substantial morbidity, mortality and resource consumption. Currently, two approaches are acceptable: maintaining sinus rhythm by AADs vs. controlling the VR. However, the optimal treatment strategies for AF for different subgroup of patients remain unclear and await results from further ongoing randomized controlled trials. Independent of the use of rate control or rhythm control strategy, the risk of thrombo-embolic complications in high risk patients remains, and anti-thrombotic therapy should be considered in all AF patients with high stroke risk. Decisions for immediate or delayed cardioversion, pharmacologically or electrically, and anticoagulation have to be made based on the clinical presentation and the individual patient's need for restoration and maintenance of sinus rhythm.

The chance of maintaining sinus rhythm and the risk of adverse side effects should be considered when long term AADs therapy is used to suppress AF. In some patients, VR control by drugs or catheter ablation with pacemaker and anti-thrombotic prophylaxis may be preferable to cardioversion and long term AAD therapy. The limited efficacy and risk of pharmacological therapy for preventing AF have stimulated interest in non-pharmacological approaches to maintain sinus rhythm. In particularly, further technological advances in the catheter ablation technique for restoration and maintenance of sinus rhythm appear promising and may play a more important role in the treatment of AF in the near future.

References

1 Benjamin EJ, Wolf PA, Kannel WB. The epidemiology of atrial fibrillation, pp. 1–22. In: Falk RH, Podrid PJ, Editors, Atrial Fibrillation: Mechanisms and Management, 2nd edition. Lippinott-Raven Publishers, Philadelphia; 1997.
2 Lok NS, Lau CP. Prevalence of palpitations, cardiac arrhythmias and their associated risk factors in ambulant elderly. Int J Cardiol 1996;54:231–236.
3 Braunwald E. Shattuck lecture: Cardiovascular medicine at the turn of the millennium: Triumphs, concerns and opportunities. N Engl J Med 1997;337:1360–1369.
4 Levy S, Maarek M, Coumel P et al. Characterization of different subsets of atrial fibrillation in general practice in France: The ALFA study. The College of French Cardiologists. Circulation 1999;99:3028–3035.
5 Moe GK, Abildskov JA. Atrial fibrillation as a self-sustaining arrhythmia independent of focal discharge. Am Heart J 1959;58:59–70.
6 Tse HF, Lau CP. Electrophysiological properties of the fibrillating atrium:implications for therapy. Clin Exp Pharm Physiol 1998;25:293–302.
7 Haïssaguerre M, Jaïs P, Shah DC et al. Spontaneous initiation of atrial fibrillation by ectopic beats originating in the pulmonary veins. N Engl J Med 1998;339:659–666.
8 Allessie MA, Lammers WJEP, Bonke FIM et al. Experimental evaluation of Moe's multiple wavelet hypothesis of atrial fibrillation, pp. 265–275. In: Zipes EP, Jalife J, editors. Cardiac Electrophysiology and Arrhythmias. Fla:Grune & Stratton, Inc, Orlando; 1985.

9 Cox JL, Canavan TE, Schuessler RB *et al.* The surgical treatment of atrial fibrillation. J Thorac Cardiovasc Surg 1991;101:406–426.

10 Wijffels MC, Kirchhof CJ, Dorland R *et al.* Atrial fibrillation begets atrial fibrillation: A study in awake chronically instrumented goats. Circulation 1995;92:1954–1968.

11 Daoud EG, Bogun F, Goyal R *et al.* Effect of atrial fibrillation on atrial refractoriness in humans. Circulation 1996;94:1600–1606.

12 Tse HF, Lau CP, Ayers GM. Heterogeneous changes in electrophysiologic properties in the paroxysmal and chronically fibrillating human atrium. J Cardiovas Electrophysiol 1999;10:125–135.

13 Li D, Faseh S, Leung TK *et al.* Promotion of atrial fibrillation by heart failure in dogs. Atrial remodelling of a different sort. Circulation 1999;100:87–95.

14 Morillo CA, Klein GJ, Jones DJ *et al.* Chronic rapid atrial pacing:structural functional, and electrophysiological characteristics of a new model of sustained atrial fibrillation. Circulation 1995;91:1588–1595.

15 Goette A, Honeycutt C, Langbery JJ. Electrical remodeling in atrial fibrillation. Time course and mechanisms. Circulation 1996;94:2968–2974.

16 Coumel P. Paroxysmal atrial fibrillation: A disorder of autonomic tone? Eur Heart J 1994;15 (Suppl A):9–16.

17 Tomika T, Takei M, Saikawa Y *et al.* Role of autonomic tone in the initiation and termination of paroxysmal atrial fibrillation in patients without structural heart disease. J Cardiovasc Electrophysiol 2004;14:559–564.

18 Jung F, DiMarco JP. Treatment strategies for atrial fibrillation. Am J Med 1998;104:272–286.

19 Fuster V, Ryden LE, Asinger RW *et al.* ACC/AHA/ESC guidelines for the management of patients with atrial fibrillation:executive summary. A Report of the American College of Cardiology/American Heart Association Task Force on Practice Guidelines and the European Society of Cardiology Committee for Practice Guidelines and Policy Conferences (Committee to Develop Guidelines for the Management of Patients With Atrial Fibrillation):developed in Collaboration With the North American Society of Pacing and Electrophysiology. J Am Coll Cardiol 2001;38:1231–1266.

20 Hohnloser SH, Kuck KH, Lilienthal J *et al.* Rhythm or rate control in atrial fibrillation – Pharmacological Intervention in Atrial Fibrillation (PIAF): A randomized trial. Lancet 2000;356:1789–1794.

21 Van Gelder IC, Hagens VE, Bosker HA *et al.* A comparison of rate control and rhythm control in patients with recurrent persistent atrial fibrillation. N Engl J Med 2002;347:1834–1840.

22 The AFFIRM Investigators. A comparison of rate control and rhythm control in patients with atrial fibrillation. N Engl J Med 2002;347:1825–1833.

23 Carlsson J, Miketic S, Windeler J *et al.* Randomized trial of rate-control versus rhythm-control in persistent atrial fibrillation: The Strategies of Treatment of Atrial Fibrillation (STAF) trial. J Am Coll Cardiol 2003;41:1690–1696.

24 Opolski G, Torbicki A, Kosior DA *et al.* Rate control vs. rhythm control in patients with nonvalvular persistent atrial fibrillation. The results of the Polish How to Treat Chronic Atrial Fibrillation (HOT CAFÉ) Study. Chest 2004;126:476–486.

25 Wyse DG. Rate control vs rhythm control strategies in atrial fibrillation. Prog Cardiovasc Dis. 2005;48:125–138.

26 Chung MK, Shemanski L, Sherman DG *et al.* Functional status in rate- versus rhythm-control strategies for atrial fibrillation: results of the Atrial Fibrillation Follow-Up Investigation of Rhythm Management (AFFIRM) Functional Status Substudy. J Am Coll Cardiol 2005;46:1891–1899.

27 Marshall DA, Levy AR, Vidaillet H *et al.* CoST-effectiveness of rhythm vs. rate control in atrial fibrillation. Ann Intern Med 2004;141:653–661.

28 Corley SD, Epstein AE, DiMarco JP *et al.* Relationships between sinus rhythm, treatment, and survival in the Atrial Fibrillation Follow-Up Investigation of Rhythm Management (AFFIRM) Study. Circulation 2004;109:1509–1513.

29 Vora A. Management of atrial fibrillation in rheumatic valvular heart disease. Curr Opin Cardiol 2006;21:47–50.

30 Rawles JM. What is meant by a "controlled" ventricular rate in atrial fibrillation? Br Heart J 1990;63:157–161.

31 DiBianco R, Morganroth J, Freitag JA *et al.* Effects of nadolol on the spontaneous and exercise–provoked heart rate of patients with chronic atrial fibrillation receiving stable dosages of digoxin. Am Heart J 1984;108:1121–1127.

32 Tse HF, Lam YM, Lau CP, Cheung BM, Kumana CR. Comparison of digoxin versus low-dose amiodarone for ventricular rate control in patients with chronic atrial fibrillation. Clin Exp Pharmacol Physiol 2001;28:446–450.

33 Farshi R, Kistner D, Sarma JS *et al.* Ventricular rate control in chronic atrial fibrillation during daily activity and programmed exercise: A crossover open–label study of five drug regimens. J Am Coll Cardiol 1999, 33:304–310.

34 Tse HF, Lau CP. Advances in Internal and External Cardioversion, pp. 419–435. In: Israel CW, Barold SS, editors. Advances in the Treatment of Atrial Tachyarrhythmias, Pacing, Cardioversion and Defibrillation. Futura Publishing Co, Inc., Armonk, NY; 2001.

35 Goldschlager N, Epstein AE, Naccarelli G *et al.* Practical guidelines for clinicians who treat patients with amiodarone. Practice Guidelines Subcommittee, North American Society of Pacing and Electrophysiology. Arch Intern Med 2000;160:1741–1748.

36 Lip GY, Edwards SJ. Stroke prevention with aspirin, warfarin and ximelagatran in patients with non-valvular atrial fibrillation: A systematic review and meta-analysis. Thromb Res 2006;118:321–333.

37 Lip GY, Boos CJ. Antithrombotic treatment in atrial fibrillation. Heart 2006; 92:155–161.

38 Gage BF, Waterman AD, Shannon W *et al.* Validation of Clinical Classification Schemes for Predicting Stroke: Results From the National Registry of Atrial Fibrillation JAMA 2001;285:2864–2870.

39 Levine MN, Raskob G, Beyth RJ *et al.* Hemorrhagic complications of anticoagulant treatment: The Seventh ACCP Conference on Antithrombotic and Thrombolytic Therapy. Chest. 2004;126 (suppl):287S–310S.

40 Singer DE, Albers GW, Dalen JE *et al.* Antithrombotic therapy in atrial fibrillation: The Seventh ACCP Conference on Antithrombotic and Thrombolytic Therapy. Chest 2004;126 (suppl):429–456S.

41 Gage BF, van Walraven C, Pearce L *et al.* Selecting patients with atrial fibrillation for anti-coagulation: stroke risk stratification in patients taking aspirin. Circulation 2004; 110:2287–2292.

42 Hart RG, Palacio S, Pearce LA. Atrial fibrillation, stroke, and acute antithrombotic therapy: Analysis of randomized clinical trials. Stroke. 2002;33:2722–2727.

43 Jaffer AK, Ahmed M, Brotman DJ *et al.* Low-molecular-weight-heparins as periprocedural anticoagulation for patients on long-term warfarin therapy: A standardized bridging therapy protocol. J Thromb Thrombolysis 2005;20:11–16.

44 Ostermayer SH, Reisman M, Kramer PH. Percutaneous Left Atrial Appendage Transcatheter Occlusion (PLAATO System) to Prevent Stroke in high-Risk Patients With non-Rheumatic Atrial Fibrillation Results From the International multi-Center Feasibility Trials J Am Coll Cardiol 2005;46:9–14.

45 Crystal E, Lamy A, Connolly SJ *et al*. Left Atrial Appendage Occlusion Study (LAAOS): A randomized clinical trial of left atrial appendage occlusion during routine coronary artery bypass graft surgery for long-term stroke prevention. Am. Heart J 2003;145:174–178.

46 Cox JL. Cardiac surgery for arrhythmias. J Cardiovasc ElectroPhysiol 2004;15:250–262.

47 Khargi K, Hutten BA, Lemke B, Deneke T. Surgical treatment of atrial fibrillation; a systematic review. Eur J Cardiothorac Surg 2005;27:258–265.

48 Reston JT, Shuhaiber JH. meta-analysis of clinical outcomes of maze–related surgical procedures for medically refractory atrial fibrillation. Eur J Cardiothorac Surg 2005;28:724–730.

49 Knight BP, Gersh BJ, Carlson MD *et al*. Role of permanent pacing to prevent atrial fibrillation: science advisory from the American Heart Association Council on Clinical Cardiology (Subcommittee on Electrocardiography and Arrhythmias) and the Quality of Care and Outcomes Research Interdisciplinary Working Group, in collaboration with the Heart Rhythm Society. Circulation 2005;111:240–243.

50 Lau CP, Tse HF, Yu CM *et al*. New Indication for Preventive Pacing in Atrial Fibrillation (NIPP–AF) Investigators. Dual-site atrial pacing for atrial fibrillation in patients without bradycardia. Am J Cardiol 2001;88:371–375.

51 Sweeney MO, Prinzen FW. A new paradigm for physiologic ventricular pacing. J Am Coll Cardiol 2006;47:282–288.

52 Tse HF, Lau CP. Future prospects for implantable devices for atrial defibrillation. Cardiol Clin 2004;22:87–100.

53 Wood MA, Brown-Mahoney C, Kay GN, Ellenbogen KA. Clinical outcomes after ablation and pacing therapy for atrial fibrillation: A meta-analysis. Circulation 2000;101:1138–1144.

54 Doshi RN, Daoud EG, Fellows C *et al*. Left ventricular-based cardiac stimulation post AV nodal ablation evaluation (the PAVE study). J Cardiovasc ElectroPhysiol 2005;16:1160–1165.

55 Verma A, Natale A. Should atrial fibrillation ablation be considered firST-line therapy for some patients? Why atrial fibrillation ablation should be considered firST-line therapy for some patients. Circulation 2005;112:1214–1222.

56 Padanilam BJ, Prystowsky EN. Should atrial fibrillation ablation be considered firST-line therapy for some patients? Should ablation be firST-line therapy and for whom? the antagonist position. Circulation 2005;112:1223–1229.

57 Tse HF, Lau CP. Catheter ablation for persistent atrial fibrillation: Are we ready for "prime time"? J Cardiovasc ElectroPhysiol 2005;16:1148–1149.

58 Hsu LF, Jais P, Sanders P *et al*. Catheter ablation for atrial fibrillation in CHF. N Engl J Med 2004;351:2373–2383.

59 Wazni OM, Marrouche NF, Martin DO *et al*. Radiofrequency ablation vs antiarrhythmic drugs as firST-line treatment of symptomatic atrial fibrillation: A randomized trial. JAMA 2005;293:2634–2640.

60 Cappato R, Calkins H, Chen SA *et al*. Worldwide survey on the methods, efficacy, and safety of catheter ablation for human atrial fibrillation. Circulation 2005;111:1100–1105.

61 Pappone C, Vicedomini G, Manguso F *et al*. Robotic Magnetic Navigation for Atrial Fibrillation Ablation J Am Coll Cardiol 2006;47:1390–1400.

62 Healey JS, Baranchuk A, Crystal E, Morillo CA, Garfinkle M, Yusuf S, Connolly SJ. Prevention of atrial fibrillation with angiotensin-converting enzyme inhibitors and angiotensin receptor blockers: A meta-analysis. J Am Coll Cardiol 2005;45(11):1832–1839.

63 Fuster V, Ryden LE, Cannon DS *et al*. ACC/HAH/ESC 2006 Guidelines for the management of patients with atrial fibrillation. J Am Coll of Cardiol 2006;48:854–906.

CHAPTER 11

Mitral Regurgitation

Jui-Sung Hung, Kean-Wah Lau, Zee-Pin Ding, Do Doan Loi, Pham Manh Hung and Thach N. Nguyen

Introduction

Mitral regurgitation (MR) is the most common valvular disease. Modern management of patients with chronic MR requires a concerted consideration of various factors. These include the etiology, pathophysiology, severity of the valvular lesion, natural history, complications of the disease, and efficacy of the various therapeutic modalities. The mitral valve is a complex structure, and therefore the etiology of MR is diverse. Clinical presentations of MR depend on the severity and speed of development of the regurgitation MR, and complications of the valve disease. While the detection of MR is usually simple, understanding of its underlying pathophysiology and its consequences are vital in formulating management strategies (Table 11.1). The established treatments of MR include

Table 11.1 Management strategies for mitral regurgitation.

1. Detect MR and underlying problem at the earliest
2. Prevent LV remodeling
3. Treat MR
4. Mitral repair if feasible

LV, left ventricular; MR, mitral regurgitation.

Table 11.2 Etiology of mitral regurgitation.

Mitral valve leaflets
Myxomatous degeneration – mitral valve prolapse
Rheumatic fever
Connective tissue disorders – systemic lupus, scleroderma
Infective endocarditis
Neoplasm – left atrial myxoma
Trauma – chest injury, valvuloplasty (balloon or mechanical device)
Hypertrophic cardiomyopathy
Drug – fenfluramine/phentermine
Congenital – cleft/fenestrated mitral valve, endocardial cushion defects etc.

Chordae tendineae
Myxomatous degeneration
Infective endocarditis
Rheumatic heart disease
Rupture – spontaneous, infective endocarditis, trauma

Papillary muscles
Papillary muscle dysfunction – ischemia, myocardial infarction
Papillary muscle rupture – myocardial infarction, trauma

Mitral annulus
Calcification – idiopathic, chronic renal failure, hyperparathyroidism, rheumatic heart disease
Dilatation – connective tissue disorder, dilated cardiomyopathy

Structurally normal mitral valve
Functional/ischemic MR

Prosthetic value dysfunction
Paravalvular leak, infective endocarditis, ring or strut fracture, disc or ball dysfunction or dislodgement, tissue valve attrition

MR, mitral regurgitation.

both medical and surgical approaches. Percutaneous techniques to repair the mitral valve are being developed.

The mitral valve apparatus is a complex structure whose function depends not only on the integrity of the valve leaflets but also their supporting structures including the left atrium (LA), mitral annulus, chordae tendineae, papillary muscles and left ventricle, especially at the base of the papillary muscles. Hence, abnormalities of any component of the mitral apparatus, whether structural or functional, may lead to MR. The etiology of MR are listed in Table 11.2. More commonly causes of MR are discussed in detail in page 319 of the "Echocardio-graphic evaluation section". These include rheumatic heart disease, mitral valve prolapse, flail mitral valve, infective endocarditis and ischemic/functional MR.

Mitral Regurgitation Begets Mitral Regurgitation

Abnormality of one structural component of the mitral valve may adversely affect other related structures, thereby aggravating the severity of MR and creating a vicious cycle. Left ventricular (LV) dilatation develops as the MR progresses regardless of the etiology of MR. The ventricular dilatation leads to: (1) mitral annulus dilation, which causes further leaflet mal-cooptation; and (2) restricted mitral leaflet motion. In the latter, papillary muscles are displaced downwards, increasing the distance between the apices of the papillary muscles and the mitral orifice. This process places undue tension on the chordae and leaflets, thus restricting the degree of upward excursion of the latter structure. LA dilatation tends to displace the posterior mitral leaflet, thereby increasing the degree of regurgitation; this in turn leads to further atrial enlargement.

Functional Mitral Regurgitation

MR may also occur in the presence of a structurally normal mitral valve. In this type of functional MR, the mitral valve is rendered incompetent because of ventricular remodeling that has disturbed the geometric relationship between the subvalvular apparatus and the valve leaflets. For example, in dilated cardiomyopathy the dilated LV leads to downward displacement of the papillary muscles and enlarges the mitral annulus; these changes result in MR. In a substantial number of patients with ischemic cardiomyopathy, the MR is due to ventricular remodeling that is initiated by either a myocardial infarction or severe ischemia.

Pathophysiologic and Hemodynamic Basis for Clinical Presentations

The hemodynamics in patients with chronic MR is a function of interrelated factors including the preload, afterload and myocardial contractility, and the hemodynamic alterations in turn determine the nature and severity of clinical presentations in these patients.

Preload

In chronic MR, increased left ventricular preload is primarily related to the severity of MR. In the presence of moderate to severe MR, longstanding volume overload of the LV results in eccentric hypertrophy of the LV in which the degree of ventricular dilation is out of proportionate to the degree of the hypertrophy. This ventricular dilatation allows accommodation of increased preload to maintain effective forward cardiac output even in the presence of severe MR. However, this compensatory mechanism fails when there is a reduction in preload (e.g. hypovolemia due to dehydration, blood loss or overdiuresis), myocardial failure or dysrhythmia (commonly bradycardia or atrial fibrillation).

Afterload/Left Atrial Compliance

When the systemic vascular resistance is normal and in the absence of LV failure, LA compliance predominantly dictates the degree of reduction in LV afterload, and the hemodynamic and clinical picture in patients with severe MR. In most of these patients, the LA compliance is moderately increased and the LA pressure is significantly elevated, leading to a rise in pulmonary vascular resistance and pulmonary arterial pressure. However, the degree of elevation in mean LA pressure is generally less than that encountered in patients with severe mitral stenosis. In this group of patients with severe MR, cardiac output is usually well maintained until the onset of LV dysfunction.

Less commonly, in patients with severe MR, the LA compliance is markedly increased in the presence of gross LA enlargement. Thus, the LA pressure is normal or only slightly elevated, and pulmonary arterial pressure and pulmonary vascular resistance are normal or only slightly elevated at rest; these hemodynamic changes are usually accompanied by a low cardiac output. The longstanding structural remodeling in the grossly dilated LA invariably results in permanent atrial fibrillation.

In contrast, in acute severe MR – from chordal/papillary muscle rupture or dysfunction, or mitral leaflet perforation as a consequence of trauma or endocarditic – the LA compliance is relatively normal. The lack of increase of LA compliance, however, causes a marked increase in LA pressure with a giant V wave, and severe pulmonary congestion. In acute MR, the LV size is also relatively preserved with the result that preload is relatively limited; this in turn causes a marked decrease in forward cardiac output and hypotension.

Myocardial Contractility

In severe chronic MR, myocardial contractility ultimately determines prognosis, surgical risk and postoperative outcome. Unfortunately, there is a lack of direct clinical parameters in assessing contractility. Currently, the two best and simple parameters that are used as indirect reference indices of contractility are the LV ejection fraction (EF) and LV end-systolic volume.

Ejection fraction

The ejection fraction (EF), a simple ejection phase index, is a function of contractility, preload and afterload. In severe chronic MR, the absence of isovolumetric contraction phase and reduced afterload allows a greater proportion of the contractile energy of the LV to be expended in shortening than in tension development, thereby enabling the LV to adapt to the increased preload imposed by the MR. This increased preload and the reduced afterload permit maintenance of EF in the normal or even in the supranormal range as long as contractility remains unimpaired. Hence, when there is a reduction in EF to subnormal levels, it usually indicates impairment in myocardial function and *ipso facto*, contractility. Moderately reduced EF of 40–50% generally signifies severe, often irreversible, impairment of contractility, and identifies patients who may do poorly after surgical correction of the MR. An EF of <35% in patients with severe MR usually represents advanced myocardial dysfunction; these patients are at high operative risk and may not experience satisfactory clinical and cardiac improvement after mitral valve surgery.

End-systolic volume
LV end-systolic volume, which is relatively independent of preload, increases as myocardial contractility falls. Measurement of end-systolic diameter has been found to be a useful predictor of function and survival following mitral valve surgery. In general, the surgical outcome is excellent when the end-systolic diameter is <45 mm or 26 mm/m^2.

Echocardiographic evaluation

Echocardiography provides detail assessment of the morphology of the mitral valve, detects and grades the severity of MR and thus provides insight into the etiology and mechanism of MR. These together with its non-invasive nature make it an ideal imaging tool in MR. Importantly, it also allows serial studies to assess progression of MR, and plays a critical role in risk stratification of the patients with MR as well as in decision making for their medical and surgical managements.

When transthoracic images are suboptimal, transesophageal approach usually yields excellent images of the mitral valve and complements transthoracic imaging in the grading of MR severity. It is also an important tool to guide the surgical mitral valve repair.

How to Evaluate Mitral Regurgitation Severity
Complete evaluation of the regurgitant mitral valve by echocardiography provides accurate anatomical and functional status of the valve. Severity of MR is best determined by Doppler methods. 2-D echocardiography has limited roles in the assessment of MR severity but provides supportive evidence of significant MR. As each method has its own limitations, final decision on the grading of MR should be based on integration of all the variables used in the assessment of MR severity (Tables 11.2 and 11.3).

Doppler Color Flow Imaging
This method is routinely used for detection, as well as for grading MR severity. Estimation of the jet area in the LA, width of the vena contracta and the color flow evaluation of the flow convergence can accurately grade severity of MR [1].

Specific Signs of Mitral Regurgitation Severity

Table 11.3 Grading of mitral regurgitation severity (specific signs): usefulness and limitations*.

	Mild	Moderate	Severe	Usefulness	Limitations
Doppler Jet area	<4 cm²		>10 cm²	Easy and fast evaluation; reliable in central jets	Underestimation in eccentric jets and acute MR
Jet area/LA area (%)	<20%	20–40%	>40%		
Vena contracta (cm)	<0.3	0.3–0.7	≥0.7	Simple and differentiates mild from severe MR; useful in acute and eccentric jets	Not useful in multiple jets; meticulous attention to measurement due to small value
EROA PISA method (cm²)	<0.20	0.20–0.29 0.30–0.39	>0.40	Quantitative; provides prognostic information; reliable in trained hands; accurate in central jets	Less accurate in eccentric jets; angle correction required in eccentric jets
EROA Quantitative Doppler (cm²)	<0.20	0.20–0.39 0.30–0.39	>0.40	Useful in eccentric and multiple jets	Technically challenging

*Quantitative parameters can subdivide moderate MR into mild–moderate and moderate–severe groups.
Adapted from Zoghbi *et al.* [1].
EROA, effective regurgitant orifice area; LA, left atrium; MR, mitral regurgitation; PISA, proximal isovelocity surface area.

Left Atrial Jet Area

This simple method for estimating jet area in the LA provides rapid screening for the presence of MR, as well as semi-quantitative assessment of MR severity. Jet area $<4\,cm^2$, or 20% of the LA area, is usually associated with mild regurgitation. A large central jet of more than $10\,cm^2$, or 40% of the LA area, is generally associated with severe MR [1].

Pitfalls – Factors Affecting the Jet Area

While the jet area is the easiest and most rapid method for assessing MR severity, one should remember that the jet area can be affected by a number of factors. These include instrument and hemodynamic factors as well as the jet characteristic [2].

Instrument factors

The jet size is affected by pulse repetition frequency (PRF) and color gain. The jet area is inversely proportional to the PRF. It is recommended that the Nquist limit (aliasing velocity) be set at 50–70 m/s. Higher and lower settings can give rise to erroneous grading of the severity of MR. The color gain should be optimized by increasing the gain until the appearance of color speckles, and then reducing it until the speckles completely disappear from the non-moving areas.

Hemodynamic factors

Jet area is affected by the flow rate as well as the driving pressure. Hence, the jet area may appear larger by increasing the driving force across the mitral valve, such as in patients with hypertrophic cardiomyopathy, severe aortic stenosis, and hypertension where the LV systolic pressure is elevated. The effect of driving pressure on the jet area is especially important in the operating theatre. The jet area may be reduced causing underestimation of MR severity due to preload and afterload reduction by effects of general anesthesia. In patients with acute severe MR the jet area may not reflect MR severity. The size of the jet area is limited by the high LA pressure and reduced compliance of the LA.

Jet characteristic

Eccentric and wall impinging jets appear to be significantly smaller than centrally directed jets of the same MR severity [3,4]. This is because the central jet is able to entrain the red blood cells on all sides of the regurgitation jet while the eccentric jet is only able to entrain red blood cells on the side away from the wall of the receiving chamber (Coanda effect).

Vena contracta method

The vena contracta is the narrowest portion of the MR jet and occurs at the origin or just downstream from the orifice. The width of the vena contracta is a surrogate of the effective regurgitant orifice [5,6].

This method is simple and useful to differentiate mild from severe MR. Vena contracta width of 0.3 cm or less is associated with mild MR, while 0.7 cm or more is associated with severe MR [1].

Advantages

The advantage of evaluating MR severity by this method is its independence of flow rates and the driving force across the fixed orifice. Vena contracta is also less affected by technical factors such as PRF compared to the jet area in the receiving chamber. As discussed previously, in patients with eccentric jets and those with acute MR in whom jet areas are less reflective of regurgitant severity, the severity of MR can be reliably evaluated by the vena contracta method.

Limitations

As the width of vena contracta is small, less than 1 cm, slight errors in measurement may result in misclassification of the grading of MR severity. This error in measurement can be minimized by using the zoom mode to enlarge the image of the vena contracta. To improve lateral and temporal resolution, the color flow sector should also be as narrow as possible (to increase the frame rate). This method is also not reliable in the presence of multiple jets. The width of the vena contracta in patients with multiple jets cannot be added to grade MR severity.

Proximal Isovelocity Surface Area or Flow Convergence Method

Estimation of the effective regurgitant orifice area (EROA) by the proximal isovelocity surface area (PISA) method provides quantitative assessment of MR severity. The calculation of the effective mitral regurgitant orifice is based on the assumption that the PISA is a hemisphere. The formula for this is $EROA = 2\pi R^2 \times$ (aliasing velocity)/(peak MR velocity). As the calculation of the PISA is based on that of a hemisphere, the aliasing velocity must be chosen so that the flow convergence has a hemispheric shape. Using color flow imaging, the continuous wave Doppler cursor should be aligned with the color flow jet in order to obtain the maximum MR velocity. If the MR velocity is underestimated, the EROA may be erroneously larger. Meticulous care should be taken in measuring the radius of the PISA. As this is small, the image of the PISA should be optimized with high-resolution zoom view for the largest obtainable PISA. Angle correction is necessary when the base of the hemisphere is not flat.

Limitations

This method is simple, reliable and reproducible in trained hands. It is more accurate for central jets and those with a circular orifice [7]. It is less accurate in eccentric jets and not valid in the presence of multiple jets.

Pulse Doppler Quantitative Method

Doppler derived flow rates across the mitral valve and another valve without significant regurgitation can be used to calculate the effective regurgitant orifice area. This method, however, is challenging and requires considerable degree of expertise but offers an advantage in patients with eccentric or multiple

Supportive Signs of Mitral Regurgitation Severity

Table 11.4 Grading of mitral regurgitation severity (supportive signs): usefulness and limitations.

	Mild	Moderate	Severe	Usefulness	Limitations
Structural parameters					
LA size	Normal	Normal or dilated	Usually dilated	Normal excludes chronic significant MR	Seen in other conditions
LV size	Normal	Normal or dilated	Usually dilated	Normal excludes chronic significant MR	Seen in other conditions
Mitral leaflets or support apparatus	Normal or abnormal	Normal or abnormal	Abnormal/flail		
Doppler parameters					
Mitral inflow, PW Doppler	Dominant mitral A wave		Dominant E wave >1.2 m/s	Simple	Dominant E wave can be seen in other conditions with elevated LAP and LVEDP
Pulmonary venous flow	Dominant systolic flow	Blunting of systolic flow	Reversed systolic flow	Simple	Blunting of systolic flow is also seen in other causes of elevated LAP and LVEDP
CW Doppler density	Faint	Dense	Dense	Simple	Qualitative
CW jet contour	Parabolic	`Parabolic	Triangular	Simple	Qualitative

Adapted from Zoghbi et al. [1].

CW, Continuous wave; LA, left atrium; LV, left ventricle; LAP, left atrial pressure; LVEDP, left ventricular end diastolic pressure; PW, pulsed wave.

regurgitant jets where the PISA method is less accurate and measurement of the width of the vena contracta cannot be applied in the latter situation.

Indirect markers of MR severity provide insight into the hemodynamic impact of the regurgitation on LA pressure, LV end-diastolic pressure and left atrial and ventricular volumes. These provide supportive evidence for the MR severity.

Doppler Methods
Mitral inflow velocities
For patients over 50 years of age, the mitral E and A velocities are reversed so that the E velocity is less than the A velocity, as a result of abnormalities in relaxation in older individuals. In severe chronic MR, the E velocity is more than 1.2 m/sec [8]. The presence of predominant A velocity usually indicates that the MR is not severe.

Continuous wave Doppler spectral display
The density of the spectral display of any regurgitant jet is proportional to the number of red blood cells in the regurgitant jet. This can be used semi-quantitatively in the assessment of MR severity. In moderate and severe MR the jet is dense and approaches or equals the density of the antegrade mitral inflow spectral Doppler. The contour of the continuous wave spectral display may also provide clue to the degree of MR. The shape of the continuous wave spectral Doppler display is parabolic in mild and moderate MR. It is, however, triangular in severe MR. This is due to the rapid rise of the LA pressure during systole.

Pulmonary venous flow
The normal pulmonary venous flow is characterized by a higher systolic flow velocity and a lower velocity in diastole. As the degree of MR increases there is progressive decrease in the systolic velocity. In patients with moderate MR, the systolic velocity may be blunted and in severe MR systolic flow is reversed [9]. The blunting of the systolic pulmonary venous flow may also be seen in any situation with elevated LA pressure. The pulmonary venous systolic flow reversal is specific but is not a sensitive marker of severe MR. This sign is dependent on the presence of V wave which is often absent in chronic severe MR.

2-D Echocardiography – Left Atrial and Left Ventricular Size and Mitral Leaflet Pathology
Mild MR does not lead to remodeling of the LV or LA. Presence of dilatation of LA and LV is associated with at least moderate MR. It should be remembered, however, that there are many other causes of dilatation of the LA and LV. Pathology of the mitral valve may provide a clue to the MR severity. Flail mitral valve usually indicates that the MR is at least moderately severe.

Grading of Mitral Regurgitation Severity

Evaluation of MR severity should be based on integrating all variables used in assessing MR severity as each has its own limitation with technical and measurement errors. Thomas *et al.* [10] developed an index of MR severity using six variables. Each of the variables can be scored on a scale of 0 to 3 and then averaged. These variables include color Doppler regurgitant jet width and penetration, color Doppler PISA radius, continuous wave (CW) Doppler characteristics of the regurgitant jet, pulmonary artery pressure, pulmonary venous flow pattern and LA size. In the study all patients with a score of 1.7 or less have mild MR, while all patients with severe MR have a score of 1.8 and above. A value of 2.2 and above identified patients with severe MR with sensitivity, specificity and positive predictive accuracy of 90%, 88% and 79% respectively. This study emphasizes the need for integration of MR variables in the MR grading.

Risk Stratification

Quantitation of MR is recommended in patients with moderate and severe MR as it has impact on prognosis and management. This will help to risk stratify patients and define which group of patients will need closer follow-up and which group may benefit from surgery. Patients with functional MR with EROA of $20\,mm^2$ and above have adverse prognosis [11]. In this group of patients who are undergoing coronary artery bypass surgery, mitral valve surgery is usually advised. On the other hand, in patients with organic valve disease, adverse outcome is seen even in asymptomatic patients with EROA of $40\,mm^2$ and above [12]. Early surgery may be recommended in patients with repairable valve and performed only in centers with such expertise.

Etiology and Mechanism of Mitral Regurgitation

Rheumatic Mitral Regurgitation

The inflammatory changes associated with the rheumatic process transforms the mitral valve into a stiff funnel-shaped unit. Changes brought on by the rheumatic process results in thickening of the leaflets, tethering of the leaflets due to shortening, and thickening of the subvalvular apparatus as well as fusion of the commissures. This can result in a predominantly stenotic valve, predominantly regurgitant valve, or a valve with mixed stenotic and regurgitant lesions. The classical features of a rheumatic mitral valve on 2-D echo are well known. They include thickened leaflets particularly at the tips, elbowing of the anterior mitral leaflet and markedly restricted or immobile posterior leaflet. Shortening of the subvalvular apparatus results in apical displacement of the coaptation point. These features are best appreciated in the parasternal long axis view. In the short axis view, commissural fusion is seen but this is only minimal in predominantly regurgitant lesions. It is in this view that the mitral valve area can be accurately assessed by planimetry. In patients with predominant regurgitant valve, there is significant retraction of the leaflets, resulting in failure of coaptation. This is best appreciated in the short axis as well as the parasternal long axis views. The extent of the mal-coaptation of the leaflets is proportional to the MR severity.

Mitral Valve Prolapse

The gold standard for the diagnosis of mitral valve prolapse (MVP) is 2-D echocardiography. MVP is seen as displacement of the mitral leaflets, into the LA beyond the line connecting the annular-hinge points, of 2 mm or more. The diagnostic criteria have been refined in light of 3-D echocardiography data by Levine *et al.*, which showed the mitral annulus to be saddle shaped and not planar [13]. This diagnostic criteria has avoided over-diagnosis of MVP. Early studies have estimated the prevalence of MVP to be 5–15%. Recent observational studies using more rigorous criteria have demonstrated a more accurate prevalence of 1.6–2.4% [14].

The refined diagnosis criterion allow the diagnosis of MVP to be made only from the parasternal long axis and the apical long axis views. This is because these imaging views pass through the highest point of the annulus while in the apical four-chamber view the imaging plane passes through the lowest point of the annulus. The apparent displacement of the leaflets into the LA in the apical four-chamber view does not represent prolapse of the mitral valve.

MVP is not a single disease entity but rather a spectrum of disease processes with different pathologies. Echocardiography enables differentiating the classic from the non-classic mitral valve prolapse and thus provides useful prognostic information. In classic MVP where there is myxomatous degeneration of the valve, there is thickening (5 mm or more) as well as redundancy of the leaflets. The classic MVP is associated with risk of complications and sudden cardiac death [14]. Non-classic variety is defined as displacement of >2 mm and maximal thickness of <5 mm. The risk of complications is no more than that of the general population and has been recommended to be considered as normal variants.

Flail Mitral Valve

The most common cause of flail mitral valve is ruptured chordae usually in association with MVP. It may also be caused by endocarditis or a blunt chest trauma. A less common cause of flail mitral leaflet is rupture of the papillary muscle in the setting of an acute myocardial infarction. On 2-D echocardiography the flail segment is seen as a portion of the leaflet that is bent backwards with the tip pointing towards the LA. This differentiates flail valve from a prolapsed valve where the tip of the prolapsed leaflet points towards the LV. In patients with ruptured papillary muscle, the detached portion of the papillary muscle is seen as a mass attached to the ruptured chordae being flung into and out of the LA.

It is important to identify a flail valve as it is usually associated with at least moderately severe MR. The classic natural history study by Ling *et al.* [15] has shown adverse prognosis associated with flail mitral valve with over 90% of patients with cardiac related complications including death at 10 years.

Mitral Valve Infective Endocarditis

The Duke criteria for the diagnosis of infective endocarditis have incorporated echocardiographic findings as major criteria [16]. Vegetation is seen as an oscillating mass on a valve or apparatus on the upstream path of the jet. There may be other accompanying abnormalities such fistulas, abscesses and pseudoaneurysm, prosthetic dehiscence and paravalvular regurgitation that support the diagnosis of infective endocarditis.

Ischemic/Functional Mitral Regurgitation

In ischemic or functional MR the mitral valve is morphologically normal. The MR is brought about by the abnormal geometry of the valve caused by remodeling of the LV causing displacement of the papillary muscles and mitral annulus dilatation. This leads to malcoaptation of the leaflets with resultant regurgitation. In contrast to primary mitral valve regurgitation, ischemic or functional MR results from an abnormal LV whereas in primary valve disease, it is the chronic impact of the regurgitation that leads to dilatation and eventual impairment of LV function. In ischemic or functional MR the 2-D echocardiographic appearance of the mitral valve consists of tethering of the leaflets with a characteristic bent in the anterior leaflet caused by the lifting of the mid portion of the mitral leaflet by the displaced papillary muscle. The point of coaptation is apically displaced. These results in the characteristic tenting appearance of the mitral valve. The larger the tenting area of the mitral valve, the more severe the regurgitation [17]. The height of the tenting area also reflects the MR severity.

Decision-making for Surgery

Timing of Mitral Valve Surgery

Echocardiography provides useful information on the impact of chronic volume overload on the heart and thus help in the decision on the timing of mitral valve surgery. These include end systolic diameter of the LV cavity (≥ 4.0 cm), ventricular ejection fraction (EF) ($\leq 60\%$), the presence of pulmonary hypertension as well as the size of the effective regurgitant orifice. Recent work by Enriquez-Sarano et al. [12] showed that asymptomatic patients with EROA of 0.40 cm^2 have an adverse prognosis with 5 year cardiac event rate of $33 \pm 3\%$ and suggest surgery in this group of patients.

Selection of Surgical Candidates for Mitral Valve Repair

Selection of candidates for valve repair is based on preoperative echocardiographic findings. Patients with MVP, in particular those with posterior leaflet, are usually amenable to valve repair. On the other hand, when a mitral valve is ravaged by infection, it is an unlikely candidate for repair. The mitral valve in ischemic or functional MR, is intrinsically normal but geometry is altered by remodeling of the LV. Such patients benefit from mitral annuloplasty while undergoing concomitant coronary artery bypass surgery. These patients usually improve symptomatically with improvement in functional class post surgery.

Localization of Mitral Regurgitation Lesion

Echocardiographic localization of the MR lesion guides the surgeon to the site for repair [18,19]. This is important as identification of the regurgitation site can be difficult during surgery. Localization will also aid the surgeon in the planning of mitral valve surgery and assessing the likelihood of repair. Anterior leaflet repairs are generally more difficult than posterior leaflet repairs but ultimately the likelihood of successful repair depends on the expertise of the surgeon. The localization of MR can be made on good quality transthoracic examinations. The color flow imaging of the mitral valve in the parasternal short axis view is often helpful in the identification of the site of regurgitation. An anteriorly directed jet indicates a posterior leaflet pathology while a posteriorly directed jet is due to anterior leaflet abnormality [18,19]. Most patients will require transesophageal echo, which allows scallop-by-scallop analysis to identify the site of the MR lesion [20].

Cardiac Catheterization
Routine cardiac catheterization is usually not necessary for the evaluation of chronic MR, particularly if surgery is not contemplated, as all the necessary information and manifestations can be obtained from echocardiography. However, it may be performed when there is discrepancy between clinical and non-invasive findings, and when there is a need to determine the presence and severity of associated valvular diseases or coronary artery disease, especially prior to mitral valve surgery [21].

Risk stratification
In general, symptom severity and status of myocardial function are used in risk stratification of patients with chronic MR. Symptom severity associated with chronic MR is determined by the degree of MR, its rate of progression, the pulmonary artery pressure, atrial fibrillation and the presence of any co-existing structural heart disease. Management strategy for patients with severe, chronic MR is based on this principle (Figure 11.1). Most patients are relatively asymptomatic, even with severe MR. Symptoms generally develop only when there is LV failure, significant pulmonary hypertension, or the onset of atrial fibrillation. In such situations, the patient is considered at high-risk and thus a surgical candidate. However, the patient may be placed in a high-risk category even in the absence of symptoms when myocardial dysfunction becomes evident.

As discussed previously, the LVEF and end-systolic dimension assessed by echocardiography are used as surrogates of contractility to define the various stages of chronic MR. The compensated stage of MR is indicated by a LV end-diastolic dimension <60 mm, an end-systolic dimension <40 mm, and EF >60%; it augurs a benign prognosis and does not warrant surgical intervention. The decompensated stage is defined by an end-diastolic dimension >70 mm, an end-systolic dimension >45 mm and EF <50–55%; surgery in patients at this stage is at risk of suboptimal short- and long-term outcome. The EF in these patients may further decline when the advantage of afterload reduction is lost after surgical correction of MR. The natural history of the transitional stage between the compensated and decompensated stages is less precise; it is generally associated with a good clinical outcome when surgery is performed at this time [22–31].

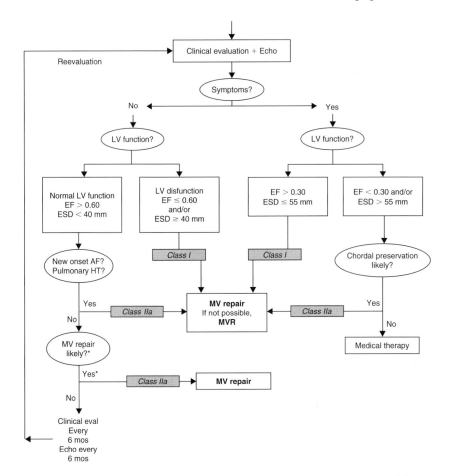

Figure 11.1 Management strategy for patients with chronic severe mitral regurgitation. *Mitral valve (MV) repair may be performed in asymptomatic patients with normal left ventricular (LV) function if performed by an experienced surgical team and if the likelihood of successful MV repair is greater than 90%. AF indicates atrial fibrillation; Echo, Echocardiography; Ejection fraction; ESD, end-systolic dimension; eval, evaluation; HT, hypertension; MVR, mitral valve replacement. (Adapted from reference 21)

Chronic Mitral Regurgitation

Medical Management

Modern management of patients with chronic MR requires a concerted consideration of various factors. These include the pathophysiology, severity of the valvular lesion, natural history of the disease, complications of the disease, efficacy of the various therapeutic modalities and endocarditis prophylaxis.

Physical Activity

Asymptomatic patients with normal LV function can probably exercise without restriction. In contrast, those with mild symptoms, LV dysfunction or atrial fibrillation should be limited to low-to-moderate-demand activities [21,32,33].

Vasodilator Therapy

In asymptomatic patients with normal ventricular function, vasodilator therapy is of no benefit and may even mask the indication for surgery by limiting the development of symptoms associated with decreasing LV function, so this mode of therapy is probably not indicated for these patients. Hence, chronic vasodilator therapy, in combination with digoxin and diuretics, should be reserved for candidates not suited for surgery [34–39].

Anticoagulation

The risk of cardioembolism is increased in patients with MR, particularly when there is co-existing atrial fibrillation. Long-term oral anticoagulation therapy with warfarin (target international normalized ratio (INR) 2.0–3.0) is indicated for patients with MR and a history of systemic embolism, atrial fibrillation, and those with sinus rhythm and an enlarged LA (diameter >5.5 cm). If recurrent embolism occurs despite adequate anticoagulation, low-dose aspirin, dipyridamole or clopidogrel should be added [40].

Endocarditis Prophylaxis

Prophylaxis for infective endocarditis is highly desirable for certain dental and surgical procedures in patients with MR associated with structural mitral valve disease [41].

Acute Mitral Regurgitation

In acute MR, the goal of non-surgical therapy is to diminish the amount of MR, in turn increasing forward output and reducing pulmonary congestion. If there is adequate mean arterial pressure, pharmacological therapy with afterload reducing agents may temporarily stabilize the acute MR prior to surgery. Intra-venous nitroprusside [42] and nitroglycerin can reduce pulmonary pressure, LV end-diastolic pressure and volume, and reduce regurgitant flow and concomitantly, increase forward flow. In hypotensive patients, nitroprusside should not be used alone, but in combination with an inotropic agent (such as dobutamine or dopamine). If an operation is not needed immediately, afterload-reducing agents, especially angiotensin-converting enzyme inhibitors (ACEI) and direct-acting vasodilators (such as hydralazine), may help to reduce the regurgitant fraction and increase the forward output. For such patients with acute hemodynamically significant MR, especially from postinfarction papillary muscle rupture, placement of an intra-aortic balloon pump can serve as a temporary stabilizing measure until surgical repair can be undertaken. The majority of patients with acute severe MR will need urgent surgical intervention.

Surgical Treatment

In the management of MR, the cardiologist-in-charge is faced with two important decisions: (1) Is the magnitude of the MR severe enough to be causing symptoms or LV dysfunction and therefore necessitating surgical therapy? If it is, (2) When and what type of surgical therapy should be performed? As discussed earlier, advances in echocardiography have facilitated the physicians in decision-making with more precision. Unlike vasodilator therapy, surgical valve repair or replacement is substantially more effective in the treatment of chronic severe MR in improving clinical status and survival in those with symptoms and LV dysfunction.

Indications for Corrective Surgery

The optimal timing for corrective surgery is determined by a number of variables: (1) the severity of MR; (2) severity of symptoms; (3) mitral valve repair feasibility; (4) LV function; and (5) preference and expectations of the patient.

Corrective surgery is usually indicated in patients with severe MR and ventricular dysfunction; the prime determinant of postoperative outcome. The goal of treatment is to avert the development of irreversible LV dysfunction that precludes an optimal outcome, by operating on these patients before an advanced state is reached. Age (>75 years) *per se* should not be considered a contraindication to surgery, provided the patient's overall health is reasonable; surgical risk, however, is higher than for younger patients. Guidelines for recommendations of mitral valve surgery in non-ischemic, severe chronic MR are shown in Table 11.5.

Asymptomatic Patients

Management decisions in this scenario rest largely on echocardiographic parameters. In the presence of normal LV systolic function (EF $\geq$ 60%), the management is usually conservative with recommendation for 6- to 12-monthly clinical and serial echocardiographic follow-up assessments. If there is progressive LV enlargement or LA enlargement, progressive deterioration in LV function, pulmonary hypertension (defined as pulmonary arterial systolic pressure >50 mmHg at rest or >60 mmHg with exercise), and/or onset of atrial fibrillation, then early surgery should be considered, particularly if the likelihood for successful repair is high [21,33,43].

The threshold for surgical intervention is lower if the valve appears to be repairable rather than replaced. In contrast to the asymptomatic patients with normal LV function, most would now agree that those with documented depressed LV function (EF < 60% and/or an LV end-systolic diameter >40 mm), even in the absence of symptoms should be considered for surgery. Surgery, repair or replacement, performed at this time will likely prevent further deterioration in LV function and improve longevity [30].

Patients with Mild Symptoms

Surgery is indicated in mildly symptomatic patients (NYHA class II) with normal or borderline LV function, if it appears that valve repair is feasible and the operative risk is low. If EF < 55%, surgery is recommended even if valve replacement is necessary [21,43,44].

Table 11.5. Recommendations for mitral valve surgery in non-ischemic severe mitral regurgitation.

Indication	Level of evidence
Class I	
Mitral surgery is recommended to:	
1. Symptomatic patients with acute severe MR	(B)
2. Patients with NYHA class II, III, or IV symptoms in the absence of severe LV dysfunction (EF < 30% or EDD > 55 mm)	(B)
3. Asymptomatic patients with mild to moderate LV dysfunction (EF 50–60%, and/or ESD > or = 40 mm)	(B)
Mitral repair is recommended for over MV replacement (MVR) in the majority of patients with severe chronic MR who requires surgery	(C)
Class IIa	
Mitral repair is reasonable in experienced center for	
1. Asymptomatic patients with preserved LV function (EF > 60%, and ESD < 40 mm) in whom the likelihood of successful repair without residual MR > 90%	(B)
Mitral surgery is reasonable for the following patients:	
1. Asymptomatic patients with preserved LV function and (1) new onset of atrial fibrillation or (2) pulmonary hypertension (PASP > 50 mmHg at rest or >60 mmHg with exercise	(C)
2. Patients with chronic severe MR due to a primary abnormality of the mitral apparatus, NYHA functional class II, III, or IV symptoms and severe LV dysfunction (EF < 30% or EDD < 55 mm) in whom MV repar is highly likely.	
Class IIb	
Mitral repair may be considered for patients with chronic severe MR due to severe LV dysfunction (EF < 30%) who have persistent NYHA functional class III0IV symptoms despite optimal therapy for heart failure including biventricular pacing	(C)
Class III	
1. **Mitral surgery** is not indicated for patients with preserved LV function (EF < 60% and EDD < 40 mm) in whom significant doubt about the feasibility of repair exists	(C)
2. Isolated mitral surgery is not indicated for patients with mild or moderate MR	(C)

ACC/AHA guidelines for classifying indications for diagnostic and therapeutic procedures.
Class I   Conditions for which there is evidence and/or general agreement that a given procedure or treatment is useful and effective
Class II   Conditions for which there is conflicting evidence and/or a divergence of opinion about the usefulness/efficacy of a procedure or treatment
Class IIa   Weight of evidence/opinion in favor of usefulness/efficacy
Class IIb   Usefulness/efficacy less well established by evidence/opinion
Class III   Conditions for which there is evidence and/or general agreement that the procedure/treatment is not useful and in some cases may be harmful
Level of evidence A: Multiple (3-5) population risk strata evaluated. General consistency of direction and magnitude of effect
Level of evidence B: Limited (2-3) population risk strata evaluated
Level of evidence C: Very limited (1-2) population risk strata evaluated
ESD, end-systolic dimension; EDD, end-diastolic dimension; EF, ejection fraction; NYHA, New York Heart Association; MV, mitral valve; MR, mitral regurgitation; PASP, pulmonary artery systolic pressure.
Adapted from Bonow et al. [21]

Patients with Moderate to Severe Symptoms

Most patients with NYHA class III or IV and LVEF >30% are candidates for corrective surgery, preferably valve repair. Surgery in these patients, although unlikely to normalize the LV function postoperatively, will probably improve symptoms and may prevent further deterioration in LV function. However, when LV dysfunction (EF < 30%) is far-advanced, surgery is unlikely to afford optimal outcome due to long-term irreversible LV damage. There are data to indicate that surgery should not be delayed until severe symptoms develop in patients with severe chronic MR. In patients with severe chronic MR, the severity of their symptoms are directly related to their perioperative and long-term postoperative mortality rates; this relationship appears to be independent of the baseline EF [22,30,45,46].

Mitral Valve Repair

Mitral valve repair, particularly if the valve assessed echocardiographically is suitable for it, and if the surgical expertise is available, is preferred to valve replacement because the former procedure circumvents the potential complications associated with a prosthetic valve, and provides superior clinical, functional and survival benefits compared to valve replacement. Valve calcification, rheumatic valve disease and anterior leaflet involvement decrease the likelihood of successful repair, whereas uncalcified posterior leaflet disease is almost always reparable. A decremental success rate for mitral valve repair is observed for severe chronic MR secondary to degenerative myxomatous valves, ischemia, endocarditis, and rheumatic disease [21,33,47–50].

Intraoperative transesophageal color flow Doppler mapping, if available, should be used routinely as it is extremely useful in assessing the adequacy of the valve repair; it allows for immediate corrective surgery (valve replacement if necessary) if the valve repair is deemed inadequate.

Surgery in Functional Mitral Regurgitation

Although surgical mitral valve repair or replacement in patients with functional MR (FMR) has been reported to reduce symptoms and improve exercise tolerance, no randomized prospective controlled trials have been performed to assess the efficacy of the surgical procedure. The available clinical data, which are supported by recent laboratory work, strongly suggest that the surgical treatment of FMR results in little, if any, survival benefit or reverse remodeling.

Percutaneous Mitral Valve Repair

The technique of percutaneous mitral valve repair is still evolving but appears quite promising. Short-term preliminary results demonstrate the non-surgical approach to mitral valve repair to be safe and effective. There are two approaches – edge-to-edge repair, and mitral annuloplasty methods. The percutaneous edge-to-edge repair technique is an adaptation of the Alfieri surgical method for repairing mitral valve. The latter method has been proven effective for the treatment of MR without producing mitral stenosis and has been shown to preserve the dynamic annular function during exercise [51,52]. Instead of apposing the two leaflets of the mitral valve with the use of sutures in the surgical approach, researchers have developed a modified percutaneous method using a clip.

EMERGING TREND

The EVEREST trial 24 patients with degenerative myxomatous mitral valve of at least moderately severe MR underwent the procedure, which approximated the middle scallops of the mitral leaflets to create a double orifice with improved leaflet cooptation [53].

27 patients had six-month follow-up. Clips were implanted in 24 patients. There were no procedural complications and four 30-day major adverse events: partial clip detachment in three patients who underwent elective valve surgery, and one patient with post-procedure stroke that resolved at one month. Three additional patients had surgery for unresolved MR, leaving 18 patients free from surgery. In 13 of 14 patients with reduction of MR to ≤2+ after one month, the reduction was maintained at six months. Percutaneous edge-to-edge mitral valve repair can be performed safely and a reduction in MR can be achieved in a significant proportion of patients to six months. Patients who required subsequent surgery had elective mitral valve repair or intended replacement.

Annular dilation results in papillary-chordal dysfunction and poor leaflet coaptation; these changes in turn causes MR. Surgical mitral annuloplasty when necessary, is often performed during mitral valve repair with good outcome [54]. The second percutaneous method to repair MR uses a deformable constraining ring that is introduced and deployed in the coronary sinus. Because the coronary sinus encircles the mitral annulus, in particular the posterior segment of the sinus, implanting a device in the coronary sinus allows for partial mitral annuloplasty. This approach, however, has the potential to compress the left circumflex artery (with resultant myocardial ischemia) because of its proximity to the coronary sinus, and coronary sinus thrombosis or fibrosis. There is also a deep concern regarding the durability of the device that is currently available [55].

Real World Question: How to Manage Anticoagulation Regimen in Pregnant Women with Mechanical Prosthetic Valves ?

Warfarin (vitamin K antagonist (VKA) crosses the placenta and has been associated with an increased incidence of spontaneous abortion, prematurity, and stillbirth. Warfarin can also cause bleeding in the fetus, and fetal cerebral hemorrhage can complicate labor and delivery, especially if forceps evacuation is necessary. Warfarin is probably safe during the first 6 weeks of gestation, but there is a risk of embryopathy if warfarin is taken between 6 and 12 weeks of gestation. For women requiring long-term warfarin therapy who are attempting pregnancy, it seems wise to perform frequent pregnancy tests with the substitution of unfractionated heparin (UFH) or low-molecular-weight heparin (LMWH) for warfarin when pregnancy is achieved. Warfarin is also relatively safe during the second and third trimesters of pregnancy but must be discontinued and switched to a heparin compound several weeks before delivery.

Unfractionated Heparin (UFH) Heparin does not cross the placenta and does not have the potential to cause fetal bleeding or teratogenicity. Thus, heparin is generally considered safer than warfarin during pregnancy in terms of the development of embryopathy. However, bleeding at the utero-placental junction is possible, and numerous case series and patient registries attest to a high incidence of thromboembolic complications (12% to 24%), including fatal valve thrombosis, in high-risk pregnant women managed with subcutaneous UFH or LMWH. Unfortunately, the efficacy of adjusted dose subcutaneous heparin has not been definitively established. During pregnancy, the activated partial thromboplastin time (aPTT) response to heparin is often attenuated because of increased levels of factor VIII and fibrinogen. Adjusted dose subcutaneous UFH can cause a persistent anticoagulant effect at the time of delivery, which can complicate its use before labor. Bleeding complications appear to be very uncommon with LMWH.

Low-Molecular-Weight Heparins (LMWHs) have potential advantages over UFH during pregnancy because they 1) cause less heparin-induced thrombocytopenia; 2) have a longer plasma half-life and a more predictable dose response than UFH; 3) have greater ease of administration, with lack of need for laboratory monitoring and the potential for once-daily dosing administration; 4) are likely associated with a lower risk of heparin-induced osteoporosis; and 5) appear to have a low risk of bleeding complications. They do not cross the placenta and are likely safe for the fetus. As the pregnancy progresses (and most women gain weight), the potential volume of distribution for LMWH changes. It is thus necessary to measure plasma anti-Xa levels 4 to 6 h after the morning dose and adjust the dose of LMWH to achieve an anti-Xa level of approximately 0.7 to 1.2 units per ml.

Although LMWHs have been used successfully to treat deep venous thrombosis in pregnant patients, there are no data to guide their use in the management of patients with mechanical heart valves (810). Reports of LMWH use in pregnant women with prosthetic heart valves are becoming more frequent, and many physicians now prescribe these agents during pregnancy in women with mechanical valves, but treatment failures have been reported. The 2006 guidelines by the ACC/AHA are highlighted below.

Table 11.6 Selection of Anticoagulation Regimen in Pregnant Patients With Mechanical Prosthetic Valves.

Class I

1. All pregnant patients with mechanical prosthetic valves must receive continuous therapeutic anticoagulation with frequent monitoring. (Level of Evidence: B)
2. For women requiring long-term warfarin therapy who are attempting pregnancy, pregnancy tests should be monitored with discussions about subsequent anticoagulation therapy, so that anticoagulation can be continued uninterrupted when pregnancy is achieved. (Level of Evidence: C)

(Continued)

Table 11.6 (*Continued*)

3. Pregnant patients with mechanical prosthetic valves who elect to stop warfarin between weeks 6 and 12 of gestation should receive continuous intravenous UFH, dose-adjusted UFH, or dose-adjusted subcutaneous LMWH. (Level of Evidence: C)
4. For pregnant patients with mechanical prosthetic valves, up to 36 weeks of gestation, the therapeutic choice of continuous intravenous or dose-adjusted subcutaneous UFH, dose-adjusted LMWH, or warfarin should be discussed fully. If continuous intravenous UFH is used, the fetal risk is lower, but the maternal risks of prosthetic valve thrombosis, systemic embolization, infection, osteoporosis, and heparin-induced thrombocytopenia are relatively higher. (Level of Evidence: C)
5. In pregnant patients with mechanical prosthetic valves who receive dose-adjusted LMWH, the LMWH should be administered twice daily subcutaneously to maintain the anti-Xa level between 0.7 and 1.2 U per ml 4 h after administration. (Level of Evidence: C)
6. In pregnant patients with mechanical prosthetic valves who receive dose-adjusted UFH, the aPTT should be at least twice control. (Level of Evidence: C)
7. In pregnant patients with mechanical prosthetic valves who receive warfarin, the INR goal should be 3.0 (range 2.5 to 3.5). (Level of Evidence: C)
8. In pregnant patients with mechanical prosthetic valves, warfarin should be discontinued and continuous intravenous UFH given starting 2 to 3 weeks before planned delivery. (Level of Evidence: C)

Class IIa
1. In patients with mechanical prosthetic valves, it is reasonable to avoid warfarin between weeks 6 and 12 of gestation owing to the high risk of fetal defects. (Level of Evidence: C)
2. In patients with mechanical prosthetic valves, it is reasonable to resume UFH 4 to 6 h after delivery and begin oral warfarin in the absence of significant bleeding. (Level of Evidence: C)
3. In patients with mechanical prosthetic valves, it is reasonable to give low-dose aspirin (75 to 100 mg per day) in the second and third trimesters of pregnancy in addition to anticoagulation with warfarin or heparin. (Level of Evidence: C)

Class III
1. LMWH should not be administered to pregnant patients with mechanical prosthetic valves unless anti-Xa levels are monitored 4 to 6 h after administration. (Level of Evidence: C)
2. Dipyridamole should not be used instead of aspirin as an alternative antiplatelet agent in pregnant patients with mechanical prosthetic valves because of its harmful effects on the fetus. (Level of Evidence: B)

References

1 Zoghbi WA, Enriquez-Sarano M, Foster E *et al*. Recommendations for Evaluation of the severity of native Valvular Regurgitation with Two-dimensional and Doppler Echocardiography. J Am Soc Echocardiogr 2003;16:777–802.
2 Sahn DJ. Instrumentation and physical factors related to visualization of stenotic and regurgitant jets by Doppler color flow mapping. J Am Coll Cardiol 1988;12:1354–1365.
3 Cape EG, Yoganathan AP, Weyman AE, Levine RA. Adjacent solid boundaries alter the size of regurgitant jets on Doppler color flow maps. J Am Coll Cardiol 1991;17:1094–1102.
4 Chen C, Thomas JD, Anconina J *et al*. Impact of impinging wall jet on color Doppler quantification of mitral regurgitation. Circulation 1991;84:712–720.
5 Heinle SK, Hall SA Brickner ME, Willett DL, Grayburn PA. Comparison of vena contracta width by multiplane transesophageal echocardiography with quantitative Doppler assessment of mitral regurgitation. Am J Cardiol 1998;81:175–179.

6 Tribouilloy C, Shen WF, Quere JP *et al*. Assessment of severity of mitral regurgitation by measuring regurgitant jet width at its origin with transesophageal Doppler color flow imaging. Circulation 1992;85:1248–1253.

7 Enriquez-Sarano M, Miller FA Jr, Hayes SN *et al*. Effective mitral regurgitant orifice area: clinical use and pitfalls of the proximal isovelocity surface area method. J Am Coll Cardiol 1995;25:703–709.

8 Thomas L, Foster E, Schiller NB. Peak mitral inflow velocity predicts mitral regurgitation severity. J Am Coll Cardiol 1998;31:174–179.

9 Pu M, Griffin BP, Vandervoort PM *et al*. The value of assessing pulmonary venous flow velocity for predicting severity of mitral regurgitation: a quantitative assessment integrating left ventricular function. J Am Soc Echocardiogr 1999;12:736–743.

10 Thomas L, Foster E, Hoffman JI, Schiller NB. The mitral regurgitation index: an echocardiographic guide to severity. J Am Soc Echocardiogr 1999;33:2016–2022.

11 Grigioni F, Enriquez-Sarano M, Zehr K *et al*. Ischaemic mitral regurgitation: long term outcome and prognostic implications with quantative Doppler assessment. Circulation 2001;103:1759–1764.

12 Enriquez-Sarano M, Avierinos JF, Messika-Zeitoun D *et al*. Quantitative Determinants of the Outcome of Asymptomatic Mitral Regurgitation. N Engl J Med 2005;352:875–883.

13 Levine RA, Triulzi MO, Harrigan P *et al*. The relationship of mitral annular shape to the diagnosis of mitral valve prolapse. Circulation 1987;75:756–767.

14 Freed LA, Levy D, Levine RA *et al*. Prevalence and Clinical Outcome of Mitral Valve Prolapse. New Engl J Med 1999;341:1–7.

15 Ling H, Enriquez-Sarano M, Seward J *et al*. Clinical outcome of mitral regurgitation due to flail leaflets. N Eng J Med 1996;335:1417–1423.

16 Durack DT, Lukes AS, Bright DK. New criteria for diagnosis of infective endocarditis: utilization of specific echocardiographic findings. Am J Med 1994;96:200–209.

17 Yiu SF, Enriquez-Sarano M, Tribouilloy C *et al*. Determinants of the degree of functional mitral regurgitation in patients with systolic left ventricular dysfunction: a quantitative clinical study. Circulation 2000;102:1400–1406.

18 Stewart WJ, Currie PJ, Salcedo EE *et al*. Intraoperative Doppler color flow mapping for decision–making in valve repair for mitral regurgitation: technique and results in 100 patients. Circulation 1990;81:556–566.

19 Stewart WJ, Salcedo EE, Cosgrove DM. The value of echocardiography in mitral valve repair. Cleve Clin J Med 1991;58:177–183.

20 Foster GP, Isselbacher EM, Rose GA *et al*. Accurate localization of mitral regurgitant defects using multiplane transesophageal echocardiography. Ann Thorac Surg 1998;65:1025–1031.

21 Bonow RO, Carabello B, Chatterjee K, de Leon AC *et al*. ACC/AHA 2006 practice guidelines for the management of patients with valvular heart disease. A report of the American College of Cardiology/ American Heart Association Task Forces on practice guideline (Committee on management of patients with valvular heart disease). J Am Coll Cardiol 2006:598–675.

22 Schuler G, Peterson KL, Johnson A *et al*. Temporal response of left ventricular performance to mitral valve surgery. Circulation 1979;59:1218–1231.

23 Borow KM, Greeen LH, Mann T *et al*. end-systolic volume as a predictor of postoperative left ventricular performance in volume overload from valvular regurgitation. Am J Med 1980;68:655–663.

24 Carabello BA, Stanton NP, McQuire LB. Assessment of preoperative left ventricular function in patients with mitral regurgitation:value of the end-systolic wall stress-end-systolic volume ration. Circulation 1981;64:1212–1217.

25 Phillips HR, Levine FH, Carter JE *et al*. Mitral valve replacement for isolated mitral regurgitation: analysis of clinical course and late postoperative left ventricular ejection fraction. Am J Cardiol 1981;48:647–654.

26 Zile MR, Gaasch WH, Carroll JD *et al*. Chronic mitral regurgitation: predictive valve of preoperative echocardiographic indices of left ventricular function and wall stress. J Am Coll Cardiol 1984;3:235–242.

27 Ross J Jr. Afterload mismatch in aortic and mitral valve disease;implications for surgical therapy. J Am Coll Cardiol 1985;5:811–826.

28 Crawford MH, Souchek J, Oprian CA *et al*. Determinants of survival and left ventricular performance after mitral valve replacement. Circulation 1990;81:1173–1181.

29 Wisenbaugh T, Skudicky D, Sareli P. Prediction of outcome after valve replacement for rheumatic mitral regurgitation in the era of chordal preservation. Circulation 1994;89:191–197.

30 Enriquez-Sarano M, Tajik AJ, Schaff HV *et al*. Echocardiographic prediction of survival after surgical correction of organic mitral regurgitation. Circulation 1994;90:830–837.

31 Enriquez-Sarano M, Tajik AJ, Schaff HV *et al*. Echocardiographic prediction of left ventricular function after correction of mitral regurgitation: results and clinical implications. J Am Coll Cardiol 1994;24:1536–1543.

32 Cheitlin MD, Gouglas PS, Parmley WW. 26th Bethesda conference: recommendations for determining eligibility for competition in athletes with cardiovascular abnormalities. Task Force 2: Acquired valvular heart disease. J Am Coll Cardiol 1994;24:874–880.

33 Lung B, Gohlke-Barwold C, Tornos P *et al*. Recommendations on the management of the asymptomatic patient with valvular heart disease. Eur Heart J 2002;23:1252–1266.

34 Greenberg BH, Massie BM, Brundage BH *et al*. Beneficial effects of hydralazine in severe mitral regurgitation. Circulation 1978;58:273–279.

35 Levine HJ, Gaasch WH. Vasoactive drugs in chronic regurgitant lesions of the mitral and aortic valves. J Am Coll Cardiol 1996;28:1083–1091.

36 Greenberg BH, DeMotts H, Murphy E *et al*. Arterial dilators in mitral regurgitation: effects on rest and exercise hemodynamic and long term clinical follow up. Circulation 1982;65:181–187.

37 Wisenbaugh T, Sinovich V, Dullabh A *et al*. Six month pilot study of captopril for mildly symptomatic severe isolated mitral and isolated aortic regurgitation. J Heart Valve Dis 1994;3:197–204.

38 Marcotte F, Honos GN, Walling AD *et al*. Effect of angiotensin-converting enzyme inhibitor therapy in mitral regurgitation with normal left ventricular function. Can J Cardiol 1997;13:479–485.

39 Dujardin KS, Enriquez-Sarano M, Bailey KR *et al*. Effect of losartan on degree of mitral regurgitation quantified by echocardiography. Am J Cardiol 2001;87:570–576.

40 Fuster V, Ryden LE, Asinger RW *et al*. ACC/AHA/ESC guideline for the management of patients with atrial fibrillation:executive summary. Circulation 2001;104:2118–2150.

41 Dajani AS, Taubert KA, Wilson W *et al*. Prevention of bacterial endocarditis. Recommendations by the American Heart Association. JAMA 1997;277:1794–1801.

42 Horstkotte D, Shulte HD, Niehues R *et al*. Diagnostic and therapeutic consideration in acute, severe mitral regurgitation: experience in 42 consecutive patients entering the intensive care unit with pulmonary edema. J Heart Vae Dis 1993;2:512–522.

43 Otto CM. Clinical practice. Evaluation and management of chronic mitral regurgitation. N Engl J Med 2001;345:740–746.

44 Dalrymple–Hay MJ, Bryant M, Jones RA *et al*. Degenerative mitral regurgitation: when should we operate/ Ann Thorac Surg 1998;66:1579–1584.

45 Bonow RO, Nikas D, Elefteriades VA. Valve replacement for regurgitant lesions of aortic or mitral valve in advanced left ventricular dysfunction. Cardiol Clin 1995;13:73–83.

46 Carabello BA. Is it ever too late to operate on the patient with valvular heart disease? J Am Coll Cardiol 2004;44:376–383.

47 Enriquez-Sarano M, Schaff HV, Orszulak TA *et al.* Valve repair improves the outcome of surgery for mitral regurgitation: a multivariate analysis. Circulation 1995;91:1022–1028.

48 Cooper HA, Gersh BJ. Treatment of chronic mitral regurgitation. Am Heart J 1998;135:925–936.

49 Yau TM, El-Ghoneimi YA, Armstrong S *et al.* Mitral valve repair and replacement for 0. rheumatic disease. J Thorac Cardiovasc Surg 2000;119:53–60.

50 Mohty D, Orszulak TA, Schaff HV *et al.* Very long-term survival and durability of mitral valve repair for mitral valve prolapse. Circulation 2001;104:11–17.

51 Maisano F, Torracca L, Oppizzi M *et al.* The edge-to-edge technique: a simplified method to correct mitral insufficiency. Eur J Cardiothorac Surg 1998;12:240–245.

52 Umana JP, Salehizadeh B, DeRose JJ *et al.* Bow-tie mitral valve repair: an adjuvant technique for mitral regurgitation. Ann Thorac Surg 1998;66:1640–1646.

53 Feldman T, Wasserman HS, Herrmann HC *et al.* Percutaneous mitral valve repair using the edge–to–edge technique: six-month results of the EVEREST Phase I clinical trial. J Am Coll Cardiol 2005;46:2134–2140.

54 Bach DS, Boiling SF. Improvement following correction of secondary mitral regurgitation in end-stage cardiomyopathy with mitral annuloplasty. Am J Cardiol 1996;78:966–969.

55 Webb JG, Harnek J, Munt BI *et al.* Percutaneous transvenous mitral annuloplasty. Initial human experience with device implantation in the coronary sinus. Circulation 2006;113: 851–855.

CHAPTER 12

Stroke

Thach N. Nguyen, Marc Simaga, Sundeep Mangla, Rajiv Kumar and Sanjeev V. Maniar

Introduction

The study and treatment of cerebrovascular disease is undergoing rapid evolution as new techniques, new medications, further understanding of the underlying pathophysiology of neuronal injury, and new concepts for protecting the brain are being developed across the world. The clinical diagnosis, management, and therapy of stroke is evolving, as is the role of public education in making sure patients and their families have access to these new life- and brain-saving techniques by the quick recognition of stroke symptoms. New imaging techniques, especially MRI diffusion and perfusion-weighted imaging, take away some of the uncertainties and may help guide the diagnostic considerations and therapies. We have an improving understanding of risk factors, and the role of risk-reduction in minimizing stroke's impact on our patients. Neurologic rehabilitation is also keeping step with new techniques and rational treatments to return those affected by stroke to productive lives.

Strokes are classified generally into two types: ischemic (71%) or hemorrhagic (26%) with 3% from other etiologies (Table 12.1). The term "stroke" is most generally applied to the phenomenon of brain ischemia, ultimately resulting in irreversibly injured brain tissue. The process can be linked to general hypoperfusion of brain tissue do to hemodynamic insufficiency, vascular thrombosis of intracerebral or craniocervical arteries, or an embolic event. Bleeding into the brain in hemorrhagic strokes is usually caused by rupture of an artery (secondary to hypertension or amyloid angiopathy), leading to intra-cranial hemorrhage (ICH), or bleeding around the brain surface (usually by a ruptured aneurysm or arteriovenous malformation) into the subarachnoid space (subarachnoid hemorrhage, SAH) and the cerebrospinal fluid (CSF). Therapeutic considerations are vastly disparate in these conditions, and recognition of ischemic vs. hemorrhagic stroke via clinical and diagnostic testing is critical.

Table 12.1 Classification of strokes.

Ischemic events	Hemorrhagic events
Vascular thrombosis in:	Intracerebral hemorrhage
Intracerebral arteries	Bleeding into brain parenchyma
Craniocervical arteries	
Venous sinuses	Subarachnoid hemorrhage
	Bleeding around the brain into the
Embolism from	subarachnoid space and CSF
heart (endocardium, valves)	Arteriovenous malformation
aorta, great vessels	
veins (paradoxical from a patent foramen ovale)	
Systemic hypoperfusion due to	
cardiac failure	
anemia, hypovolemia	
lacunar infarct (lipohyalinosis) mainly caused by	
hypertension, diabetes, dyslipidemia	

CSF, cerebrospinal fluid.

Once a stroke has occurred, the therapies currently available may lessen its ultimate effect on the patient or quicken recovery. Prevention of these events is ultimately the goal of our efforts, as many of the important risk factors, such as smoking, diabetes or hypertension etc., can be controlled through education and medical intervention (Table 12.2). Those at risk should receive adequate information to make intelligent decisions on lifestyle and recognize the importance of compliance with medical therapy.

Table 12.2 Risk factors for stroke.

Unmodifiable risk factors
1. **Age** (incidence increases after age 55, but ¼ of stroke patients are younger than 65)
2. **Gender** (risk higher in men, but more women over 65 die of stroke than men)
3. **Race** (African Americans >2 × risk compared to whites)
4. **Prior stroke** (highest in first 30 days; cumulative risk 5–14% at 1 year, 25–40% at 5 years)
5. **Heredity** (family history of stroke, complicated by common risk factors, life style)

Modifiable risk factors
1. **Hypertension** (decreasing blood pressure (BP) by 10 mmHg can reduce risk by 35–40%)
2. **Smoking** (which affects BP, accelerates atherosclerosis, and alters platelet function)
3. **Transient ischemic attacks** (5% of patients will develop a completed stroke by 1 month)
4. **Heart disease** (atrial fibrillation, valvular disease, myocardial infraction, congestive heart failure all increase risk)
5. **Diabetes mellitus** (accelerates atherosclerosis, microvascular changes)
6. **Hypercoagulopathy** (anticardiolipins, protein S and C deficiency, Leiden factor V abnormalities, hyperhomocystinemia, prothrombin gene abnormalities, cancer, pregnancy)
7. **Polycythemia** (increases vascular resistance and slows blood flow)
8. **Sickle cell anemia** (causes intravascular clumping of red blood cells)
9. **Carotid bruit** (an indicator for carotid stenosis)

Transient ischemic attack (TIA) is a manifestation of brain ischemia lasting minutes to hours. The time limit is arbitrarily set at 24 hours for complete resolution of symptoms. These patients may appear normal at neurologic examination, however, they have a ten-fold increase in risk for a fully completed stroke compared with those who never had a TIA. Clearly, proper management of the patient with TIA will reduce the likelihood of stroke. The recognition of TIA symptoms by the patient will require more public education and a heightened awareness of stroke symptoms, which will eventually lead to appropriately urgent diagnostic testing. The reduction of modifiable risk factors, consideration of carotid endarterectomy or carotid stenting in appropriate patients, and the use of antiplatelet agents or anticoagulation can reduce the risk of stroke considerably [1]. The diagnosis of stroke should be considered in anyone with a sudden onset of focal neurological deficits or alteration of consciousness, with the differential diagnosis considering possible mechanisms for the event (Table 12.3).

Table 12.3 Differential diagnoses for stroke.

1. Meningitis/encephalitis
2. Hypertensive encephalopathy
3. Intracranial mass (tumor, hematoma)
4. Cerebral/cervical trauma (closed head injury, arterial dissection)
5. Seizure
6. Migraine
7. Metabolic derangement (hyperglycemia, hypoglycemia, drug overdose, hypoxia, hypercarbia, renal and hepatic disease)
8. Subdural hematoma

The management of stroke requires a chain of events to occur in rapid succession in order for the patient to benefit from the newest therapies. As with the *chain of survival* recognized for improving survival in the case of sudden cardiac death, so to does the stroke *chain of survival and recovery* require rapid recognition of stroke symptoms, rapid activation of the emergency service (EMS) system, rapid transport with pre-hospital evaluation and treatment, pre-notification of the receiving facility, and rapid diagnosis and definitive care with potential thrombolytic medications and other emerging interventional techniques [1]. Unfortunately, many stroke patients deny their symptoms, delay transport to the hospital for hours, and deny themselves access to these new technologies.

Initial Assessment

The initial assessment of patients with stroke, including preliminary determination of the time of onset of the stroke, should be performed by EMS personnel prior to arrival at the emergency room (ER). The time of onset of the stroke is defined as the time the patient was last known to be without clinical deficit or, if the ischemic stroke occurred on awakening, the time the patient went to bed is considered the time of onset. If the findings suggest a possible stroke, the paramedics should contact the ER about their expected arrival with a possible candidate for thrombolysis. This information would allow the ER to mobilize the team for acute aggressive stroke treatment. When the patient arrives at the ER, a complete physical examination should include all of the components for a thorough neurological and neurovascular assessment.

The general initial evaluation should assess the patient's airway, ventilation, and circulation, providing supplement oxygen, and then sending initial serum tests and establishing intravenous (IV) access. The neurological exam at this point need not be exhaustive [2], and usually can be done in 5–10 minutes. Clinical data should be obtained through careful history taking of the patient or their family, with emphasis on the points described in Table 12.4.

Cervicocranial trauma, cardiac murmur, and arterial bruits are assessed. The presence of ocular hemorrhage or meningismus predicts intracranial bleeding. Other diagnoses can be considered with findings of coma, papilledema, or fever suggesting SAH, tumor, infection, or toxic/metabolic derangements. If consciousness is impaired, stroke-related or idiopathic seizure, hemorrhage,

Table 12.4 Pertinent details in the history.

1. Personal and family illnesses, past and present
2. History of past TIA's or CVA's
3. Time of onset of the current stroke symptoms
4. Patient's activity at onset of symptoms
5. Course of the symptoms through time
6. Accompanying symptoms since onset [3]

CVA, Cerebrovascular accident; TIA, Transient ischemic attack.

hypoxia, increased intracranial pressure, or brain stem involvement must be considered. Visual changes, speech or memory disturbances, or signs of neglect can be assessed in the alert patient. Gait can also be tested in some patients to give insight into cerebellar function as well as motoric evaluation.

CLINICAL PEARLS

Differential diagnoses of strokes The patient with hemorrhagic stroke usually presents a picture of more serious illness, with a more rapidly deteriorating course than ischemic lacunar events. These patients more frequently present with severe headache, nausea, vomiting, and declining level of consciousness.

The patient with subarachnoid hemorrhage may present with "the worst headache of my life" after exertion, with rapid onset of pain, which quickly reaches maximum severity, but without focal neurological deficit. There may be transient loss of consciousness, and pain radiating to the face or neck, photophobia, nausea, and subtly altered mental status. Subhyaloid retinal hemorrhage can be an important sign of SAH. The presence of papilledema, and/or loss of venous pulsation in the fundus are infrequently present as signs of increased intracranial pressure. Meningismus with nuchal rigidity, photo- and phonophobia also suggests the diagnosis of SAH, although the patient may not develop these signs for several hours. (Movement of the neck should not be attempted until cervicocranial instability is ruled out.) About one quarter of patients with SAH due to aneurysm will have minor or moderately severe symptoms to slight bleeding prior to the actual rupture of the vessel: a sentinel or warning leak [4].

Patients with ICH usually have even more profound deficits, decreased level of consciousness, nausea and vomiting. In both conditions, the pattern of presentation, timing, and history will help guide the work-up and treatment. The majority of the patients with ICH, if they survive, tend to have favorable prognosis as far as disability is concerned.

Localization of Ischemic Stroke

Precise localization of ischemia is not necessary [5]. However, general information regarding an area of ischemia would help to map a strategy for work-up. The differential diagnosis between anterior and posterior circulation is shown in Table 12.5 [6].

1 Is the ischemia in the anterior (carotid, middle cerebral, or anterior cerebral artery) or posterior (vertebrobasilar) circulation? This information is important in determining which circulation to image, as well as to pertaining to prognosis [6].

2 Is the event cortical or subcortical? Cortical events are more likely to be embolic or due to large vessel abnormalities.

3 Is the stroke embolic or lacunar? (Cardio-embolic, thrombo-embolic or a lacunar stroke.) Cardio- or thrombo-embolic strokes are rapid in progression compared to lacunar stroke which has slow progression.

Table 12.5 Differences between stroke from the anterior vs. posterior circulation.

Function	Anterior circulation	Posterior circulation
Motor dysfunction	Contralateral faces	Ipsilateral faces
		Ipsilateral cranial nerves sign such as double vision, decreased gag, tongue deviation, etc
	Contralateral extremities	Contralateral extremities
	*Clumsiness	*Clumsiness
	*Weakness	*Weakness
	*Paralysis	*Paralysis
	*(Dysarthria)	*(Dysarthria)
Loss of vision fields	Ipsilateral eye	In one or both homonymous visual
	Homonymous hemianopia	
Sensory deficit	Contralateral faces	Ipsilateral faces
	Contralateral extremities	Contralateral extremities
	*Numbness or loss of sensation	*Numbness or loss of sensation
	*Paresthesia	*Paresthesia
Speech	Dysphasia (dominant hemisphere)	

*Typical signs but non-diagnostic in isolation: ataxia, vertigo, diplopia, dysphasia, dysarthria.

Ideally at this point in the work-up, localization of the event to the anterior or posterior circulation and some insights into potential mechanism should be possible. If hemorrhage is ruled out and clinical localization is established, further imaging is not essential. However, because of transient symptoms, poor description, or symptoms that may localize to either the anterior or the posterior circulation, it may not be possible to localize the event (e.g., isolated dysarthria).

Once the patient is bought to the ER, logistics and time frame for the initial assessment are listed in Table 12.6 [5].

Table 12.6 Logistics in the ER: 7 (D's) steps to stroke identification and treatment.

Procedure	Time frame
1. Detection	
2. Dispatch (911)	10 minutes from detection
3. Delivery	20 minutes from detection
4. Door	30 minutes from detection
5. Data*	40 minutes from detection
6. Decision	50 minutes from detection
7. Drug therapy	60 minutes from detection

*(CBC with platelet count, prothrombin time, partial thromboplastin time, serum electrolytes, blood glucose, 12 lead ECG and insert two IV lines).

Imaging for Diagnosis and Interventions

New imaging techniques are adding to our ability to assess the stroke patient quickly and non-invasively. Under ideal conditions, the technical staff will be on site or on call with very rapid response as soon as the patient has started his trip to the hospital. A non-contrast CT scan of the brain should be the initial diagnostic imaging test, with chest and/or cervical spine films performed if indicated. The CT scan needs to be reviewed immediately for the presence of hemorrhage (either ICH or SAH). The non-contrast CT scan of the head is 100% sensitive in detecting ICH and 95% sensitive in detecting SAH. The findings may be normal in patients with acute ischemic stroke when performed early enough [6]. If there are early CT changes, it is not only indicative of severe disease, but is also a check on the true time of event onset. Then without ICH, in an acceptable time frame for treatment, the patient could undergo revascularization therapy. Transcranial Doppler (TCD) study in acute events where time is a major factor is not a good diagnostic tool and accuracy is somewhat questionable.

On the cellular level, ischemic stroke is not a single fixed event, but rather a dynamically evolving process. It is caused by an abnormal decrease of blood flow to a particular region of the brain. Some areas with very low blood flow go to infarction in a short period of time. Other sections, however, may exhibit dysfunction for extended periods before becoming irreversibly damaged. Other sections with similar occlusions stay healthy or hibernating through the collaterals from the contralateral side.

To achieve optimal recovery, the physicians must identify the location and extent of the ischemic core (irreversible damage) as well as the ischemic penumbra (potentially reversible) before mapping a strategy and implementing a course of therapy. Because the clinical findings are diverse and fluctuate according to the presence and adequacy of the collateral system, they are not always helpful in pinpointing the acutely occluded artery. Although cerebral angiography is considered the gold standard for identifying an intracranial vascular occlusion, it is not without great risk and it may delay the treatment process. Diffusion- and perfusion-weighted imaging is an evolving MRI technique that detects perfusion and random diffusion of water in a brain territory [6].

Perfusion-Weighted Imaging

Once contrast agent is rapidly injected to the cerebral vascular system, the passage of intravascular contrast material will decrease the brain signal intensity. This is caused by changes in magnetic susceptibility within vessels that result from a high concentration of contrast. The first few scans will show darkening of the cortical gray matter, then the next scans will show the same change in the white matter. At the end, when the circulation time through the brain concludes, the parenchymal signal intensity reverts to baseline intensity [7–10]. In simple terms, perfusion-weighted imaging (PWI) gives the information about the blood perfusion of a brain territory.

Diffusion-Weighted Imaging

Diffusion is a random motion occurring on a microscopic scale. The diffusion coefficient of water is a physical property based on the local environment of the water molecules. In a container of pure water, the diffusion of water is more rapid than within the cells of the brain. This principle is also applied in diffusion-weighted imaging (DWI), producing an image of the brain with diffusion contrast [10]. The failure to maintain ionic equilibrium induces a net flux of water from the extracellular space into the intracellular space; this phenomenon is commonly known as "cytotoxic edema." The diffusion coefficient of intracellular water is much less than its extracellular coefficient, which is likely due to restricted movement of water caused by the large number of intracellular structures. This change in the ratio from intracellular to extracellular water results in an overall apparent decrease in the diffusion of water [10]. In simple terms, PWI gives information about the integrity of the cells in an area where injury is suspected.

Clinical-Imaging Correlations

In the perfusion/diffusion MRI evaluation of patients with acute stroke, there are typically three patterns.

1 Recent full recovery: diffusion abnormality > perfusion defect.
2 Completed injury: diffusion abnormality = perfusion abnormality.
3 Fresh injury: diffusion abnormality < perfusion defect.

1 Diffusion abnormality without a perfusion defect

In cases where the cause of the ischemic injury has resolved at the time of imaging, a diffusion abnormality might be present without an associated perfusion defect. An embolus to a major vessel may occlude a branch of that vessel long enough to cause an infarction. Subsequent initiation of autothrombolysis by the body's own mechanisms can result in restoration of flow, preventing further ischemic damage.[10]

2 Diffusion abnormality with a matching perfusion defect

The second type of pattern, a DWI abnormality with a matching perfusion defect, usually results in an ultimate infarct size that is slightly larger than the original DWI abnormality. In this situation, reperfusion to the area most severely injured has not occurred by the time of imaging. An increase in the volume of the infarct often takes place over the next several days. The physiological basis for this observation is not completely understood. One hypothesis is based on the production of excitotoxic chemicals by the infarcted tissue. Diffusion of these substances into surrounding tissues may trigger a cascade of events that culminates in secondary infarction. This observation points to a therapeutic window for prevention of further brain injury that may last for several days [10].

3 Diffusion abnormality with a larger perfusion defect

The third and most common pattern seen when imaging cases of acute stroke with this technique occurs when the perfusion abnormality is significantly larger than the diffusion abnormality. Often, if therapeutic intervention is not undertaken, the DWI abnormality will increase in size to match or nearly match the perfusion defect. However, timely intervention can prevent this deterioration [11].

At the present time, perfusion and diffusion MRI studies are playing a critical role in guiding patient management decisions. These studies highlight the difference between perfusion and diffusion imaging and the microscopic changes in flow can be detected in advance of a soon-to-be completed infarction, which opens a window of opportunity resulting in timely clinical intervention to reverse the injury process in areas at risk. This information helps to triage viable candidates with ischemic areas that may or may not be salvaged by thrombolytic therapy (TT), neuroprotective agents, or mechanical manipulations [7–11].

There is not always a need for both PWI and DWI. DWI appears to have the greatest sensitivity to early changes seen in the infarcted brain. It will probably become the standard imaging technique for stroke, as it becomes more widely available. Whatever technique is used, the emergent evaluation's goal is to confirm if the cause of the patient's neurological change is due to ischemic stroke, to further guide therapy for reversible causes, and, if possible, elucidate the etiology of the stroke and predict any possible complications.

Management

Management of ischemic stroke includes conservative treatment, IV/intra-arterial (IA) thrombolytic agents and percutaneous mechanical techniques. The goal is to recanalize the acutely occluded arteries in order to preserve the ischemic penumbra, which is defined as the relatively less ischemic anatomical area surrounding the profoundly ischemic center [12] (Table 12.7).

Unfortunately, all interventions carry substantial risks and complications. Failure of pharmacological thrombolysis or mechanical manipulation in the coronary system for acute myocardial infarction (MI) ends with an inability to revascularize the vessel, or failure to salvage the myocardium. By contrast, both successful and unsuccessful pharmacological or catheter-based revascularizations in the intracranial vasculature may be accompanied by shattering complications, including cerebral hemorrhage. Although the potential benefits of treatment are great, its complications are also debilitating and devastating.

Table 12.7 Options in the treatment of ischemic stroke.

1. Conservative treatment with heparin
2. IV thrombolytic therapy
3. Local intracerebral IA thrombolysis
4. Mechanical reperfusion (angioplasty or mechanical breakup of thrombus)
5. Pharmacological neuroprotective agents (investigational)
6. Anti-platelets therapy-aspirin, clopidogrel or dipyridamole/ASA

ASA, acetylsalicyic acid; IA, intra-arterial; IV, intravenous.

IV Thrombolysis

Following the success of TT in acute MI (AMI), pharmacological rescue was suggested for the treatment of acute ischemic stroke. There was no scientifically supported effective method to actively treat or reopen the blockage causing acute stroke until 1995, when the National Institute of Neurologic Disorders and Stroke (NINDS) reported the results of the first of many multicenter prospective trials. These first randomized clinical trials (RCTs) of IV thrombolysis succeeded in clarifying many aspects of this complex problem, including the efficacy and safety of different fibrinolytic agents, the therapeutic window to reverse the injury process, and the benefits or complications in different subsets of patients.

Evidence-based Medicine: The NINDS trial

In the National Institute of Neurological Disorders and Stroke trial, 333 patients were randomized within 3 hours of symptom onset to receive IV tissue plasminogen activators (t-PAs) (0.9 mg/kg; maximum 90 mg) or placebo. This trial tested the hypothesis that IV administration of tPA would facilitate thrombolysis of an intravascular thrombus and subsequently improve clinical neurologic outcomes. The study found that carefully selected acute ischemic stroke patients receiving IV TT within 3 hours from symptoms onset benefited over traditional medical therapy (30% relative benefit over placebo for improved neurologic outcome). The mortality was similar in the t-PA arm (17%) or in the placebo arm (21%) ($P = 0.30$). Symptomatic ICHs were more frequent with t-PA (6.4%) compared with placebo (0.6%) ($P < 0.001$) and out of these ICHs, approximately 50% were fatal [13].

Ischemic strokes can become further disabling or catastrophic if delayed bleeding occurs into the damaged brain tissue. Hemorrhagic conversion of an ischemic hemorrhage is shown to occur more often when thrombolytic medication is administered [13,14]. Despite the increased risk of hemorrhagic conversion secondary to thrombolytic administration, the mortality remained stable relative to traditional treatments and the percentage of patients returning to a level of independent survival was significantly enhanced. The number of patients required to treat for one patient to benefit from this therapy is seven. Even with this exciting breakthrough, only a small percentage (1–5%) of stroke patients are currently deemed eligible for treatment [3]. Factors limiting greater applicability include the extremely short therapeutic window (less than 3 hours, beyond which risk of cerebral hemorrhage will surpass the benefit) and numerous high-risk exclusion criteria [13].

Evidence-based Medicine: The ECASS II trial

The Second European Cooperative Acute Stroke Study randomized patients within 6 hours of symptom onset. Approximately 80% received therapy after 3 hours. The primary end-point was a favorable outcome (score of 0 or 1) on the modified Rankin scale 90 days after treatment. The results did not confirm the statistical efficacy of t-PA but showed a trend in its favor. A *post hoc* analysis of the Rankin scale scores dichotomized for death and dependence revealed a statistically significant 8.3% absolute reduction in death or significant disability in the t-PA group. The overall mortality was similar in two groups at 10.6% and the ICH rate was 8.8% in the t-PA arm vs. 3.4% in the placebo arm (*P* value was not reported) [15].

Once the patient is planned to have IV thrombolysis, the patient's condition needs to be evaluated by an impairment scale. The National Institutes of Health stroke scale is most commonly used (Table 12.8). This scale can help to triage potential thrombolytic candidates as well as predict outcomes. Use of IV recombinant tissue type plasminogen activator (rt-PA) should be avoided in patients with a score of less than 4 (unless there is global aphasia) or greater than 22 (because risk of hemorrhage is increased with such severe cerebral infarction). A score of 16 or more is predictive of severe disability or death. A score of 6 or less predicts good recovery. Score 9 should not be counted in the total NIH score. For limbs with amputation, joint fusion, etc., give a score of 9 and explain the reason. For intubated patient or other physical barriers to speech, give a score of 9 and explain the reason. An expanded version is available at www.strokesite.org/stroke_scales/stroke_scales.html [6].

Table 12.8 The National Institutes of Health stroke scale.

Definition	Score and response	
1a Level of consciousness	0	Alert
	1	Not alert but aroused by stimulation
	2	Not alert; requires repeated stimulation
	3	Coma
1b Ask patient month and age	0	Answers both correctly
	1	Answers one correctly
	2	Answers both incorrectly
1c Ask patient to open and close eyes and hands	0	Obeys both correctly
	1	Obeys one correctly
	2	Obeys neither correctly
2 Best gaze (horizontal eye movement)	0	Normal
	1	Partial gaze palsy
	2	Forced eye deviation
3 Visual field testing	0	Normal visual field
	1	Partial hemianopia
	2	Complete hemianopia
	3	Cortical blindness

(Continued)

Table 12.8 (*Continued*)

Definition	Score and response	
4 Facial paresis	0	Normal
	1	Minor paralysis
	2	Partial paralysis
5a Right arm motor function	0	Normal
	1	Drift
	2	Some effort against gravity
	3	No effort against gravity
	4	No movement
	9	Not testable
5b Left arm motor function	0	Normal
	1	Drift
	2	Some effort against gravity
	3	No effort against gravity
	4	No movement
	9	Not testable
6a Right leg motor function	0	Normal
	1	Drift
	2	Some effort against gravity
	3	No effort against gravity
	4	No movement
	9	Not testable
6b Left leg motor function	0	Normal
	1	Drift
	2	Some effort against gravity
	3	No effort against gravity
	4	No movement
	9	Not testable
7 Limb ataxia	0	None
	1	In one limb
	3	In two limbs
8 Sensory loss (pinprick test)	0	Normal
	1	Mild decrease
	2	Moderate to severe decrease
9 Best language	0	No aphasia
	1	Mild to moderate aphasia
	2	Severe aphasia
	3	Mute
10 Dysarthria (real words)	0	Normal
	1	Mild to moderate slurring
	2	Nearly unintelligible or unable to speak
	3	Intubated
11 Extinction and inattention	0	Normal
	1	Hemi-attention to one modality
	2	Hemi-attention to more than one modality

The time frame for thrombolytic therapy

At first, the NINDS trial confirmed the efficacy of IV fibrinolytic therapy if it is initiated within 3 hours of symptom onset. The ECASS trial expanded this time frame to 6 hours. Although the safety profile was not different when compared with the NINDS trial, administration of t-PA at 3–5 hours after symptom onset was no more likely than placebo to be associated with complete recovery [16]. This study's safety findings are helpful in situations when there is some uncertainty about the time of symptom onset. Since the safety of the drug has been demonstrated beyond 3 hours, the physician has some flexibility in administering t-PA beyond the 3-hour window. This is also particularly true for the anterior circulation. If the lenticulostriate arteries are directly occluded, the therapeutic window may be far less than 3–6 hours; the danger of hemorrhage from these vessels increases exponentially after 5–9 hours. For cortical vessels, the time window for rescue may be from 8–24 hours, depending on how good the pial collateral supply is [17]. If the CT scan suggested of more than one-third infarction in the MCA territory, the incident of hemorrhagic conversion is higher. Initial studies and current FDA approved treatment strategies are based primarily on strict *clinical* inclusion and exclusion criteria. Several research protocols are now exploring application of new *imaging* techniques using MRI diffusion and perfusion criteria to expand the treatment window beyond the initial 3 hour window. The hypothesis is that each individual has a unique therapeutic window, based on their own cerebrovascular collaterals and physiologic tolerance for ischemia. By imaging the unique physiologic characteristics of each individual patient, previous clinical stratification strategies may be enhanced and a greater number of stroke patients may be eligible for therapy rather than relegating them to generalized temporal limits [7–9].

Types of thrombolytic agents

t-PA (Activase™) was successfully evaluated in the NINDS trial and subsequently approved by the FDA for the treatment of acute ischemic stroke. This is the only fibrinolytic drug available in the US that is FDA-approved for ischemic stroke. Other trials continue to use t-PA as the study drug (ECASS, ATLANTIS, STARS, etc.).

Streptokinase was given in a Multicenter-Acute Stroke Trial in Europe (MAST-E). Recruitment was terminated early because of the high incidence of ICH and mortality [18]. A second study, the Australian Streptokinase Trial (ASK), was likewise terminated [19].

Urokinase was studied in many trials and is no longer available in the US.

Ancrod was given to patients with acute stroke in the Stroke Treatment with Ancrod Trial (STAT). It is a serine protease derived from the Malaysian pit viper venom that removes fibrinogen from the blood. The starting dose of ancrod was calculated on the basis of body weight and initial fibrinogen level. The drug was administered continuously for 3 days then intermittently for 2 days for a total of 5 days. It was monitored and its dose adjusted to maintain a fibrinogen level within the target range of 40–69 mg/dL. As seen with other thrombolytic trials, significantly more patients achieved the positive end-point with the treatment drug (41.4% vs. 35%, respectively, $P < 0.05$). The mortality was equal at 10% in both groups. The rate of ICH was related to the fibrinogen level between 9 and 72 hours after therapy (5.2% for the ancrod arm vs. 2% in the placebo arm). The highest rate of ICH (13.8%) was seen in the group of patients with fibrinogen level <40 mg/dL [20].

Glycoprotein IIb-IIIa inhibitor (Abciximab, Reopro™) was given to patients with acute ischemic stroke to measure the risk of fatal and non-fatal ICH within 5 days of therapy. No major fatal or non-fatal cases of ICH were identified. 19% of abciximab patients and 5% of placebo patients had asymptomatic hemorrhage. The mortality was 17% and 15%, respectively [21].

Discussing the risk of thrombolysis with patients and families

Before the treatment, the patient and family need to be informed of the benefits and risks of the IV TT. If the benefits outweigh the risks, then the patient should receive aggressive therapy. The most feared complication is ICH. The risk of ICH (in the NINDS trial) was 6.4% in patients receiving rt-PA and 0.6% in patients receiving placebo. ICH was associated with more severe stroke, evidence of infarction on the pre-treatment CT scan of the head, and uncontrolled hypertension. Despite the increased risk of ICH, the overall mortality at 3 months was equal in both groups. The benefit is that the patients treated with rt-PA are at least 30% more likely to have minimal or no disability at 3 months.

After a stroke, a patient's ability to fully comprehend the risks and benefits of treatment may be compromised by apprehension, aphasia, visuo-spatial neglect, or altered consciousness. In addition, a 3-hour therapeutic window leaves little time to counsel patients before therapy. The social problem can also be aggravated because this encounter may be the first ever between the physician assigned to see the patient who presents at the ER without a regular family physician. In this case, the doctor–patient relationship is very preliminary and the communication between the two sides needs further strengthening and trust. Therefore, in any case, when talking to patients and their families, the physician needs to be direct and frank and should invite questions. After the patients and their families agree to proceed with TT, receipt of verbal consent should be documented in the medical records [5].

All of the guidelines on TT are based on the NINDS trial. The indications are listed in Table 12.9; the contraindications are listed in Table 12.10. Management protocol is listed in Table 12.11 and the algorithm for high blood pressure management is shown in Table 12.12.

Table 12.9 Indications for thrombolytic therapy in ischemic stroke.

1. Clinical diagnosis of ischemic stroke causing a measurable neurological deficit. Time of symptom onset well established to be <180 min before treatment would begin
2. Age greater than or equal to 18 years

Table 12.10 Contraindications and warnings for thrombolytic therapy in ischemic stroke.

Present illness
1. Only minor or rapidly improving stroke symptoms*
2. Clinical presentation suggestive of subarachnoid hemorrhage, even with normal CT*
3. More than 3 hours after symptom onset

Past medical or surgical history
1. History of gastrointestinal or urinary tract hemorrhage or MI within 21 days
2. Within 3 months any intra-cranial surgery, serious head trauma, or previous stroke
3. Previous major surgery or serious trauma in the previous 14 days
4. Recent arterial puncture at a non-compressible site
5. Recent lumbar puncture within 7 days
6. History of ICH
7. Known arterio–venous malformation or aneurysm
8. Seizure at the onset of stroke

Physical examination
1. On repeated measurements, systolic BP >185 mmHg or diastolic BP >110 mmHg at the time treatment is to begin, and patient requires aggressive treatment to reduce BP to within these limits
2. Post-myocardial infarction pericarditis
3. Rapid resolving of minor deficits
4. Obtunded or comatose condition

Computed tomography
1. Evidence of intracranial hemorrhage on pretreatment CT scan.
2. Involvement of more than ⅓ of the MCA on CT scan indicates a high chance of hemorrhagic transformation with thrombolysis
3. Intracranial tumor

Laboratory studies
1. Known bleeding diathesis
2. Platelet count <100,000/mm
3. Patient has received heparin within 48 hours and has an elevated PTT
4. Current use of oral anticoagulant (e.g., warfarin)
5. Recent use with an elevated PT >15 sec or INR >1.7
6. Abnormal blood glucose (<50 or >400 mg/dL)

BP, blood pressure; ICH, intra-cranial hemorrhage; INR, international normalized ratio; MCA, middle cerebral artery; MI, myocardial infarction; PT, prothrombin time; PTT, partial thromboplastin time.

Table 12.11 Protocol guidelines: sequence of events.

1. **Determine whether time** is available to start treatment with rt-PA before 3 hours
2. Draw blood for tests while preparations are made to perform non-contrast CT scan
3. Start recording BP

4. **Neurological examination**
5. **CT scan without contrast**
6. Determine whether CT has evidence of hemorrhage
   If the patient has severe head or neck pain or is somnolent or stuporous, be sure there is no evidence of SAH. If there is a significant abnormal lucency suggestive of infarction, reconsider the patient's history, since the stroke may have occurred earlier
7. **Review required test results**
   Hematocrit
   Platelets

(Continued)

Table 12.11 (*Continued*)

Blood glucose
PT or PTT (in patients with recent use of oral anticoagulants or heparin)

8. *Review patient selection criteria*
9. *Infuse rt-PA*
   Give 0.9 mg/kg 10% as a bolus IV then the rest is (maximum of 90 mg) infused over 60 min
   with 10% of the total dose administered as an initial IV bolus over 1 min
   Do not use the cardiac dose
   Do not exceed the 90 mg maximum dose
   Do not give aspirin, heparin, or warfarin for 24 hours

10. *Monitor* the patient carefully, especially the BP, follow the BP algorithm
    Monitor neurological status (see sample orders)
    Adjunctive therapy
    No concomitant heparin, warfarin, or aspirin during the first 24 hours after symptoms onset.
    If heparin or any other anticoagulant is indicated after 24 hours, consider performing a non-
    contrast CT scan or other sensitive diagnostic imaging method to rule out intracranial
    hemorrhage before starting an anticoagulant

BP, blood pressure; IV intravenous; PT, prothrombin time; PTT, partial thromboplastin time; rt-PA,
recombinant tissue type plasminogen activator?; SAH, subarachnoid hemorrhage.

Table 12.12 Algorithm for blood pressure control.

Monitor blood pressure every 15 min (should be <185/110 mmHg)

*Before treatment with thrombolytic drug, if for two readings apart, the systolic pressure is
between 185 and 230 mmHg or the diastolic pressure is between 105 and 120 mmHg:*
1. Give labetolol 10 mg IV over 1–2 min. The dose may be repeated and/or doubled every
   10–20 min up to 150 mg. Monitor BP every 15 min during treatment. Observe for hypotension.
   If these measures do not reduce BP <185/110 and keep it down, the patient should not be
   treated with rt-PA

*After thrombolytic drug was given, if for two readings apart, the systolic pressure is
between 185 and 230 mmHg or the diastolic pressure is between 105 and 120 mmHg:*
1. Give labetolol 10 mg IV over 1–2 min. The dose may be repeated and/or doubled every
   10–20 min up to 150 mg. Monitor BP every 15 min during treatment. Observe for hypotension

*If the systolic pressure is greater than 230 mmHg or the diastolic pressure is between 120
and 140 mmHg:*
1. Give labetolol 10 mg IV over 1–2 min. The dose may be repeated and/or doubled every
   10–20 min up to 150 mg. If satisfactory response is not obtained, use nitroprusside. Monitor
   BP every 10 min during treatment. Observe for hypotension

If the diastolic pressure is greater than 140 mmHg:
1. Infuse sodium nitroprusside (0.5–10 mcg/kg/min)
2. Monitor BP every 15 min during treatment. Observe for hypotension

During and after treatment:
1. Monitor BP for the first 24 hours after starting treatment
2. Every 15 min for 2 hours after starting the infusion, then
3. every 30 min for 6 hours, then
4. every hour for 18 hours

BP, blood pressure; IV, intravenous; rt-PA, recombinant tissue type plasminogen activator; PT,
prothrombin time.

Intracranial hemorrhage

In case of either success or failure with TT, or even without receiving a thrombolytic drug, a significant percentage of ischemic and infarcted brains will undergo hemorrhagic transformation. If reperfusion is accomplished too late, the infarcted brain can be exposed to direct arterial pulse pressure, which may precipitate devastating hemorrhage in the presence of anticoagulant and thrombolytic agents. So the goal of reperfusion, therefore, is to open occluded vessels while their endothelium and territories are still viable [7–10].

CLINICAL PEARLS

Management of Intra-cranial Hemorrhage Patients who have an abrupt decline in neurological status within the first 24 hours after initiation of TT should be considered to have an ICH until it is proven otherwise. Practically, TT should be stopped.

An emergency CT scan of the head is done and neurosurgery consultation is requested if there is ICH.

Hematoma evacuation or external ventricular drainage, or both, may be life-saving. This is why the patient or families should be informed so they understand that possible significant neurological morbidity may be expected in patients who survive hematoma evacuation.

A prothrombin time (PT), partial thromboplastin time (PTT), hematocrit, and serum fibrinogen level should be obtained.

If the effect of rt-PA needs to be reversed, the patient should be given cryoprecipitate or fresh frozen plasma (6 units) or single donor platelets (1 unit).

Local Intra-arterial Thrombolysis

The concept of IV thrombolysis represented a significant advance over traditional conservative medical management of stroke patients, however, as described above, patient eligibility and benefits remain limited to a small subpopulation of the overall afflicted population. The therapeutic strategy to administer a smaller dose of thrombolytics IA directly within the intraluminal thrombus represented a significant potential advance over IV therapy.

Evidence-based Medicine: The PROACT II trial

In the Prolyse in Acute Cerebral Thromboembolism trial II, the patients were randomized to receive heparin alone or heparin with intra-arterial recombinant prourokinase in patients with angiogram-proven middle cerebral artery occlusion in an expanded treatment window up to 6 hours from symptom onset. At 90 days, 40% of patients with therapy had slight or no disability compared with 25% treated by heparin alone ($P = 0.04$). Even within this prolonged therapeutic window, and in more severely injured patients, intra-arterial thrombolysis demonstrated a 58% relative benefit over placebo for improved clinical outcomes. The recanalization rate at 2 hours (complete plus partial patency, TIMI grades 2 (48%) or 3 (19%)) was 67% in the prourokinase group vs. 18% in the control group. As seen in other trials, the mortality rate at 90 days was similar in the two groups (25%) and the rate of ICH was 10.2% in the treatment arm and 1.8% in the control arm [14].

Despite the modest rate of recanalization (complete recanalization ~19%) and the increased risk of hemorrhagic conversion (10%) [14], IA thrombolysis represented a significant advance over IV TT with improved clinical outcomes in a prolonged therapeutic window in more critically affected patients. Unfortunately, a reported manufacturing quality assurance deficiency of urokinase resulted in suspension of urokinase production, and FDA approval for Prourokinase was never granted (www2.kumc.edu/druginfo/ drugsafety/ drgsafe99-2.html). The therapeutic benefit over IV and conservative medical therapy remains significant, and compassionate off-label use of similar thrombolytics (tPA, urokinase) is performed throughout the world in clinical stroke treatment centers where the resources and expertise have been adequately developed.

The inclusion criteria for direct intracranial intra-arterial thrombolysis are listed in Table 12.13.

Table 12.13 Indications and exclusion criteria of intra-arterial thrombolysis.

Indications
1. Fibrinolytic therapy within 6 hours from onset of symptoms
2. Symptoms appropriate to the location of the occlusion
3. No history of recent infarct

Exclusion criteria
1. Rapidly improving clinical symptoms
2. Very severe onset symptoms (e.g., seizures)
3. Recent stroke (<6 weeks)
4. Bleeding disorder
5. Certain types of recent surgery
6. CT scan evidence of intracranial bleed, large area of edema, or mass effect

Arterial infusion techniques

If a patient meets the criteria for emergency intracranial fibrinolysis, a diagnostic angiogram is performed in the antero-posterior and lateral projections [22]. If possible, angiography of the opposite carotid artery and one vertebral artery should be done to determine the status of anterior and posterior communicating arteries and leptomeningeal anastomoses. All intracranial vasculature is evaluated, beginning with theuninvolved vessels to assess the collateral supply to the ischemic territory. The target vessel is studied last for direct evidence of vessel occlusion. If the study is positive, heparin is given intravenously, generally recommended at a relatively low dose as used in PROACT II trial, 2000 units initially [14,17].

Isotonic contrast is very slowly injected because the capillary endothelium is ischemic and there is no significant run-off or reflux if the vessel is occluded. This may theoretically increase the risk for contrast related endothelial injury, and more concerning, acute vessel rupture and sudden death secondary to high intravascular pressure. The thrombus is laced with rt-PA, injected as the catheter is withdrawn; the catheter tip is left at the thrombus. A continuous infusion is begun at the rate of 30 mL per hour [14,17].

The progress is checked every 15 min by contrast injection through the guide around the microcatheter. The microcatheter position is adjusted as thrombolysis progresses to maintain the tip of the catheter as close to the thrombus as possible. If an underlying stenosis is encountered, angioplasty may be required to prevent acute re-thrombosis. The decision to stop therapy is based on the response, the duration and depth of ischemia, and the location of the occlusion. The heparin infusion is stopped at the end of the procedure [17].

Post-procedural management includes control of blood pressure if elevated, neurological monitoring, and routine supportive care. Control of hypertension (intravenous labetalol and/or nitroprusside if needed) is indicated if reperfusion of a large ischemic area has been achieved and the BP is above 180/110 bpm. Otherwise, a modest physiological increase in BP is therapeutic for the ischemic area and should not be aggressively treated. Neurological progression should be monitored closely and other co-morbidity appropriately treated [17].

Complications

The major complication of this procedure is symptomatic intraparenchymal hemorrhage. In addition, reperfusion edema can worsen an already bad situation. Factors that affect the incidence of bleeding conversion are included in Table 12.14 [17].

Table 12.14 Factors influencing the incidence of bleeding conversion.

1. The length of time of occlusion
2. The status of the lenticulostriate arteries
3. When and if reperfusion was accomplished
4. The systemic BP
5. The presence or absence of very early ischemic changes on CT scan

BP, blood pressure.

Intra-arterial or intravenous thrombolysis?

Both IV and IA thrombolytic treatments showed improvement of outcome when given within 3 hours of symptom onset. However, there are logistical advantages and disadvantages between the two modalities as listed in Table 12.15.

Table 12.15 Comparison between intravenous and intra-arterial thrombolytic therapy.

Intravenous therapy	Intra-arterial therapy
Access: advantage	**Access: disadvantage**
1. Quick initiation of treatment (10–15 min)	Cerebral angiogram is performed
2. No need for skilled personnel	Placement of microcatheter in clot
3. No need for special equipment	(Time: 45 min or more)
Assessment: disadvantage	**Assessment: advantage**
1. Clinical diagnosis	Direct visualization of thrombus
2. CT scan to rule out ICH	Correlation of lesion with clinical findings
Infusion: disadvantage	**Infusion: advantage**
1. Blind fixed dose treatment	Lytic agent may not be necessary if clot cleared
2. Systemic thrombolytic state	Lytic agent given until clot is cleared
	Less systemic thrombolytic state because agent is given locally

IA, intra-arterial; ICH, intra-cranial hemorrhage; IV, intravenous.

The techniques of cerebral angiography are discussed in the next section as a rescue intervention during an endovascular procedure.

IA Mechanical Thrombolysis

The utilization of thrombolytics for acute stroke (intravenous and intra-arterial), have resulted in a significant benefit for patients over traditional conservative medical therapy, however the hemorrhagic conversion rates remained relatively high and the number of patients excluded from eligibility secondary to the numerous high-risk exclusion criteria limits applicability. This has led to a search for a mechanical method of clot retrieval that may increase the number of patients eligible for therapy, enhance recanalization efficacy, minimize the potential for hemorrhagic conversion, and further improve the rate of independent survival for stroke victims.

The wire

The embolus can be fragmented with several passages of guidewire and catheter through its length; by twisting the curved end of the wire within the thrombus while the wire is pulled back; and by saline injection into the thrombus through the micro catheter [23]. Vessel perforation with excessive manipulation can be a concern.

Balloon angioplasty

When anatomically possible or with a failure of pharmacologic thrombolysis, mechanical thrombolysis using a soft high-compliance neurovascular balloon may be performed in an attempt to macerate the thrombus and enhance low-dose pharmacologic therapy. Balloon inflations should be limited to less than 20–30 seconds and should be performed at very low pressures (less than

1 atm.) when attempting to macerate intraluminal thrombus. If an underlying stenosis is observed following successful thrombolysis, primary angioplasty of the stenotic segment may be required acutely to maintain vascular patency. This can be performed using a low-compliance atherosclerotic angioplasty balloon, with short duration (10–30 secs) and low pressure (1–5 atm.) inflations in an attempt to stretch the stenotic intracranial vascular segment [24–26]. The short balloon inflation and low pressure are to avoid compromising the perforating arteries, flow limiting dissections, and vessel rupture [27]. Post-angioplasty angiogram should be performed to assess for success, distal embolization, and intimal or medial damage to the artery. The combination of TT and mechanical disruption usually helps to achieve vessel recanalization faster than thrombolysis alone. It also decreases the need for a large amount of thrombolytic agent, thus decreasing the possibility of reperfusion ICH [23].

Intra-arterial clot retrieval or mechanical thrombolysis

The FDA has approved the Mechanical Embolus Removal in Cerebral Ischemia (MERCI) retrieval system, a corkscrew-like apparatus, to remove blood clots from the brain in patients experiencing an ischemic stroke within 8 hours of onset of stroke symptoms.

Evidence-based Medicine: The MERCI trial

In the MERCI 1 study successful recanalization occurred in 12 patients (43%) with the retriever alone, and in 18 (64%) with additional IA tPA. No symptomatic ICH occurred. In the full MERCI trial, in which the device was deployed in 141 of 151 patients, recanalization with the device occurred in 68 patients (48%), which was significantly better than the rate in placebo arm of the Prolyse in Acute Cerebral Thromboembolism (PROACT) II trial of patients with MCA occlusions ($P < 0.0001$). Additional adjuvant therapy led to recanalization in 85 (60%). Symptomatic ICH occurred in 7 (8%) [28].

The initial safety and efficacy studies demonstrated promising early results in a very critically ill population of patients in a further prolonged therapeutic window of 8 hours. Recanalized patients experienced a higher rate of functional neurologic recovery (46%) and decreased mortality (32%) compared to persistently occluded patients (10% functional recovery, 54% mortality). Nevertheless, the rate of recanalization remained modest (46%) and procedural complications occurred at a significant rate (7.1%). In spite of the prolonged therapeutic window, the symptomatic hemorrhagic conversion rate remained relatively low (7.8%) compared with trials utilizing pharmacologic thrombolytics within a similar therapeutic window [28], further supporting the hypothesis that minimizing thrombolytic administration during attempted recanalization may improve clinical outcomes [10].

Adjunct Pharmacotherapy

Nicardepine and/or adenosine, 200–400 mcg, is very useful for treating distal spasm. Glycoprotein 2b3a inhibitors are promising drugs. When good flow has been rapidly re-established, protamine may be given to reverse anticoagulation or intravenous heparin can be discontinued to hopefully lessen the risk of hemorrhagic conversion.[23]

Complications

The most feared post-embolic recanalization complication is intracranial hemorrhage [23]. It may be part of a natural pathological process that degrades the integrity of the vascular system and the exudation of blood components into the cerebral environment. Spontaneous or facilitated reperfused ischemic brain parenchyma is very prone to hemorrhagic conversion. Ischemically damaged terminal branches, especially the lenticulostriate basal ganglionic arteries, are also very prone to rupture, without recourse from collaterals [23]. When the horizontal M1 segment of the MCA is recanalized and reperfused, it is the combination of ischemic brain parenchyma and ischemic damage to the small vessels that causes the highest post-recanalization hemorrhage into the basal ganglia [23].

Difficult Problems and Suggested Solutions

Real World Question How to Treat Iatrogenic Periprocedural Acute Thromboembolic Stroke?

Embolization of thrombotic or atherosclerotic material can be caused by instrumentation through the aortic arch, in the ventricle, or in the supra-aortic vessels, including the carotid arteries. It is an uncommon but important complication from endovascular intervention. Experienced operators with meticulous and compulsive attention to techniques, coupled with careful patient selection, should encounter this problem in less than 1% of coronary angioplasty or 13% of carotid interventions [29]. It is important to assess the neurological status of the patient after every step of the procedure. Even minute changes in the level of consciousness, minimal confusion, slurred speech, or other changes in the neurological status can indicate distal embolization [22]. During endovascular interventions, especially in the carotid territory, a change in neurological status should initiate the actions listed in Table 12.16 [22].

Table 12.16 General care of patients with periprocedural ischemic stroke.

1. General care of the patient should be instituted
2. Maintaining normal BP, heart rate
3. Maintaining airways and administration of oxygen
4. In case of carotid procedure, the stenting should be quickly and efficiently completed, including stent deployment. Additional maneuvers will involve working through the stented segment to access distal vasculature
5. If the patient becomes uncooperative or agitated, and especially if there are compromised airways, the intervention of an anesthesiologist is required

BP, blood pressure.

A diagnostic angiogram is done in the anteroposterior and lateral projections. The angiograms are carefully examined to determine the site and extent of intracranial vessel embolism. Because of anatomical arrangements and flow pattern, the most likely site of intracranial embolism is the distal internal carotid artery and the middle cerebral artery and its branches. Large vessel occlusion is usually obvious (especially in lateral projection), but embolism in the smaller branches requires careful scrutiny. Acute small branch vessel occlusion may be noted only in comparison with preprocedural angiography. The availability of a good preprocedural intracranial angiogram is therefore essential in all patients undergoing supra-aortic vessel stenting. Change of neurological status can ensue not only from occlusive phenomena such as embolus, but also from intracerebral hemorrhage or hyperperfusion syndrome (especially if very tight stenosis or an occluded artery is opened). If on the diagnostic angiogram there are no signs of embolism, a CT scan should be performed forthwith. If there are signs of localized expanding phenomenon indicating ICH, heparin should be reversed and a CT scan performed [2].

Equipment and Adjunctive Medications Needed for Neurovascular Rescue

The sheath within the common carotid artery is the basic support for advancement of the variable-stiffness microcatheter into the intracranial circulation. Through this sheath, a guide catheter is advanced into the ICA over a wire. This guide should not be advanced deeply into the internal carotid artery if there are tortuosities or coils in this vessel. This would produce spasm or even dissection. Through this guide catheter (5 or 6 French), a variable-stiffness microcatheter (2.3–3.0 French) is advanced. All of these catheters should be continuously perfused with heparinized saline, which should be appropriately prepared, dripped, and filtered without air to avoid stroke producing air emboli. The variable-stiffness microcatheter is advanced over the wire into the intracranial segment of the internal carotid artery. There are a variety of neurovascular guiding wires that are now commercially available from a variety of vendors. Choice of wire is based an individual patient's vascular anatomy, favoring wires with good torqability, adequate stiffness, and atraumatic malleable tips. If the position of the embolus is obvious (in the internal carotid artery or horizontal M1 segment of the middle cerebral artery), no additional arteriography is needed. If the occlusive lesion is within the trifurcation of the middle cerebral artery or distally, an angiogram through the variable-stiffness microcatheter is performed (using 1–3 cm syringe) in both projections, so the occluded branch of the middle cerebral artery is identified and subsequently entered. Road mapping is useful. Before the recanalization is attempted, the length of the occluded vessel segment should be determined. This can be done by careful analysis of the diagnostic angiogram by looking for retrograde flow into the occluded artery. If there is no retrograde flow, the variable-stiffness microcatheter is passed through the embolus over the wire distally. Rotating movement of the distal curved end of the wire usually shows a patent vessel. The wire is withdrawn and slow injection of contrast through the microcatheter is undertaken, while the catheter is slowly pulled back simultaneously. This determines the distal end of the embolus, which can be both "soft" and "hard." The soft one consists of blood coagulation and is prone to lysis. The hard one consists of stenotic debris (part of the plaque with cholesterol and calcium) and cannot be lysed, but it can be mechanically disrupted. There are three techniques to reopen an acutely occluded intracranial artery: thrombolysis, mechanical disruption, and removal of the embolus [22].

Take Home Message

When taking care of patients with ischemic stroke, the non-neurologist interventionalists should remember that the clinical findings of stroke are very diverse and fluctuating according to the presence and adequacy of the collaterals. The therapeutic window remains very short: the best is less than 3 hours; this is why only 1.6% of patients with stroke are currently eligible for interventional treatment. During treatment, the clinical recovery is not brisk. There is no dramatic improvement as in primary angioplasty for AMI where the symptoms and the ECG changes improve in a matter of seconds, because rescue intervention in ischemic stroke deals with recovery of neurons (not muscle) and their unknown interaction with the CSF environment.

Patients with very severe strokes, prolonged time to presentation, and high stroke scale scores (>20), may have an increased risk for poor outcomes despite intervention, perhaps secondary to large irreversible infarct size and limited ischemic penumbra [28].

Patients imaged with MR perfusion and diffusion possessing a perfusion defect significantly larger than the diffusion abnormality may be most likely to benefit from revascularization, and at lowest risks for hemorrhagic complications. (Hypothesis currently being tested in several trials – both IV and IA).

IA neurovascular intervention remains technically challenging, requiring significant experience within the delicate environment of the intracranial vasculature, which is at high risk and low tolerance for vessel injury, flow-limiting dissection, perforation, secondary branch occlusions, and associated morbidity and mortality. Mechanical thrombolysis or clot retrieval may offer significant advantages over pharmacologic therapy, limiting thrombolytic dosage and accelerating the time to revascularization, perhaps offering a greater opportunity for patient recovery and limiting therapeutic adverse events.

After successful and unsuccessful interventions, the clinical outcome may remain poor as the brain is an organ very sensitive to injury. Unlike the heart, where minimizing infarcted myocardium may result in a diminished EF and further cardiovascular decompensation without significant functional morbidity, even a small region of persistent brain ischemia/infarct may result in devastating functional morbidity (coma, blindness, language deficit, etc.) despite successful recanalization.

Hemorrhagic conversion can present as a disease process or secondary to timely or delayed reperfusion injury as a result of successful therapeutic interventions. Neurovascular intervention remains a high risk arena, with a high mortality and morbidity rate despite successful therapy. The best mortality is 10% compared with 3% mortality for primary angioplasty. The best long-term result is a 58% relative clinical benefit with IA thrombolysis [11,14].

Just as coronary bypass surgery was in its infancy 30 years ago or percutaneous angioplasty was in its infancy 20 years ago, rescue intervention in ischemic stroke is in its preliminary steps, despite rapid progress over the last decade. With time, patience, and more studies, hopefully the mechanism of ischemic stroke will continue to be better elucidated and the rescue interventions will continue to evolve with greater technical and clinical efficacy, and enhanced application to an appropriately risk-stratified population. This continues to be the challenge for the next decade and beyond.

References

1 North American Symptomatic Carotid Endarterectomy Trial Collaborators. Beneficial effect of carotid endarterectomy in symptomatic patients with high-grade carotid stenosis. N Engl J Med 1991;325:445–453.

2 Bamford J. Clinical examination in diagnosis and subclassification of stroke. Lancet 1992;339:400–402.

3 Caplan LR. Stroke: A Clinical Approach. 2nd edition. Boston, Butterworth-Heinemann, 1993.

4 Hauerberg J, Andersen BB, Eskesen V, Rosenorn J, Schmidt K. Importance of the recognition of a warning leak as a sign of a ruptured intracranial aneurysm. Acta Neurol Scand 1991;83:61–64.

5 Meschia JE. Management of acute ischemic stroke. Postgrad Med 2000;107:85–93.

6 Flemming KD, Brown Jr RD. Cerebral infarction and transient ischemic attacks. Postgrad Med 2000;107:55–79.

7 Thomalla G, Schwark C, Sobesky J, et al. Outcome and Symptomatic Bleeding Complications of Intravenous Thrombolysis Within 6 Hours in MRI-Selected Stroke Patients. Comparison of a German Multicenter Study With the Pooled Data of ATLANTIS, ECASS and NINDS tPA Trials. Stroke 2006;37(3):852–858.

8 Hjort N, Butcher K, Davis SM, et al. UCLA Thrombolysis Investigators. Magnetic resonance imaging criteria for thrombolysis in acute cerebral infarct. Stroke 2005;36(2):388–397.

9 Derex L, Nighoghossian N, Hermier M, et al. Influence of pretreatment MRI parameters on clinical outcome, recanalization and infarct size in 49 stroke patients treated by intravenous tissue plasminogen activator. J Neurol Sci 2004;225(1–2):3–9.

10 Schaefer P, Gonzalez G. Perfusion and diffusion MRI of acute stroke. Berlex Laboratories, May 1998.

11 Nguyen TN, Vu QT, Simaga M, et al. Interventions in ischemic stroke, pp. 351–378. In Nguyen T, editor. Practical handbook of advanced interventional cardiology. Futura Publishing, 2001.

12 Heiss WD, Graf R, Weinhard J, *et al.* Dynamic penumbra demonstrated by sequential multitracer PET after middle cerebral artery occlusion in cats. J Cereb Blood Flow Metab 1994;14;892–902.

13 The National Institute of Neurological Disorders and Stroke rt-PA Stroke Study Group. Tissue plasminogen activator for acute ischemic stroke. NEJM 1995;333:1581–1587.

14 Furlan A, Higashida R, Wechsler L, *et al.* intra-arterial prourokinase for acute ischemic stroke. The PROACT II study: A randomized controlled trial. Prolyse in Acute Cerebral Thromboembolism. JAMA 1999;282(21):2003–2011.

15 Hacke W, Kaste M, Fieschi C, *et al.* Randomized, double-blind placebo-controlled trial of TT in IV alteplase in acute ischemic stroke (ECASS II). Lancet 1998;352:1245–1251.

16 Clark WM, Wissman S, Albers GW, *et al.* for the ATLANTIS study investigators. Recombinant t–PA (alteplase) for ischemic stroke 3 to 5 hours after symptoms onset. JAMA 1999;282:2019–2026.

17 Connors JJ. Intraarterial thrombolysis for ischemic stroke. J Invas Cardiol 1999;11:93–95.

18 Hommel M, Boissel JP, Cornu C, *et al.* Termination of trial of SK in severe acute ischemic stroke. Lancet 1994;345:57.

19 Donnan GA, Davis SM, Chambers BR, *et al.* Trials of streptokinase in severe acute ischemic stroke (author's reply). Lancet 1995;345:578–579.

20 Sherman DG, Atkinson RP, Chippendale T, *et al.* Intravenous Ancrod for treatment of acute ischemic stroke. JAMA 2000;283:2395–2403.

21 The Abciximab in Ischemic Stroke Investigators. Abciximab in acute ischemic stroke: A randomized, double-blind, placebo-controlled, dose-escalation study. Stroke 2000;31:601–609.

22 Furlan A, Higashida R, Wechsler L, *et al.* intra-arterial prourokinase for acute ischemic stroke. The PROACT study: A randomized controlled trial. JAMA 1999;282:2003–2011.

23 Choi JH, Bateman BT, Mangla S, *et al.* Endovascular recanalization therapy in acute ischemic stroke. Stroke 2006 Feb;37(2):419–24. (Epub 2005 Dec 22.)

24 Qureshi AI, Siddiqui AM, Suri MF, *et al.* Aggressive mechanical clot disruption and low-dose intra-arterial third-generation thrombolytic agent for ischemic stroke: A prospective study. Neurosurgery 2002:51(5):1319–1327; Discussion 1327–1329.

25 Gupta R, Schumacher HC, Mangla S, *et al.* Urgent endovascular revascularization for symptomatic intracranial atherosclerotic stenosis. Neurology 2003 Dec 23;61(12):1729–1735.

26 Schumacher HC, Tanji K, Mangla S, *et al.* Histopathological evaluation of middle cerebral artery after percutaneous intracranial transluminal angioplasty. Stroke 2003 Sep;34(9):e170–173. (Epub 2003 Aug 7.)

27 Barber PA, Zhang J, Demchuk AM, Hill MD, Buchan AM. Why are stroke patients excluded from TPA therapy? An analysis of patient eligibility. Neurology 2001;56(8):1015–1020.

28 Smith WS, Sung G, Starkman S, *et al.* MERCI Trial Investigators. Safety and efficacy of mechanical embolectomy in acute ischemic stroke:results of the MERCI trial. Stroke 2005;36(7):1432–1438. (Epub 2005 Jun 16.)

29 The Abciximab in Ischemic Stroke Investigators. Abciximab in acute ischemic stroke: A randomized, double-blind, placebo-controlled, dose–escalation study. Stroke 2000;31:601–609.

CHAPTER 13

Syncope

Brian Olshansky, Dayi Hu, Pham Quoc Khanh, Pham Nhu Hung, Ta Tien Phuoc and Thach N. Nguyen

Introduction

Syncope is an abrupt, transient loss of consciousness with loss of postural tone, followed by complete, rapid recovery. It is one of the most common, alarming, and challenging *symptoms* with which internists, family practitioners, pediatricians, emergency physicians, and cardiologists have to grapple [1]. Syncope remains an unresolved, often debilitating, complex and expensive medical problem that can be confused with other similar syndromes that are distinct including seizures, coma, fall and altered state of consciousness.

Syncope may have a distinct, prominent prodrome and recovery phase depending on specific causes. The frequency of syncope, and its associated mortality, varies with age, gender and cause [2–6]. The etiologies of syncope vary, often include novel and frequently surprising causes [4–5]. The differential diagnoses are extensive and ever expanding [7]. Unexpected recurrence is a problem that can be associated with serious injuries and therefore restriction may be necessary. The possibility of this restriction in activity can be psychologically and physically devastating [8].

CLINICAL PEARLS
What is important and challenging in the assessment of syncope?
Syncope, it is stated, "is the same as sudden death except that you wake up". One key to effective syncope assessment is to distinguish benign from malignant causes and to determine which patient is at long-term risk of death. Most patients with syncope have a benign cause for syncope and a benign prognosis. The main reason to treat these patients is to prevent syncope recurrence, to improve functionality and to prevent adverse consequences if syncope occurs. When there is evidence of cardiac cause in syncope, the risk of death doubles. Syncope in heart failure (HF) patients is common and is associated with an extremely poor prognosis.

The diversity in the population evaluated (outpatients, emergency room patients, hospitalized patients, the elderly), the broad definition of syncope, and differences in criteria for diagnosis (examination or questionnaire) contribute to wide variations in published data, patient outcomes and management algorithms [9–10]. Without knowledge of the cause for syncope, effective therapy is impossible to prescribe. Management of this baffling problem can become frustrating, confusing, and, often, unrewarding. The reasons of complexity in the assessment and management of syncope are listed in Table 13.1. This chapter will focus on an evaluation approach for syncope and address specific diagnostic and therapeutic issues important for the consultant cardiologist.

Table 13.1 Reasons for complexity in the assessment and management of syncope.

1. Multiple potential causes for syncope
2. No standardized diagnostic approach is possible
3. Highly variable prognosis [1]
4. Difficulty in distinguishing benign from malignant cause [2]
5. Treatment to prevent syncope differs from treatment to prevent death [2]
6. Uncertainty regarding diagnosis
7. Unclear indications and usefulness of hospitalization
8. Difficulty in determining benefits of treatment

Classification

Syncope is generally classified as cardiovascular, non-cardiovascular, and syncope of unknown origin (SUO). The reason for classifying syncope in this way is to provide prognostic data and determine the need for aggressive management [9,11,12]. Those patients who have an underlying cardiovascular problem associated with syncope have a high mortality in the 1–2 years following the episode. The total mortality rate in this group is 30% at 2 years and over 80% at 5 years. Arrhythmic deaths, now potentially treatable, account for over half the deaths of patients with cardiac-related syncope.

When a non-cardiovascular cause for syncope is diagnosed, the mortality is low (1–6% at 2 years). Almost all non-cardiovascular causes are associated with an excellent prognosis. Patients in this category are generally young and healthy as opposed to an older, more ill population who are more likely to have potentially life-threatening cardiovascular disease.

Patients with SUO have a low projected annual mortality ($<6\%$) [12]. This suggests that after a careful evaluation, if no cause for syncope can be found, while recurrences may occur (and they occur at the same rate whether or not a diagnosis is secured), the overall likely survival is excellent.

CLINICAL PEARLS

Caveats on the diagnosis of syncope The ascribed cause for syncope may be incorrect. Even if it is correct, the mechanism by which it occurs can be obscure (e.g., asystole may be autonomically mediated or due to sinus node disease leading to different treatment options). The danger is that a patient may be treated for the wrong condition with subsequent consequences of this treatment and the real cause for syncope may be missed. A patient diagnosed as having neurocardiogenic syncope, following a positive tilt table test, can also have long QT interval syndrome, as there is an association between the two. One condition is life threatening and the other is not. A patient with syncope is diagnosed with hypertrophic cardiomyopathy and has an implanted cardioverter defibrillator (ICD) implanted for this reason, but the cause for syncope turns out to be related to a hemodynamic effect of the cardiomyopathy and it recurs. Syncope may be related to several physiologic mechanisms in this disorder. Furthermore, while an ICD may prevent death, it may not prevent syncope due to ventricular arrhythmias.

Table 13.2 Common causes of syncope.

Non-cardiovascular disease
Reflex mechanisms
1. Neurocardiogenic
2. Micturition
3. Deglutition
4. Post-tussive
5. Defecation
6. Glossopharyngeal
7. Postprandial
8. Carotid sinus hypersensitivity
9. Hyperventilation
10. Dysautonomic storms ("Ganglionitis")
11. Valsalva

Orthostatic hypotension
1. Dysautonomia
2. Fluid depletion
3. Illness, bed rest
4. Drugs

Psychogenic
1. Hysterical
2. Panic disorder
3. Anxiety disorder

Metabolic
1. Hypoglycemia
2. Hypoxia
3. Dehydration (intentional?)
4. Hyperventilation

Neurological
1. Undiagnosed seizures
2. Improperly diagnosed – confusional states hypoglycemia, stroke, etc.
3. Drug induced loss of consciousness (consider alcohol)

Cardiovascular disease
Arrhythmic etiology
1. AV block with bradycardia (due to structural changes or drugs)
2. Sinus pauses, bradycardia (vagal, sick sinus syndrome, drugs)
3. VT due to structural heart disease

Non-arrhythmic etiology: obstructive/reflex etiologies
1. Hypertrophic cardiomyopathy
2. Aortic stenosis

Syncope of unknown origin – about 50% of patients

AV, atrio-ventricular; VT, ventricular tachycardia.

Table 13.3 Uncommon causes of syncope.

Cardiovascular disease
Arrhythmic etiology
1. Supraventricular tachycardia (AVNRT, accessory pathway (WPW syndrome), etc.)
2. The long QT interval syndrome(s)
3. Idiopathic VT (Bellhassen, RVOT tachycardia)
4. Myocardial infarction causing bradycardias and tachycardias
5. Right ventricular dysplasia
6. Brugada syndrome
7. Hypertrophic cardiomyopathy

Non-arrhythmic etiology
1. Pulmonary embolus
2. Pulmonary hypertension
3. Dissecting aortic aneurysm (Marfan's syndrome)
4. Subclavian steal
5. Cardiac tumors – atrial myxoma
6. Cardiac tamponade – cardiovascular
7. Cardiomyopathies (idiopathic, sarcoidosis, amyloidosis)
8. Myocarditis
9. Coronary anomalies: hypoplasia, spasm, bridging, aberrant ostia, anomalous origin
10. Congenital heart diseases

Non-cardiovascular disease
Circulating mediators
1. Carcinoid syndrome
2. Systemic mastocytosis
3. Drugs/supplements – hormones (steroid), drugs (cocaine), Ma Huang, diuretics

Environmental
1. Heat stroke, cold exposure

Blunt trauma
1. Contusion and coronary thrombosis

AVNRT, atrio-ventricular nodal reentrant tachycardia; ROVT, right outflow tract; VT, ventricular tachycardia; WPW, Wolff-Parkinson-White.

The list of causes and their treatments is long but whatever the mechanism, syncope is not a gradual process, but an abrupt change in physiology suggesting that if there is an underlying trigger, it must work with another paroxysmal change in the physiology whether it is autonomic, vascular or arrhythmic. Modern data indicate that at best, only 50–70% of syncope patients will have a tentative diagnosis secured, even with appropriate electrophysiology testing and tilt table testing. Causes for syncope (not exhaustive) are listed in Tables 13.2 and 13.3.

Differential Diagnoses

Orthostatic hypotension [13,14], as well as, mistakenly, epilepsy, is commonly cited causes for syncope [15,16]. The rate of epilepsy diagnosis in a syncope population varies and is based on the population evaluated, the person who is evaluating the symptom and the ability to assess the cause of syncope with certainty. Dysfunction of the cortical centers (seizure, stroke, transient ischemic attack

(TIA), chemical/metabolic disruption (i.e., hypoglycemia, drug use, alcohol intoxication) may mimic some of the features of syncope and therefore be confused with "true" syncope, as opposed to a "gray out": visual changes, presyncope, near syncope, collapse, or light-headedness; but these episodes are distinctly different. It may be difficult to obtain a history to distinguish these rather vague symptoms, and other, potential mechanisms. Other conditions can lead to apparent loss of consciousness, including confusion, dementia and falls.

Evaluation

Syncope can be a diagnostic conundrum: the cause is rarely obvious and the individual at highest risk for recurrence and death can be difficult to detect. Even in the best of circumstances, arrival at a diagnosis requires a "leap of faith", that is, assumptions must be derived from the evaluation regarding actual responsible causes. In the past, no specific evaluation scheme was proper for all patients with syncope so a uniform diagnostic approach is difficult to formulate and challenging for even the best clinicians [17].

Guidelines from the AHA/ACCF

In an attempt to help guiding the work-up process, the American Heart Association/American College of Cardiology foundation (AHA/ACCF) released a statement on the evaluation of syncope [18]. The stated purpose of the evaluation of patients with syncope is shown in Table 13.4.

The AHA/ACCF statement suggests an algorithm for evaluation. As part of the assessment, an attempt is made to evaluate (transient) orthostatic syncope or (functional) neurocardiogenic syncope, and assess for structural heart disease. If the above work-up is negative, then in the case of single episode of syncope, the work-up is complete. In the case of recurrent problems, then long-term follow-up for bradycardias and tachycardias is necessary [18]. However, there are better ways to proceed on the diagnostic process. These are suggested in Figure 13.1.

With better monitoring tools now being developed, it is likely that the management approaches to assess patients with syncope are improving dramatically. The identification of the cause for syncope depends on the certainty of the diagnosis, the tests performed and the patient. Repeated unfocused testing is

Table 13.4 Goals of evaluation for syncope.

1. Determine whether the patient is at increased risk of death
   Structural heart disease
   Myocardial ischemia
   Genetic heart disease (WPW, long QT syndrome, Brugada syndrome, polymorphic VT)
2. Improve quality of life
3. Prevent injury to patients and others

VT, ventricular tachycardia; WPW, Wolff-Parkinson-White.

useless. Even if a tilt table test is not diagnostic, when no definite diagnosis is apparent, and cardiovascular disease is ruled out, syncope most often has a benign, frequently dysautonomic (neurocardiogenic or other abnormal autonomic reflex) origin. Dysautonomic syncope can be provoked by transient, obscure and non-reproducible triggers.

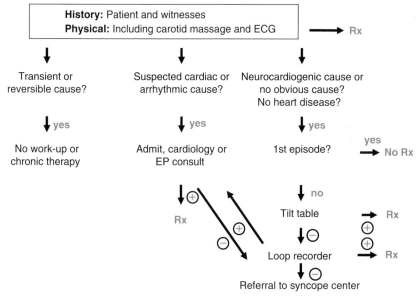

Figure 13.1 Evaluation and management strategies for patients with syncope. Adapted from [86].

History

An effective approach requires careful integration of clues provided in the history and physical examination, combined with keen clinical acumen and judicious use of diagnostic testing. A careful, detailed, and perceptive history cannot be overemphasized, as this is the basis upon which all of the subsequent diagnostic work-up depends. While the patient's recall is invariably incomplete, preceding activities, feelings, and symptoms may be important. A precise characterization of the symptom complex can be crucial to the diagnosis. First, the episodes must be defined. Is it really syncope? The problem must be confirmed to be syncope and not epilepsy, hysteria, light-headedness or dizziness, or gradual loss of vision and/or motor tone. Specific sensory and/or motor auras suggest a seizure. Syncope, when viewed in its most broad definition of global hypoperfusion, can present itself, (especially in the elderly) with isolated transient loss of motor tone and hardly any impairment of consciousness. The elderly may fall or be found on the floor confused. Falls are common in the elderly but are not necessarily syncope. A carefully constructed, complete, history includes the details listed in Table 13.5.

Table 13.5 Details of a complete history.

1. All aspects surrounding the event
2. The patient's clinical characteristics
3. Other similar events
4. Medications
5. Family history
6. Witnessed accounts
7. Prodrome and post syncopal symptoms
8. Situations in which the event occurred
9. Concomitant medical conditions
10. Concomitant symptoms

Examination of the events surrounding the syncopal episode is also important: a patient with abrupt loss of consciousness (no prodrome) who recovers quickly ("classic" Stokes Adams attack) may suffer from an arrhythmia. Neurocardiogenic syncope is usually associated with nausea, vomiting, pallor, sweating, shivering, and the urge to defecate or urinate. Fatigue or depression can follow the episode. The presence of such symptoms, however, does not rule out arrhythmia as a cause of syncope and their absence can occur in so-called malignant neurocardiogenic syncope.

History alone can positively identify characteristic "situational" syncope syndromes such as deglutition syncope, emotional syncope, cough syncope, micturition syncope, trumpet players' syncope, carotid sinus syncope, etc. No further testing may be required. The history can provide needed corroborating clues to narrow the scope of causes.

The presence of structural heart disease: a patient with left ventricular (LV) dysfunction is at high risk of death but other patients with no LV dysfunction can also have a malignant cause of syncope (examples: right ventricular (RV) dysplasia, long Q-T interval syndrome).

Family History

This is especially important in the young, apparently healthy, patient, where the initial reflex of the physician is to dismiss the events as due to a benign vasovagal cause. However, a family history of Wolff–Parkinson–White (WPW) syndrome, familial cardiomyopathy, long QT syndrome, arrhythmogenic right ventricular dysplasia, hypertrophic cardiomyopathy (HCM), Brugada syndrome and especially sudden cardiac death (SCD) at a young age should be treated with extreme concern.

Drug History

Vasoactive medications can cause hypotension and orthostatic hypotension, but anti-arrhythmic and psychotropic drugs, diuretics, and even antihistamines and antifungals, can lead to serious ventricular (generally polymorphic) arrhythmias related to QT prolongation. There is a long list of medications that can cause brady- and tachycardias [19,20].

Age

The prognostic assessment of syncope should consider age along with the differential diagnosis, category, and other risk factors. In younger patients, the cause of isolated syncope is generally neurocardiogenic, psychiatric, or situational (e.g. stress, prolonged standing, and dehydration). While such diagnoses may entail their own therapeutic challenges, these are non-life-threatening problems that often resolve without elaborate evaluation or medical therapy. Young patients with frequent, recurrent episodes may need treatment to prevent debilitating consequences. Syncope in a young patient rarely has a life-threatening cause but there are situations in which concern lingers (exercise-induced syncope, for example), and there are conditions that need to be considered and excluded: hypertrophic cardiomyopathy, long QT interval syndrome, and the Wolff–Parkinson–White syndrome, Brugada syndrome.

Middle-aged patients (40–65 years), similar to younger patients, can have neurocardiogenic syncope, but a potentially serious cardiovascular cause must be considered as well.

The elderly are most likely to pass out, be injured from syncope, seek medical advice and be admitted [21,22]. They often have underlying cardiac causes and orthostatic hypotension so their risk of death increases precipitously. They often take many medications, some of which can cause syncope. They are especially vulnerable to hemodynamic effects of medications and often have less robust autonomic responses. Always consider, and rule out, medications as a primary cause of syncope in an elderly patient even when cardiovascular disease is present, before undertaking an aggressive, and perhaps risky, evaluation.

CLINICAL PEARLS

Causes of syncope in the young and the elderly Young patients generally have benign isolated situational causes for syncope and require no treatment but there is also a risk of a potentially life-threatening congenital arrythmia which must be ruled out. Syncope in the elderly can be a tremendous diagnostic challenge. Fifty percent are amnestic of the episodes and half of the episodes are unwitnessed. Bradycardia is often a cause for syncope in elderly patients in whom the cause is not otherwise undiagnosed. Often, the cause for syncope in the elderly is multifactorial and related to medications. Elderly patients are at greater risk of trauma when experiencing syncope.

Other Information

In all patients with syncope it is important to assess the coexisting medical conditions, concomitant symptoms, the circumstances in which syncope occurred (including prodromal and post-syncopal symptoms), whether, and in what circumstances, the patient has experienced similar episodes and witness reports of the episode of syncope. Family members may give clues to the patient's behavior that provide further insight.

CLINICAL PEARLS

Caveats on the evaluation process The key to proper evaluation and ultimate management of the patient with syncope is a complete and carefully obtained history. It is not only getting the history but listening to the patient and linking events to the syncopal episode. It is uncommon to arrive at a definitive diagnosis in a patient with syncope. The diagnosis is usually inferred from assessment of the available data and the diagnosis is generally presumptive. A trigger for syncope may be transient, obscure and not reproducible. Spontaneous remission of syncope is common. For those presenting with a single episode, 90% have no recurrence at 2 years. For those with longstanding recurrent syncope, the likelihood of syncope due to a benign cause for syncope is high.

Even a single episode of syncope in a patient with a malignant arrhythmia as cause for syncope may be associated with high risk of mortality. If a patient *were* to have a blood pressure (BP) cuff in place, an electrocardiographic (ECG) and electroencephalographic (EEG) monitor during an episode, doubts might still linger about the potential cause of the syncope. Assumptions are often made about the mechanism of syncope. A great challenge in the assessment of syncope is to avoid over-testing those at low risk of death and syncope recurrence, but avoid under-diagnosing those at high risk of sudden death.

Physical Examination

The physical examination is less likely to provide guidance in the evaluation but it can contain important diagnostic information. The following information should be collected.

Vital Signs
A resting bradycardia or an irregular pulse can indicate sick sinus syndrome, various arrhythmias, ectopy, atrio-ventricular (AV) block, premature ventricular contractions (PVC).

Orthostatic Hypotension
When orthostatic hypotension is abrupt and associated with reflex tachycardia, volume depletion should be suspected; when it is gradual and unaccompanied by increasing heart rate, autonomic dysfunction is the likely diagnosis.

Skin Turgor and Complexion
Pallor can indicate anemia, when it is associated with decreased skin elasticity, it may indicate hypovolemia due to blood loss.

The Cardiovascular Exam
This will rule in or out most "obstructive" lesions associated with syncope. It may also indicate the presence of LV dysfunction. In a patient with known hypertension, a funduscopic examination should be performed to detect

papilledema and/or retinal hemorrhages. These may be tell-tale signs of a transient hypertensive crisis causing syncope.

Carotid Sinus Massage

In elderly patients with a history suspicious for carotid hypersensitivity, carotid sinus massage should be performed as an integral part of the examination. This is an easy and cost-effective way to assess indirectly autonomic function and, specifically, carotid hypersensitivity. The results, however, should be interpreted with caution, as many older, asymptomatic patients may display long, technically abnormal, pauses (>3 seconds). A long pause is helpful only if associated with a highly suggestive history of syncope related to maneuvers that exert spontaneous pressure on the carotid sinuses (tight collars, shaving, etc.). It should be avoided if there is evidence of carotid disease (a bruit).

Diagnostic Testing

A proper diagnostic approach requires careful analysis of syncope in light of all other available clinical findings. Diagnostic tests need to be used sparingly. When used properly, they will increase the diagnostic yield compared to the history and physical exam alone. All testing must be tailored to the patient based on the findings of the history and physical examinations and with knowledge of the sensitivity and specificity of each test to identify the cause for syncope. An abnormal test result does not necessarily indicate the cause for syncope and does not necessarily sanction a "wild goose chase". The proper evaluation requires a balance of the judicious use of inpatient and outpatient diagnostic modalities. The expense and risk of the procedures and hospitalization are intensified by the possibility of causing iatrogenic harm from a diagnostic or therapeutic misadventure. A new test, the brain natriuretic peptide (BNP), was measured and showed it could differentiate between cardiac and non-cardiac syncope [23].

Observational Tests

Electrocardiogram

Every patient with syncope should receive an ECG. Although this may reveal diagnostic abnormalities in only 5–10% (such as complete heart block) and abnormalities may be non-specific, it can also provide helpful clues in another 20–30% of cases (old Q waves, various degrees and combinations of AV block and bundle branch block, pre-excitation syndrome, LV hypertrophy, non-sustained VT, etc.). The presence of left bundle branch block (LBBB) in a patient with syncope and organic heart disease is of special significance in that these patients carry a 30% rate of VT induction in the electrophysiology laboratory.

Echocardiogram

An echocardiogram alone is almost never diagnostic. It is of little help when there is no cardiac history and the physical examination and ECG are normal.

Its chief usefulness is in providing an evaluation of ventricular function in patients with suspected heart disease and assessing valvular disease. It should be performed if there are justified clinical suspicions of structural heart disease.

Signal Averaged ECG

The signal-averaged ECG (SAECG) is useful in one particular situation: in a patient with syncope, known coronary artery disease (CAD) and normal (or only mildly abnormal) LV function. An abnormal SAECG would mandate electrophysiologic testing to assess the induction of VT in this small subgroup [24].

Holter Monitoring

This is rarely diagnostic and therefore minimally helpful, as the incidence of recurrent syncope while being monitored is rare (1–5%) [25]. Further, many asymptomatic and non-specific abnormalities (such as PVCs, non-sustained VT, sinus bradycardia, sleep-related heart block and/or sinus pauses, etc.) noted may confuse the issue and lead to further unnecessary testing and therapy.

Trans-telephonic Monitoring

Trans-telephonic monitoring is becoming more advanced – a crucial aspect [26]. It enables the recording of an episode when the patient passes out. The patient must wear the monitor continuously (one such device is the size of a beeper. If the patient passes out, a button is pushed on awakening. It will store 2–3 minutes before the event. This "endless-loop recorder" is useful, but up to 35% of people use the device improperly, making it non-diagnostic.

CLINICAL PEARLS

Wise and rational testing A goal in syncope evaluation is to move from a presumptive to a definitive diagnosis. Proper assessment requires a careful assessment of the patient, an assessment based on information obtained from the history and physical examination. Some tests may provide clues to the diagnosis. These include carotid massage, ECG, tilt table test, echocardiogram, electrophysiology test, treadmill test, monitor (Holter, trans-telephonic, implantable loop recorder) but these, and all tests, must be used selectively. The more tests, the more abnormalities will be found, but these abnormalities (may be just incidental findings) may not apply to the cause for syncope. A CT scan, carotid Doppler, an EEG, cardiac enzymes and neurology consult rarely have a role in the evaluation of syncope.

Implantable Loop Recorder

An implantable monitor is inserted surgically into a subcutaneous prepectoral pocket. It is capable of recording the heart rhythm for over one year in patients with intermittent or rare episodes. The device is potentially highly cost effective as it can eliminate the need for frequent and potentially unnecessary hospitalization. The main shortcomings of this device are obviously the relative invasiveness of its implantation, and its cost. Other potentially serious drawbacks of all long-term monitoring include the fact that in order to reach a diagnosis, the patient has to be exposed to the risks of at least one more syncopal event. A more surreptitious pitfall is that monitor-obtained bradycardic manifestations of vasovagal syncope cannot be analyzed in the context of antecedent BP changes, and may therefore lead to unnecessary pacemaker implants [27].

CRITICAL THINKING

The COLAPS trial. The Comparison Of Loop Recorders Against Holter in Patients with Syncope trial is a prospective study designed to compare diagnostic utility of endless-loop recorders (ELR) and Holter monitors in the diagnosis of syncope. The results showed that among 78 patients who received ELRs, 21% of diagnoses were made within 48 hours, 50% at 15 days, and 90% at 33 days. Patients performing a successful test transmission were more familiar with technology, with ability to use a bank automatic teller machine being a significant independent predictor. Patients with a successful test transmission were, in turn, significantly more likely to record and transmit data from symptomatic episodes [28].

In general, if the symptom happens once a day, then 24–48 hour Holter is best. If the problem happens once a month, then the event monitor would be helpful. If the symptoms are very rare and erratic, then an implantable loop monitor would help to reveal the problem.

Provocative Testing

Exercise Stress Test
If the syncopal episode happens during or after exercise, then a stress test should be done to rule out ischemia as cause of arrhythmia, angina or exercise-induced syncope. Exercise stress testing is also useful for screening of catecholaminergic polymorphic VT.

Tilt Table Testing
It is useful when neurocardiogenic syncope is suspected but the diagnosis is uncertain. It should be one of the first tests considered when there is undiagnosed syncope and no structural heart disease present [29,30].

Head up tilt table (HUTT) testing can be highly effective in uncovering and/or confirming neurocardiogenic syncope. Day-to-day variability in response and induction of neurocardiogenic syncope is common, unavoidable, and simply reflects expected variability of autonomic nervous system physiology. The sensitivity of the HUTT is always in question but the sensitivity can be increased with isoproterenol or nitroglycerine, possibly by different mechanisms [31–34]. These interventions, however, will decrease the specificity, always a problem with the tilt table test. Is the arrhythmia caused during HUTT the same arrhythmia which causes syncope?

CRITICAL THINKING

Arrhythmia during syncope and HUTT test. Heart rhythm obtained during provocative condition is often used to guide therapy in vasovagal syncope. To date there was no conclusive evidence that the heart rhythm observed during a positive HUTT can predict the heart rhythm during spontaneous neurocardiogenic syncope, or that the heart rhythm observed during a spontaneous syncope will be identical to the recurrent syncope. 25 consecutive neurocardiogenic syncope patients, presenting with frequent syncope (6.9 ± 4.6 episodes/year) and a positive HUTT (cardioinhibitory in 8 patients), had an implantable loop recorder (ILR) placed. 7 also had a positive adenosine triphosphate (ATP) test. After 17.0 ± 3.6 months of follow-up, 30 neurocardiogenic episodes were observed in 12 patients. Nine episodes showed bradycardia of <40 beats/min or asystole. Progressive sinus bradycardia preceding sinus arrest was the most frequent ECG finding. Twenty-one episodes of syncope occurred without severe bradycardia. The heart rhythm observed during the first syncope was identical to the recurrence. No correlation was found between slow heart rate on the ILR interrogation and a cardioinhibitory HUTT response ($P = 1.0$) or a positive ATP test ($P = 1.0$). Therefore, in highly symptomatic patients with neurocardiogenic syncope, the heart rhythm observed during spontaneous syncope does not correlate with the HUTT. The heart rhythm during the first spontaneous syncope is identical to the recurrent syncope [35]. These results were similar to those found at the ISSUE II trial [36]. Unfortunately, asystole may occur late into the syncopal spell and thus pacing will not necessarily eliminate syncope.

Patients with fixed, true autonomic dysfunction, often have a predictable and reproducible response to HUTT. The mode of induction and the sequence of BP and heart rate changes preceding the syncopal spell can be extremely helpful when outlining specific preventive therapy. A test can be abnormal and "diagnostic" even if syncope is not induced. All HUTT results should be interpreted in light of the clinical events surrounding the syncopal spell. Although tilt testing is most helpful and yielding in young healthy adults, one has to keep in mind that the stakes are high if a malignant arrhythmia is missed. Once the electrophysiology test (EPS) is negative, HUTT does not help much [37].

Guidelines From The AHA/ACCF: Statement On Tilt Table Testing

In patients with a negative evaluation, i.e., no evidence of ischemia and a structurally normal heart, the pretest probability of the diagnosis of neurocardiogenic syncope is high, so HUTT contributes little to establishing the diagnosis. In a patient with a malignant cause of syncope, it is more important to rule out other cause of syncope such as bradyarrhythmias, supraventricular tachycardia (SVT), and VT than it is to perform a HUTT [18].

CRITICAL THINKING

A dissenting view. These authors have concerns regarding the AHA/ACCF guidelines and their recommendation concerning evaluation and treatment of patients with neurocardiogenic syncope. These authors think that the recommendation that HUTT contributes little to establishing the diagnosis is rather short-sighted and does not necessarily pertain in practical terms to patients who need to be evaluated for syncope. Moreover, other guidelines such as the European Society of Cardiology have clearly delineated a role for HUTT (Figure 13.2) [38].

Based on the complexity of the nature of syncope, the care that is required in the evaluation, the multiplicity of potential causes, and the lack of ease of performing controlled clinical trials, we do not ascribe to the ACCF/AHA guidelines as a best methodology to evaluate and treat the patient with syncope.

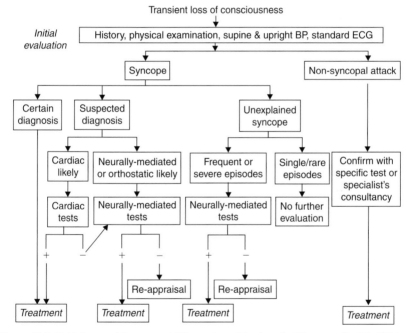

Figure 13.2 Guidelines on Management (Diagnosis and Treatment) of Syncope. Update 2004 Executive Summary: The Task force on Syncope, European Society of Cardiology. Adapted from [38].

CLINICAL PEARLS

When to do a tilt table test? Consider a tilt table test in the following situations.

1. When episodes suggest, but do not indicate, a neurocardiogenic cause.
2. If there is recurrent syncope with no apparent cause at any age.

3. When other evaluations are not revealing.
4. When therapies directed at other potential causes are ineffective.

There is no reason to perform a tilt table test when the etiology is clear from the history.

Electrophysiology Testing

The EPS is a method that uses pacing techniques to try to initiate arrhythmias by atrial and/or ventricular stimulation and to test for conduction system abnormalities. Although somewhat invasive, it is an extremely safe tool that carries a mortality and morbidity potential roughly 1/10 of that of diagnostic coronary angiography.

EPS can be useful to assess arrhythmic causes for syncope and risk for arrhythmic death. Abnormal test results are seen in 7–50% of patients with otherwise undiagnosed syncope [39]. The main use for EPS in syncope patients is to evaluate the inducibility and hemodynamic effects of monomorphic VT. If the ejection fraction (EF) < 0.40, VT can be induced in about 35% of SUO patients, whereas for those with an EF > 0.40, only 3% will have VT induced, even if structural heart disease is present [40].

EPS it most useful in: patients with CAD (and no acute ischemia); patients with a left ventricular ejection fraction (LVEF) less than 0.40; patients with LBBB; patients with an abnormal signal averaged ECG; patients with ventricular ectopy of right ventricular outflow tract origin (LBBB morphology with inferior axis).

Induction of a previously undiagnosed syncopal SVT is relatively rare (about 10%), but if induced, it can be treated by radiofrequency ablation during the same session. The induction of poorly tolerated atrial flutter of fibrillation is a much more difficult finding to interpret.

EPS are fair, at best, in evaluating bradycardias [41]. Although an abnormal sinus node recovery time can indicate sinus node disease, its presence does not necessarily mean that the syncope is caused by sinus pauses. Furthermore, sinus node recovery time is an insensitive measure of sinus node dysfunction. No test provides a direct causal link to the clinical syncopal event: the link is only a putative one. Intra- or infra-Hisian block indicates a more likely causal link to syncope. Unfortunately, the sensitivity of EPS to diagnose serious infranodal disease is only fair. Finally, EPS are also not very well suited to evaluate abnormalities in AV nodal conduction.

A negative EPS does not rule out VT as a cause of syncope especially in patients with idiopathic dilated or non-ischemic cardiomyopathies [42,43]. Further, EPS are not well suited for the evaluation of polymorphic VT.

A thorough but negative EPS, although not completely diagnostic, nevertheless indicates a generally good prognosis predicting a relatively low 2-year incidence of SCD.

If an EPS is positive for VT (the usual reason for testing in syncope), a patient will require definitive therapy for the VT. This often means insertion of an ICD if there is structural heart disease. In some instances, catheter ablation is appropriate or anti-arrhythmic drug therapy. An ICD may prevent sudden death in a patient who has syncope and inducible VT. In fact, the risk of death in patients with syncope and inducible VT at EPS is as high as the death rates in patient populations with history of aborted cardiac arrest [44]. While an ICD may prevent sudden death, it may not prevent recurrent syncope so some patients may require combination therapy including ICD with drug therapy.

The EPS lacks sensitivity in patients without CAD [45]. As such the evaluation in a patient with a dilated cardiomyopathy becomes much more complex [46–48]. A patient with dilated cardiomyopathy and syncope is at high risk for sudden death and while that risk may be due to ventricular arrhythmias alone, this is not clear and there are several other proposed mechanisms of syncope and death in this population.

CLINICAL PEARLS

Present indications of electrophysiologic studies The necessity for performing EPS has changed over the past several years and now takes a smaller role. Based on new data from multiple randomized controlled clinical trials, the risk for SCD and total mortality in patients with underlying structural heart disease, particularly when HF is present, will indicate the need for an ICD in a large number of patients who have structural heart disease and are at risk for sudden death. Thus, a patient who has syncope, has an impaired LVEF, and has congestive heart failure (CHF) may benefit from an ICD or even a cardiac resynchronization device irrespective of the results of the EPS. The reason for implanting an ICD is to reduce the risk of SCD. These patients may be at a particularly high risk of SCD if they have syncope and CHF, but it is not clear that implanting an ICD will alter the risk of syncope or improve the quality of life in these patients. However, EPS will likely not provide benefit. Further, EPS is a poor predictor of outcomes in patients who have underlying "channelopathies" such as in the long QT interval syndrome, in idiopathic polymorphic VT, in hypertrophic cardiomyopathy, in valvular heart disease or in Brugada syndrome. On the other hand, EPS may be useful to allay an arrhythmia that may be the cause for syncope. This may occur in the Wolff–Parkinson–White syndrome or even in idiopathic VT due to right ventricular outflow tract tachycardia, or left ventricular (Bellhassen's) tachycardia. In arrhythmogenic right ventricular cardiomyopathy, an EPS may not predict long-term prognosis but it may indicate the arrhythmias that are present and may have some utility in ablating some of the more recurrent episodes of VT in these patients. Nevertheless, in patients with arrhythmogenic right ventricular dysplasia, Brugada syndrome, polymorphic VT and the long QT interval syndrome, an ICD may need to be seriously considered to prevent the risk of sudden cardiac death.

Management

In general, the treatment depends on the causes of the syncope revealed in the evaluation process. If there is structural heart disease, such as aortic stenosis or hypertrophic cardiomyopathy, then the treatment is to address these obstructive lesions and assess the long-term risk for arrhythmic death. If it is due to ischemia (a highly uncommon cause for syncope), then coronary revascularization is needed but even then long-term risk assessment for SCD needs to be considered. If there is inducible monomorphic VT, in a patient with structural heart disease (*not* in a patient with idiopathic VT and normal ventricular function) then an ICD should be implanted. ICD therapy may need to be considered in patients at high risk for SCD and total mortality if there is HF present or impaired ventricular function regardless of the electrophysiology study results.

In the case of patients with CAD, syncope, and mild-to-moderate LV dysfunction (a LVEF >35%), the yield of induced VT by EPS is low. However, EPS may still be appropriate in select patients with relatively preserved ventricular function but who have structural heart disease. If there is VT induced, then an ICD is needed [18]. In the case of patients with CAD, syncope and low LVEF, and in the interest of finding a diagnosis, EPS may be helpful but it is likely not necessary. Even in the absence of syncope, in patients with CAD and an LVEF <35%, these patients have a substantial survival benefit when treated with an ICD. The rationale for the implantation of ICD is from the MADIT II, SCD-HeFT, DEFINITE and other trials [49–51].

In general, successful management of syncope depends on the proper diagnosis and on effective therapy. Every episode, and every patient with syncope, does not necessarily require therapy. Spontaneous remission is common; up to 90% with syncope pass out only once. Recurrence rates are similar whether the cause is cardiac, non-cardiac or unknown. There is a high placebo treatment response, especially if the cause for syncope is due to a neurocardiogenic mechanism.

Even if the mechanism and the diagnosis are clear, the therapy administered may be ineffective. A pacemaker, for example, will prevent syncope recurrence in a patient with acquired complete heart block but it may not in a patient with bradycardia due to neurocardiogenic syncope.

Even if a therapy is effective to prevent syncope, it may not prevent death. β-blockers may prevent recurrent syncope in patients with long QT interval syndrome, but a β-blocker may not prevent death. Alternatively, a patient with syncope due to VT could benefit from an ICD as it may prevent death but it likely will not prevent recurrent syncope. A patient could nevertheless collapse from VT before an administered shock.

Therapies for a condition such as neurocardiogenic syncope can be even more confusing. There are little controlled data available regarding treatments. A potentially effective therapy, such as a β-blockers, can actually make the problem worse ("prosyncope").

In the US two major problems in syncope are of concern: neurocardiogenic syncope and ventricular arrhythmias. Management of neurocardiogenic syncope and syncope in the athlete will be discussed below, while management of ventricular arrhythmias is discussed in the Chapter 9.

Neurocardiogenic Syncope

Neurocardiogenic syncope is used to describe the autonomic responses that may ultimately lead to inappropriate vasodilatation, relative bradycardia, hypotension, and collapse. This reflex is a final common pathway of many potential autonomic inputs [52,53]. It may present as bradycardia and hypotension (classic vasovagal), hypotension alone, postural orthostatic tachycardia syndrome (POTS) [54,55], a psychogenic or a "central" response (cerebral vasoconstriction) [56,57]. It may be an isolated, explainable event, a recurrent, poorly understood, reflex ("malignant neurocardiogenic syndrome") or present in storms that ultimately abate. The neurocardiogenic reflex can be triggered by a severe, viral syndrome or it may be due to an inherited "dysautonomic" problem. There can be a genetic predisposition and some patients are subject to multiple triggers.

The reflex involves cardiac and great vessel mechanoreceptors and the nodose ganglion. These receptors, now beginning to be understood, modulated in part by prostaglandin, endothelin, EDRF (endothelial derived growth factor [nitric oxide]), adenosine, free radicals, and paracrine cell secretions can excite vagal afferents. The vagal afferents provide input to the medulla, the nucleus tractus solitarii, the cingulate gyrus, and the hypothalamus.

Once stimulated by vagal afferents, the neurocardiogenic reflex can begin. Excessive sympathetic inhibition that follows causes inordinate and unneeded peripheral vasodilatation. An "inappropriate" bradycardia may also occur from vagal efferent stimulation and sympathetic inhibition. A negative inotropic effect may ensue with concomitant cerebral vasoconstriction. Central neurologic vasoconstriction may cause syncope without measurable bradycardia or hypotension [56,58].

Many clinical conditions may lead to this reflex. Triggers include emotion, pain, depression, fatigue, and sleep deprivation. Triggers that are more worrisome include myocardial ischemia or infarction (Bezold–Jarisch reflex), aortic stenosis and hypertrophic cardiomyopathy. Cortical centers; pain, visual, and emotional stimuli; vasopressin; the medullary cardiovascular cortical area; the adrenal glands; and cranial nerves IX, X, V, VII, VIII stimulation may trigger the response [59]. The spinal cord and unmyelinated and non-myelinated afferent fibers may become involved.

The reflex itself may have had an ontologically protective benefit. It is seen in nature frequently: the "diving reflex," the "hibernating reflex," or the "play-dead" reflex. This reflex can allow children who drown and have a cardiac arrest to unexpectedly survive. The reflex, on the other hand, can cause syncope.

CLINICAL PEARLS

Need for triggers on a susceptible terrain to ignite a neurocardiogenic syncopal episode In real world practice, the neurocardiogenic mechanism, generally benign, is the most common cause for syncope [60]. Neurocardiogenic etiologies likely explain the majority of syncopal episodes, but many neurocardiogenic mechanisms for syncope exist [61]. The neurocardiogenic reflex may be transient, self-limited, persistent or recurrent. It is there, hidden, ready to be used if there is a chance. The susceptible terrain can be related to a chronic condition (e.g. aortic stenosis) or a new acute illness (e.g. gastrointestinal bleed, dehydration from diarrhea, vasodilation from alcohol intake, etc.). Then a trigger arrives by chance, causing acute change in vascular volume due to loss of vascular volume or inappropriate vasodilation such as: new gastrointestinal bleeding, intense emotional stimuli [62], physical activity, pain or the effects of alcohol or an inotropic stimulant. A sudden trigger ignites the inappropriate bradycardia and vasodilation cascade culminating into sudden loss of BP and presented as a syncopal episode. The reflex is there from birth. The susceptible terrain is there or not. Without the susceptible terrain, even with the arrival of a trigger, there is no syncope. Neurocardiogenic syncope has to happen at the wrong time in the wrong place.

Medical Treatment

For those who have the neurocardiogenic reflex and have frequent, recurrent syncope, medical therapy may be necessary. Therapies may appear paradoxical: β-blockers to prevent bradycardia and hypotension [63,64], for example. Other potential interventions modulate the reflex, selective serotonin reuptake inhibitors (SSRIs) [65], anticholinergics (disopyramide) [66], salt loading, theophylline [67], α-stimulants (midodrine [Proamitine]) [68,69], cardiac pacing, fludrocortisone acetate (Florinef Acetate) [70], clonidine (HCl Catapres), exercise, support hose, desmopressin (DDAVP, Stimnate) and erythropoietin (Epogen Procrit), angiotensin converting enzyme (ACE) inhibitors, among others. With a better understanding of the mechanisms responsible for the neurocardiogenic response(s), better approaches to medical therapies may be achieved [70]. Many small, poorly controlled, clinical trials have shown benefits of all of the above, and other, therapies. Unfortunately, the populations tested are often highly select groups that do not necessarily represent the overall population with neurocardiogenic syncope. Many patients with neurocardiogenic syncope pass out only a few times. In this case, no therapy may be needed. For those patients who have frequent recurrent episodes of neurocardiogenic syncope, and are documented not to have psychogenic causes, long-term therapy may be needed. The autonomic nervous system, however, is relatively "plastic" and therefore any therapy given may only work temporarily. Often, therapies need to be given on a case-by-case basis and will not work for all situations or all patients. Furthermore, many of these patients respond well to the "placebo" effect of the therapy itself, confounding proper assessment of the efficacy of the therapy.

CRITICAL THINKING

The POST trial. The Prevention of Syncope Trial was a double-blind, randomized, placebo-controlled trial, for patients ≥18 years of age with a history of at least three episodes of vasovagal syncope and positive tilt test. 208 patients were randomized to either metoprolol ($n = 108$) or placebo ($n = 100$). Of the 208 patients initially entered into the study, 38% ($n = 79$) finished the 1-year study without fainting and without discontinuation of the study drug, and 35% ($n = 74$) experienced a syncopal episode while on the study drug; 26% ($n = 55$) of patients did not complete the study. At 1 year, the results showed that metoprolol was not associated with any benefit over placebo for the prevention of syncopal recurrence (efficacy analysis) [71].

Similarly, there was only an insignificant benefit associated with metoprolol over placebo with respect to syncopal recurrence or discontinuation of drug therapy (effectiveness analysis). In the prespecified analysis of age, investigators found that patients <42 years of age treated with metoprolol did significantly worse than a similar-aged cohort of patients treated with placebo. In patients 42 years of age or older, however, the difference between the metoprolol and placebo groups was not significant. With respect to the primary outcome of the effectiveness analysis (syncopal recurrence or discontinuation of drug therapy), metoprolol was associated with insignificant worsening in young patients and a nearly significant benefit in older patients compared with placebo [71].

CRITICAL THINKING

Treatment with midodrine. A double-blind, randomized, crossover trial to investigate the efficacy of midodrine, a selective α-1 adrenergic agonist that decreases venous capacitance, in preventing neurally mediated syncope triggered by passive HUTT. 12 patients with history of recurrent neurally mediated syncope, which was reproduced during head-up tilt, were randomized to receive a nonpressor dose of midodrine (5 mg) or placebo on day 1 and the opposite on day 3. One hour after drug or placebo administration, patients underwent 60-degree HUTT lasting 40 minutes (unless hypotension or bradycardia developed first). In the supine position, midodrine produced no significant change in BP or heart rate. The responses to head-up tilt were significantly different on the midodrine and the placebo day: on the placebo day, 67% (8/12) of the subjects suffered neurally mediated syncope, whereas only 17% (2/12) of the subjects developed neurally mediated syncope on the midodrine day ($P < 0.02$). These results indicate that midodrine significantly improves orthostatic tolerance during HUTT in patients with recurrent neurally mediated syncope [72].

CRITICAL THINKING

Myths and realities of β-blockade. The assessment of any medical therapy for neurocardiogenic syncope has been performed in relatively select populations. The POST trial, for example, was a group of patients having very frequent recurrent episodes of neurocardiogenic syncope [71]. This study did not demonstrate a substantial benefit of a β-blocker therapy for patients with neuro-cardiogenic syncope, and yet some patients seemed to respond to the treatment. In a patient with frequent recurrent neurocardiogenic syncope who does not respond to other therapies, a β-blocker may be considered an option but a β-blocker may also make the problem worse. A first-line therapy for neurocardiogenic syncope, after adequate hydration and avoidance approaches, is fludrocortisone. Midodrine is an option but is a complex medication to take and does not necessarily benefit all patients. While an SSRI may be beneficial, SSRIs do not universally work and are wrought with adverse effects. There are some recent data on the use of pyridostigmine for neurocardiogenic syncope and orthostatic hypotension. Midodrine and and fludrocortisone may be very useful for patients with POTS.

Training Exercises

These exercises are actually "mini-tilt table tests" which encourage the reflex and perhaps, by so doing, strengthen the individual's tolerance to it [73]. The use of tilt training is over 90% effective and while much of this response may be placebo, the safety of this approach is such that it really does not matter what the beneficial mechanism might be. The patients are instructed to tilt against a wall for 15–30 minutes a day as tolerated. This exercise may be primary therapy for some forms of neurocardiogenic syncope and it appears highly effective in preliminary studies.

CRITICAL THINKING
Intelligent and critical interpretation of clinical trials. In tilt training, there is a discrepancy between clinical results and "scientific" results. There may be a substantial benefit from tilt training but this is not clearly evident in clinical practice. Furthermore, much of the benefit may be due to a "placebo" effect. One promising approach for the patient with neurocardiogenic syncope who has a warning episode that occurs while standing, is the use of leg crossing to prevent passing out by increasing venous return and increasing afterload, forcing blood to the brain [74].

Pacing

Other data indicate that dual chamber (dual chamber pacing mode and rate adaptation (DDDR) with rate drop response) pacing may be of benefit, but the issue of "placebo" response to pacemaker implants remains debatable [75]. Many studies, including the VPS I, have shown that patients with vasovagal syncope might benefit from pacing: SAFE-PACE [76], VASIS [77], SYDIT [78], and SYNPACE [79] to name only a few). However, these were unblinded studies, and are thus subject to bias and a potential placebo effect. There are two studies which showed the contradictory results of pacing on cardioneurogenic syncope.

CRITICAL THINKING
The ISSUE II trial. The Second International Study of Syncope of Uncertain Etiology 2 trial enrolled 442 patients suspected of neurally-mediated syncope. In phase I, the patients were followed for a maximum of 24 months or until their first documented syncopal episode. Over the course of follow-up, a total of 143 patients had = 1 syncopal episode, of whom 106 had the syncopal cause documented by

ILR (57 patients had asystole (median: 11.5 seconds), four patients had bradycardia). Then 103 patients entered phase II of the study; 53 of these had pacemaker as ILR-based specific therapy due to asystole or antitachycardia therapy, based on phase I findings, and 50 patients were in sinus rhythm and received non-specific therapy. After 1 year, syncope recurrence was reduced by 80% in the ILR-based specific therapy group (41% 1-year recurrence vs. 10% in the conservative group). The subgroup of patients who received a pacemaker had a significantly lower recurrence rate of syncope compared with the patients who did not have documented bradycardia (hazard ratio (HR) = 0.20, P = 0.0005) and compared with the subgroup of 30 patients who did not receive a pacemaker despite documentation of bradycardia (HR = 0.10, P = 0.002) [36].

CRITICAL THINKING

Benefit from pacing after ILR for neurocardiogenic syncope.
Neurocardiogenic syncope has many etiologies and is only beginning to be understood. There is no one specific therapeutic approach that will work for all patients with neurocardiogenic syncope and patients with this syndrome have a diversity of causes and triggers. The tilt table test may or may not be positive in patients with presumed neurocardiogenic syncope. As shown in the ISSUE II trial [36], patients clinically may have long asystolic episodes as demonstrated by ILR even though on the tilt table test they do not have these. The actual process of neurocardiogenic syncope may differ in real life from that which occurs on a tilt table test. It is therefore uncertain which patient with neurocardiogenic syncope will benefit from a pacemaker and which will not. Further, syncope can occur before the asystolic episode. Unless the patient has evidence for long asystolic pauses that are causing syncope and the problem is not otherwise treatable but is recurrent and refractory to medical management, a pacemaker may need to be considered [36].

CRITICAL THINKING

The VPS II trial. The Second Vasovagal Pacemaker Study II is the first double-blind, randomized trial undertaken to determine whether pacing therapy reduces the risk of syncope in patients with vasovagal syncope, and is also the largest of the randomized pacemaker trials in this patient population. It enrolled 100 patients with a history of recurrent vasovagal syncope and a positive HUTT. All patients underwent implantation of a dual-chamber pacemaker and were then randomized to receive either dual-chamber pacing (DDD) with rate drop response (n = 48) or only sensing without pacing (ODO) (n = 52) as the control. The results showed that 38 patients (42% in the ODO group) and 16 patients (33% in the DDD group) experienced syncope during the follow-up period. Median duration of syncope in these patients was 2 minutes in the control group and 1 minute in the treatment group. Based on intention-to-treat analysis, the cumulative risk of syncope at 6 months was 40% in the ODO group and 31% in the DDD group (P = 0.14) [80].

CRITICAL THINKING

No benefit to pacing after positive head-up tilt table test. Unfortunately there is no clear way to judge which patient with neurocardiogenic syncope and asystolic episodes will benefit from a pacemaker. Pacemaker therapy is clearly not first-line therapy for the average patient with neurocardiogenic syncope (especially just after a positive HUTT). Pacemaker therapy may be advantageous for those patients who have long asystolic causes that appear to be the direct cause for the syncope (as proved by ILR). This could be at any age but it would mean that the episodes are recurrent, frequent, refractory to all other medical therapy and are demonstrated to be due to a systolic episodes. In this case, despite the negative results of the VPS II trial [80], a pacemaker is clearly indicated. Further, the placebo benefit of a pacemaker is hard to quantify for all patients who get pacemaker implantation for any cause, as so few placebo-controlled pacemaker trials have been performed. If the patient has clear-cut benefit from a pacemaker, as long as there is no harm, a pacemaker maybe beneficial.

When an episode of apparent neurocardiogenic syncope has no obvious cause and the patient does not have heart disease, you cannot predict whether the patient will ever experience a recurrence. Although treatment is not warranted initially in such cases, careful follow-up is needed. If another episode occurs, and evidence again suggests a neurocardiogenic mechanism, a tilt-table test may help to confirm the diagnosis and determine treatment.

CLINICAL PEARLS

Treatment of neurogenic syncope Regarding neurocardiogenic syncope, no medical therapy has proven benefit for the average patient. Treatments include lifestyle changes, avoiding things that cause syncope, adequate hydration, salt load and support hose. There can be a lack of response to hydration and salt loading, however, but prior to an event that may cause neurocardiogenic syncope, hydration, especially with ice cold water and salt loading, may be helpful. There are few controlled data for medications. Tilt training may be effective. Dual chamber (DDDR-rate drop response) pacing has little role in the average patient with neurocardiogenic syncope.

Athlete: Exercise-induced Syncope

Syncope, dizziness, collapse and loss of consciousness are among the most worrisome symptoms that occur in relation to exercise [81,82]. These dramatic symptoms can portend sudden and "unexpected" death. The cause is often uncertain and difficult to diagnose but is often related to an arrhythmia. Extensive diagnostic testing can lead to immense cost but the accuracy of such testing is subject to deserved scrutiny. Reggie Lewis, an apparently healthy, young, well-known, basketball star with syncope died of ventricular fibrillation due to a focal cardiomyopathy that some physicians felt was difficult to diagnose in life despite extensive testing. In fact, one of his physicians felt he had neurocardiogenic syncope due to the fact that he had a positive tilt table test.

The trained athlete is unique. Exercise training increases vagal tone chronically but baroreceptor adjustments reduce the possibility of a neurocardiogenic reflex. Exercise-induced enhancement of sympathetic activity is blunted. Bikers or runners (dynamic activity) rarely pass out due to hemodynamic or autonomic effects. The muscle pump increases venous return and prevents this. Marathon runners can collapse from dehydration or hypotension during prolonged exertion or at the end of exercise. Such an event is not unusual or necessarily worrisome and may not require further evaluation. When an athlete stops exercising and there is maximal peripheral vasodilatation, the muscle pump may fail, and the BP may drop to causing syncope.

It is highly unusual for an athlete to collapse from a benign cause at the onset of intense physical stress or even with prolonged, continued, activity. Syncope, during exercise, tends to be worrisome and possibly related due to a malignant, arrhythmic, cause. Reggie Lewis, for example, collapsed while dribbling down the court with uncontrollable loss of postural tone, crumpling to the floor. When something like this occurs, it is usually due to a serious arrhythmia. His death strongly emphasizes the fact that athletes who passed out in the throes of exercise have a potentially life-threatening cause for their episode, and neurocardiogenic syncope is clearly the diagnosis of exclusion.

Non-cardiac causes for syncope include neurocardiogenic responses to exercise, dehydration (sometimes intentional, e.g., wrestlers), hyperventilation, valsalva (e.g. weight lifters), and circulating mediators, (e.g., histamine, serotonin). A variant of neurocardiogenic syncope is exercise-induced neurally mediated hypotension and bradycardia. Autonomic failure and loss of peripheral muscle pump function may participate in abrupt cardiovascular collapse with syncope.

Supplements, and drugs, athletes take may cause tachy- and/or brady-arrhythmias or hemodynamic collapse. Ma Huang (from the Chinese ephedra plant), androgens and creatine, easy to obtain over-the-counter, are potentially dangerous. Illicit drugs, such as cocaine taken to enhance performance, can have serious consequences causing syncope. It is important to rule out a possibility of seizure disorder.

The cardiac causes for syncope are listed in Table 13.2. A young athlete with syncope who has significant coronary artery abnormalities will likely have other concomitant symptoms, including chest discomfort, and often has ECG myocardial abnormalities present. Ischemia should always be considered a likely trigger in those over 35 years old. Polymorphic and monomorphic VTs associated with structural heart disease can cause syncope and carry a poor prognosis in athletes. Exercise-induced "idiopathic" (no known structural heart disease) right and left VTs can cause syncope and can be ablated with a good long-term results and a good prognosis. High grade or complete AV

Table 13.6 Details of history in syncope of athlete.

1. The circumstances and timing of the episode related to exercise
2. The exercise type, sport, length and intensity of exercise
3. Hydration status
4. Medication, illicit drug and supplement use
5. Age
6. Degree of conditioning and exercise frequency
7. Presence of heart disease
8. Severity and length of episode
9. Genetic screening and family history
10. Previous surgery and implanted devices
11. The temporal relationship to exercise
12. The type of athlete ("weekend-warrior" or full-time athlete)

block or chronotropic incompetence causing syncope, during exercise, is rare in young athletes but may occur in the elderly patients treated for heart disease.

Evaluation of Syncope in the Athlete

The evaluation of syncope in the athlete is more complicated than for the non-athlete. Before allowing return to exercise, the cause of syncope should be determined and treated properly. Any syncopal episode should be considered seriously and should be carefully evaluated ruling out as needed hypertrophic cardiomyopathy, arrhythmogenic right ventricular dysplasia, coronary anomalies, and congenital long QT interval syndrome. Specific historical features to be collected are included in Table 13.6.

An adequate history can require information available from team members, the family, friends and witnesses. Symptoms must be scrutinized: Is the syncope a single or a recurrent episode? Did exercise initiate the episode? Was exercise isometric (static) or isotonic (dynamic)? In what position did syncope occur? Did syncope occur with the start of exercise, with prolonged exercise, or at the end of exercise? Were there premonitory symptoms (e.g. palpitations, impending doom, diaphoresis, or chest pain), concomitant acute illnesses, "triggers", changes in dietary habits and/or medications, or the presence of emotional stress? Was there pallor, absence of a pulse, or concomitant acute illness? Was recovery immediate or prolonged? If syncope is prolonged, consider a hemodynamic-obstructive cause, such as aortic stenosis or hypertrophic cardiomyopathy. Syncope can be mimicked by seizures and hypoglycemia. To distinguish, and exclude, these potential causes, the episode and circumstances surrounding the episode must be scrutinized carefully. The quality, severity and length of the episode and the time required for recovery can help determine potential etiologies. The physical examination should concentrate on orthostatic vital signs (squatting and standing) and a complete cardiac and neurological examination.

Diagnostic Testing for the Athlete

Any evaluation should be comprehensive, yet practical. An ECG and echocardiogram are a good place to start, and are of low risk and expense. All syncopal athletes should have at least this evaluation.

Arrhythmias can be difficult to reproduce during exercise but the mechanisms for this are understood poorly. Arrhythmias and their hemodynamic influence can be difficult to induce. Exercise testing is a standard first-line approach and may yield a diagnosis. Even so, routine exercise testing may not be an adequate method to predict cause for syncope. Sometimes, it is necessary for the individual to perform the same exercise that caused the event. An exercise test may be diagnostic even if it may not be possible to mimic the exact exercise situation that triggered the syncope. This is a useful and controlled approach to arrive at a diagnosis.

An ECG monitor can provide crucial information and may be diagnostic; it is a first line approach. Holter monitors, external endless loop recorders and implanted monitors, can help secure the diagnosis. The use of different techniques depends on the clinical situation. An exercise test may be useful, however, the specific activity associated with syncope such as soccer, basketball, or sprinting may be the only trigger for the arrhythmia. It may be necessary to monitor a patient during exercise: there may be some danger in this approach.

The tilt table test, to be diagnostic, must reproduce the symptoms exactly [83]. A tilt table test may be useful to help diagnose a neurocardiogenic cause but the results of such testing should always be considered non-specific and be interpreted cautiously. Neurocardiogenic syncope is always the diagnosis of exclusion, especially if syncope occurs during intense exertion. Children have a different center of gravity and may need a more aggressive protocol. Likewise, an athlete may need a different protocol. Compensatory mechanisms such as the skeletal muscle pump can prevent neurocardiogenic syncope during exercise although syncope may occur at exercise termination when skeletal pump is less active. Dehydration and vasodilatation may also be contributing factors.

Electrophysiology testing, while a powerful tool, can mislead in the athlete. Unless the patient has underlying CAD and LV dysfunction, an electrophysiology test lacks sensitivity and is non-specific. The test has limited, if any, use for patients with hypertrophic cardiomyopathy and right ventricular dysplasia. Electrophysiology testing results may be useful to identify, and ablate, supraventricular, and idiopathic, ventricular, tachycardias (with subsequent return of the athlete to full activity).

If all else fails and there is a high suspicion of an ischemic etiology, a cardiac catheterization may be diagnostic. The decision to proceed with this or a myocardial biopsy requires a high degree of clinical suspicion and depends on concomitant symptoms. High-resolution echocardiography can image the proximal of the coronary arteries and rule out the anomalous origin of the coronary artery ostia.

CLINICAL PEARLS

Exercise for the athlete with history of syncope Syncope during exercise may indicate a life threatening or at least an arrhythmic cause. The diagnosis will vary with the age of the patient, whether the episode occurred during isometric, isotonic, or endurance activities, and the position of patient (supine, standing, running). Consider if syncope occurred during exercise, at its onset or offset. Consider what were the associated symptoms and other conditions and was there a significant family or other medical history. Neurocardiogenic syncope is the diagnosis of exclusion in these individuals. Electrophysiology and tilt table testing may mislead. The 36th Bethesda Conference 2006 Recommendations are that athletes with syncope should not participate in sports until cause is determined and treated. If asymptomatic for 2–3 months during treatment, and the problem is not considered to recur or be life threatening, the athlete can participate. Patients who have implantable devices may require long-term restriction from some athletic activities, although the electrophysiology community is split on this [84].

Difficult Situations and Suggested Solutions

Real World Question When a Patient with Syncope Needs Hospitalization?

When to hospitalize a patient after syncope is a major concern [83]. A patient with CVD, suspected of having sustained VT, might benefit from hospitalization because it could prevent recurrent symptoms, injury, and death. Elderly patients are at high risk for underlying cardiovascular causes and should be evaluated carefully in the hospital. The elderly often live alone, often cannot care for themselves, and are especially vulnerable to injury during an episode of syncope [83].

Consider hospitalization even for an isolated episode with no suspected cardiac cause if outpatient evaluation cannot be accomplished safely and satisfactorily. A patient who loses consciousness and goes to the emergency department poses a problem. Both the patient and the physician are concerned. Although the risks may be very low, the patient may go home and die; there are medical and legal risks. Vasovagal syncope may have a malignant presentation. Patients who frequently pass out for no particular reason need to be stabilized in the hospital before going home. Dysautonomic syndromes in unstable or elderly patients require admission. Whenever a treatment is needed for syncope but it cannot be initiated safely on an outpatient basis, hospitalization is recommended. A patient with severe orthostatic hypotension requires hospitalization. Patients with syncope who should be considered for hospital admission are listed in Table 13.7.

Guidelines from the American College of Emergency Physicians: Admission of Patients with Syncope

These recommendations were stratified into three levels according to the strength of evidence. No level A recommendation was specified. The level B

Table 13.7 Indications for hospitalization.

1. Elderly
2. Structural heart disease, cardiomyopathy, valvular heart disease, hypertrophic cardiomyopathy, CAD
3. Potential arrhythmic cause of syncope without obvious structural heart disease (the young or the old with cardiac arrhythmias on monitor, a long QT interval or a delta wave)
4. Severe orthostatic hypotension
5. Unexplained syncope and significant injury
6. New neurological findings: TIA, stroke seizure disorder, or suspected neurological cause
7. Concomitant diagnoses requiring treatment
8. Frequent, severe, and difficult to control neurocardiogenic syncope

CAD, coronary artery disease; TIA, transient ischemic attack

recommendation (management strategies that reflect moderate clinical certainty) was to admit patients who had any of the following: (1) a history of CHF or a history of ventricular arrhythmias, defined as past history of premature ventricular contractions that were frequent (>10 per hour), repetitive (=2 consecutive), or multifocal; (2) associated chest pain or other symptoms compatible with acute coronary syndrome; (3) evidence of significant CHF or valvular heart disease on physical examination; or (4) ECG findings of ischemia, arrhythmia, prolonged QT interval, or bundle branch block. The level C recommendation (management based on preliminary, inconclusive, or conflicting evidence, or, in the absence of any published literature, based on panel consensus) was to consider admission for patients with syncope and any of the following: (1) age older than 60 years; (2) history of CAD or congenital heart disease; (3) family history of unexpected sudden death; or (4) exertional syncope in younger patients without an obvious, benign cause for the syncope [85].

Hospitalization may be used to perform cardiac monitoring and to formulate and undertake specific treatment plans that cannot be performed readily on an outpatient basis. Electrophysiology testing for arrhythmia evaluation is one reason to admit patients to the hospital to help determine the proper long-term treatment and to help improve the prognosis.

Take Home Message

Syncope is a common manifestation of many disease processes. The problem is recurrent and handicapping for a minority. Patients with syncope and heart disease, particularly when there is impaired LV function, bundle branch block or evidence for CHF or a positive family history, are at particularly high risk for death, require an aggressive initial approach, and may require hospitalization and aggressive therapeutic interventions (including defibrillator implantation). New diagnostic modalities are becoming available to use in patients with undiagnosed syncope. When applied judiciously, tilt testing, long-term event monitoring and

EPS emerge as the most informative techniques available. Proper treatment first involves a careful understanding of the causes for syncope based on a careful assessment of the patient initially and most importantly by the history and secondarily by the physical examination. Further diagnostic assessment should be directed based on the history and physical examination to understand the mechanisms for syncope better and to understand methods to treat that mechanism better. Once there is a diagnosis then the treatment is easier.

References

1 Kapoor WN. Syncope. N Engl J Med 2000; 343(25):1856–1862.
2 Olshansky B. Is syncope the same thing as sudden death except that you wake up? J Cardiovasc Electrophysiol 1997;8(10):1098–1101.
3 Lewis DA, Dhala A. Syncope in the pediatric patient. The cardiologist's perspective. Pediatr Clin North Am 1999;46(2):205–219.
4 Olshansky B. A Pepsi challenge. N Engl J Med 1999;340(25):2006.
5 Lempert T, Bauer M. Mass fainting at rock concerts. N Engl J Med 1995;332(25):1721.
6 Aizaki T et al. Hypokalemia with syncope caused by habitual drinking of oolong tea. Intern Med 1999;38(3):252–256.
7 Nagano M et al. Successful treatment of a patient with cardiac lymphoma who presented with a complete atrioventricular block. Am J Hematol 1998;59(2):171–174.
8 Trappe HJ, Wenzlaff P, Grellman G. Should patients with implantable cardioverter-defibrillators be allowed to drive? Observations in 291 patients from a single center over an 11-year period. J Interv Card Electrophysiol 1998;2(2):193–201.
9 Eagle KA et al. Evaluation of prognostic classifications for patients with syncope. Am J Med 1985;79(4):455–460.
10 Lee RT et al. long-term survival after transient loss of consciousness. J Gen Intern Med 1988;3(4):337–343.
11 Farrehi PM, Santinga JT, Eagle KA. Syncope: diagnosis of cardiac and noncardiac causes. Geriatrics 1995;50(11):24–30.
12 Kapoor WN et al. A prospective evaluation and follow-up of patients with syncope. N Engl J Med 1983;309(4):197–204.
13 Low PA et al. Prospective evaluation of clinical characteristics of orthostatic hypotension. Mayo Clin Proc 1995;70(7):617–622.
14 Narkiewicz K, Cooley RL, Somers VK. Alcohol potentiates orthostatic hypotension: implications for alcohol-related syncope. Circulation 2000;101(4):398–402.
15 Mathias CJ, Deguchi K, Schatz I. Observations on recurrent syncope and presyncope in 641 patients. Lancet 2001;357(9253):348–353.
16 Aysun S, Apak A. Syncope as a first sign of seizure disorder. J Child Neurol 2000; 15(1):59–61.
17 Kapoor WN. Back to basics for the workup of syncope. J Gen Intern Med 1995; 10(12):695–696.
18 Strickberger SA et al. AHA/ACCF Scientific Statement on the Evaluation of Syncope. JACC 2006;47:473–484.
19 Cherin P et al. Risk of syncope in the elderly and consumption of drugs: A case-control study. J Clin Epidemiol 1997;50(3):313–320.

20 Schoenberger JA. Drug-induced orthostatic hypotension. Drug Saf 1991;6(6):402–407.

21 McIntosh SJ, Lawson J, Kenny RA. Clinical characteristics of vasodepressor cardioinhibitory and mixed carotid sinus syndrome in the elderly. Am J Med 1993;95(2):203–208.

22 Kapoor W.N. Syncope in older persons. J Am Geriatr Soc 1994;42(4):426–436.

23 Tanimoto K, Yukiiri K, Mizushige K et al. Usefulness of brain natriuretic peptide as a marker for separating cardiac and noncardiac causes of syncope. Am J Cardiol 2004;93(2):228–230.

24 Winters SL, Stewart D, Gomes JA. Signal averaging of the surface QRS complex predicts inducibility of ventricular tachycardia in patients with syncope of unknown origin: A prospective study. J Am Coll Cardiol 1987;10(4):775–781.

25 Gibson TC, Heitzman MR. Diagnostic efficacy of 24-hour electrocardiographic monitoring for syncope. Am J Cardiol 1984;53(8):1013–1017.

26 Zimetbaum PJ, Josephson ME. The evolving role of ambulatory arrhythmia monitoring in general clinical practice. Ann Intern Med 1999;130(10):848–856.

27 Gula LJ, Krahn AD, Massel D et al. External Loop Recorders: Determinants of Diagnostic Yield in Patients With Syncope Am Heart J 2004;147(4):644–648.

28 Sivakumaran S, Krahn AD, Klein GJ, et al. A prospective randomized comparison of loop recorders versus Holter monitors in patients with syncope or presyncope. Am J Med 2003;115:1–5.

29 Grubb BP et al. Utility of upright tilt-table testing in the evaluation and management of syncope of unknown origin. Am J Med 1991;90(1):6–10.

30 Kenny RA et al. Head-up tilt: A useful test for investigating unexplained syncope. Lancet 1986;1(8494):1352–1355.

31 Bartoletti A et al. Head-up tilt testing potentiated with oral nitroglycerin: A randomized trial of the contribution of a drug-free phase and a nitroglycerin phase in the diagnosis of neurally mediated syncope. Europace 1999;1(3):183–186.

32 Brignole M et al. New classification of haemodynamics of vasovagal syncope: beyond the VASIS classification. Analysis of the pre-syncopal phase of the tilt test without and with nitroglycerin challenge. Vasovagal Syncope International Study. Europace 2000;2(1):66–76.

33 Bartoletti A et al. 'The Italian Protocol': A simplified head-up tilt testing potentiated with oral nitroglycerin to assess patients with unexplained syncope. Europace 2000;2(4):339–342.

34 Fitzpatrick AP, Zaidi A. Tilt methodology in reflex syncope: emerging evidence. J Am Coll Cardiol 2000;36(1):179–180.

35 Deharo JC, Jego C, Lanteaume A, Djiane P. An Implantable Loop Recorder Study of Highly Symptomatic Vasovagal Patients: The Heart Rhythm Observed During a Spontaneous Syncope Is Identical to the Recurrent Syncope But Not Correlated With the Head-Up Tilt Test or Adenosine Triphosphate Test. J Am Coll Cardiol 2006;47:587–593.

36 Brignole M. The Second International Study of Syncope of Uncertain Etiology (ISSUE 2) study: The implantable loop recorder allows a mechanism – based effective therapy in patients with recurrent suspected or certain neutrally mediated syncope. Program and abstracts of the European Society of Cardiology 2005 Congress; September 3–7 2005;Stockholm Sweden Hot Line II.

37 García-Civera R, Ruiz-Granell R, Morell-Cabedo S et al. Significance of Tilt Table Testing in Patients With Suspected Arrhythmic Syncope and Negative Electrophysiologic Study. J Cardiovasc ElectroPhysiol 2005;16(9):938–942.

38 Guidelines on Management (Diagnosis and Treatment) of Syncope – Update 2004 Executive Summary The Task Force on Syncope European Society of Cardiology. European Heart Journal 2004;25:2054–2072.

39 Olshansky B, Mazuz M, Martins JB. Significance of inducible tachycardia in patients with syncope of unknown origin: A long-term follow-up. J Am Coll Cardiol 1985;5(2 Pt 1): 216–223.

40 Linzer M *et al.* Predicting the outcomes of electrophysiologic studies of patients with unexplained syncope: preliminary validation of a derived model. J Gen Intern Med 1991;6(2):113–120.

41 Fujimura O *et al.* The diagnostic sensitivity of electrophysiologic testing in patients with syncope caused by transient bradycardia. N Engl J Med 1989;321(25):1703–1707.

42 Middlekauff HR, Stevenson WG, Saxon LA. Prognosis after syncope: impact of left ventricular function. Am Heart J 1993;125(1):121–127.

43 Middlekauff HR *et al.* Syncope in advanced heart failure: high risk of sudden death regardless of origin of syncope. J Am Coll Cardiol 1993;21(1):110–116.

44 Olshansky B *et al.* Clinical significance of syncope in the electrophysiologic study versus electrocardiographic monitoring (ESVEM) trial. The ESVEM Investigators. Am Heart J 1999;137(5):878–886.

45 Brembilla-Perrot B *et al.* Diagnostic value of ventricular stimulation in patients with idiopathic dilated cardiomyopathy. Am Heart J 1991;121(4 Pt 1):1124–1131.

46 Constantin L *et al.* Induced sustained ventricular tachycardia in nonischemic dilated cardiomyopathy: dependence on clinical presentation and response to antiarrhythmic agents. Pacing Clin Electrophysiol 1989;12(5):776–783.

47 Grimm W Marchlinski FE. Shock occurrence and survival in 49 patients with idiopathic dilated cardiomyopathy and an implantable cardioverter-defibrillator. Eur Heart J 1995;16(2):218–222.

48 Meinertz T, Hofmann T, Zehender M. Can we predict sudden cardiac death? Drugs 1991;41(Suppl 2):9–15.

49 Moss AJ, Zareba W, Hall WJ *et al.* for the Multicenter Automatic Defibrillator Implantation Trial II Investigators Prophylactic Implantation of a Defibrillator in Patients with Myocardial Infarction and Reduced Ejection Fraction. N Engl J Med 2002;346:877–883.

50 Bardy GH, Lee KL, Mark DB, for the Sudden Cardiac Death in Heart Failure Trial (SCD–HeFT) Investigators. Amiodarone or an Implantable Cardioverter-Defibrillator for Congestive Heart Failure. N Engl J Med 2005;352(3):225–37.

51 Kadish A, Dyer A, Daubert DP, for the Defibrillators in Nonischemic Cardiomyopathy Evaluation (DEFINITE) Investigators. Prophylactic defibrillator implantation in patients with nonischemic dilated cardiomyopathy. N Engl J Med 2004;350:2151–2158.

52 Abboud FM. Neurocardiogenic syncope. N Engl J Med 1993;328(15):1117–1120.

53 Abboud FM. Ventricular syncope: is the heart a sensory organ? N Engl J Med 1989;320(6):390–392.

54 Karas B *et al.* The postural orthostatic tachycardia syndrome: A potentially treatable cause of chronic fatigue exercise intolerance and cognitive impairment in adolescents. Pacing Clin Electrophysiol 2000;23(3):344–351.

55 Grubb BP, Klingenheben T. Postural orthostatic tachycardia syndrome (POTS): etiology diagnosis and therapy. Med Klin 2000;95(8):442–446.

56 Grubb BP *et al.* Cerebral syncope:loss of consciousness associated with cerebral vasoconstriction in the absence of systemic hypotension. Pacing Clin Electrophysiol 1998;21 (4 Pt 1):652–658.

57 Call GK *et al.* Reversible cerebral segmental vasoconstriction. Stroke 1988;19(9): 1159–1170.

58 Grubb BP. Cerebral syncope: new insights into an emerging entity. J Pediatr 2000; 136(4):431–432.

59 Mark AL. The Bezold–Jarisch reflex revisited: clinical implications of inhibitory reflexes originating in the heart. J Am Coll Cardiol 1983;1(1):90–102.

60 Grubb BP, Karas B. Diagnosis and management of neurocardiogenic syncope. Curr Opin Cardiol 1998;13(1):29–35.

61 Rea RF, Thames MD. Neural control mechanisms and vasovagal syncope. J Cardiovasc Electrophysiol 1993;4(5):587–595.

62 Engel GL. Psychologic stress vasodepressor (vasovagal) syncope and sudden death. Ann Intern Med 1978;89(3):403–412.

63 Natale A *et al*. Response to beta blockers in patients with neurocardiogenic syncope: how to predict beneficial effects. J Cardiovasc Electrophysiol 1996;7(12):1154–1158.

64 Iskos D *et al*. Usefulness of pindolol in neurocardiogenic syncope. Am J Cardiol 1998;82(9):1121–1124 (A9).

65 Grubb BP *et al*. Use of sertraline hydrochloride in the treatment of refractory neurocardiogenic syncope in children and adolescents. J Am Coll Cardiol 1994;24(2):490–494.

66 Bhaumick SK, Morgan S, Mondal BK. Oral disopyramide in the treatment of recurrent neurocardiogenic syncope. Int J Clin Pract 1997;51(5):342.

67 Natale A *et al*. Efficacy of different treatment strategies for neurocardiogenic syncope. Pacing Clin Electrophysiol 1995;18(4 Pt 1):655–662.

68 Grubb BP *et al*. Preliminary observations on the use of midodrine hydrochloride in the treatment of refractory neurocardiogenic syncope. J Interv Card Electrophysiol 1999;3(2):139–143.

69 Ward CR *et al*. Midodrine: A role in the management of neurocardiogenic syncope. Heart 1998;79(1):45–49.

70 Bloomfield DM *et al*. Putting it together: A new treatment algorithm for vasovagal syncope and related disorders. Am J Cardiol 1999;84(8A):33Q–39Q.

71 Sheldon R, Rose S, Connolly S. Prevention of Syncope Trial (POST): A randomized clinical trial of beta blockers in the prevention of vasovagal syncope;rationale and study design. Europace 2003;5:71–75.

72 Kaufmann H, Saadia D, Voustianiouk A. Midodrine in neurally mediated syncope: A double-blind randomized crossover study. Ann Neurol. 2002;52(3):342–345.

73 Reybrouck T *et al*. Tilt training: A treatment for malignant and recurrent neurocardiogenic syncope. Pacing Clin Electrophysiol 2000;23(4 Pt 1):493–498.

74 Kediet CT, Van Dijk N, Linzer M, Van Lieshout JJ, Wieling W. Management of vasovagal syncope: Controlling or aborting faints by leg crossing and muscle tensing. Circulation 2002;106:1684–1689.

75 Connolly SJ *et al*. The North American Vasovagal Pacemaker Study (VPS). A randomized trial of permanent cardiac pacing for the prevention of vasovagal syncope. J Am Coll Cardiol 1999;33(1):16–20.

76 Kenny RA, Richardson DA, Steen N *et al*. Carotid sinus syndrome: A modifiable risk factor for non-accidental falls in older adults (SAFE PACE). J Am Coll Cardiol 2001;38(5):1491–1496.

77 Sutton R, Brignole M, Menozzi C, Raviele A, Alboni P, Giani P, Moya A, for the VASIS investigators. Dual-chamber pacing is efficacious in treatment of neurally-mediated tilt-positive cardioinhibitory syncope. Pacemaker versus no therapy: A multicentre randomized study. Circulation 2000;102:294–299.

78 Ammirati F, Colivicchi F, Santini M *et al*. Permanent cardiac pacing versus medical treatment for the prevention of recurrent vasovagal syncope. A multicenter randomized controlled trial. Circulation 2001;104:52–56.

79 Raviele A, Giada F, Menozzi C *et al*. Vasovagal Syncope and Pacing Trial Investigators. A randomized double-blind placebo-controlled study of permanent cardiac pacing for the

treatment of recurrent tilt-induced vasovagal syncope. The vasovagal syncope and pacing trial (SYNPACE). Eur Heart J 2004;25:1741–1748.

80 Connolly SJ, Sheldon R, Thorpe KE *et al.* Pacemaker therapy for prevention of syncope in patients with recurrent severe vasovagal syncope. Second Vasovagal Pacemaker Study (VPS II): A randomized trial. JAMA 2003;289:2224–2229.

81 Maron BJ, Fananapazir L. Sudden cardiac death in hypertrophic cardiomyopathy. Circulation 1992;85(1 Suppl):I57–I63.

82 Maron BJ, Gohman TE, Aeppli D. Prevalence of sudden cardiac death during competitive sports activities in Minnesota high school athletes. J Am Coll Cardiol 1998; 32(7):1881–1884.

83 Rosso A, Alboni P, Brignole M. Relation of clinical presentation of syncope to the age of patients. Am J Cardiol 2005;96(10):1431–1435.

84 Lampert R, Cannom D, Olshansky B. Safety of sports participation in patients with implantable cardioverter defibrillators: a survey of heart rhythm society members. J Cardiovasc Electrophysiol 2006;17(1):11–15.

85 American College of Emergency Physicians. Clinical policy: critical issues in the evaluation and management of patients presenting with syncope. Ann Emerg Med 2001;37:771–776.

86 Grubb B, Olshansky B. (eds) (2005) *Syncope: Mechanisms and Management*. Second edition. Blackwell Publishing, Oxford.

CHAPTER 14

Congenital Heart Disease in Adults

Thach N. Nguyen, Nguyen Lan Hieu, Huynh Tuan Khanh, Zhang Shuang Chuan and Heidi M. Connolly

Introduction

In the past children with congenital heart disease (CHD) rarely reached adulthood due to limited treatment options. With the advent and progress of congenital cardiac surgery, and improvements in the medical management, the number of adults with operated CHD is increasing worldwide [1]. It is predicted that 32,000 new cases of CHD are detected per year in the US and that >85% of infants born with CHD reach adulthood. The majority of these patients had palliative or reparative surgery during childhood, but ~10% of CHD patients are not diagnosed until they are adults [1]. The increasing number of adults with CHD in the US is related not only to congenital cardiac surgery but also increased awareness and recognition of CHD, and increasing numbers of immigrants with uncorrected CHD coming to medical attention.

The majority of patients with operated CHD are not cured and thus require ongoing congenital cardiac care because of the high frequency of residua and sequelae [2]. The conditions and their expected survival are shown in Table 14.1.

Table 14.1 Survival of corrected and uncorrected congenital heart defects.

Common defects in which unoperated adult survival is expected
1. Bicuspid aortic valve
2. Pulmonary valve stenosis
3. Ostium secundum atrial septal defect
4. Small patent ductus arteriosus
5. Small ventricular septal defect

Uncommon defects in which unoperated adult survival is expected
1. Congenitally corrected transposition of the great arteries (I-TGA)
2. Ebstein's anomaly
3. Congenital pulmonary valve regurgitation
4. Lutembacher's syndrome
5. Sinus of Valsalva aneurysm
6. Coronary artery anomalies
7. Single ventricle with pulmonary stenosis

Common defects in which unoperated adult survival is exceptional
1. Large ventricular septal defect
2. Aortic forestation
3. Tetralogy of Fallot
4. Complete transposition of the great arteries

I-TGA, congenitally corrected transposition of the great arteries.

Long-term Follow-up of Adult Patients with CHD

Most patients with operated CHD require life-long informed cardiovascular follow-up. Periodic evaluation at an established adult congenital heart disease clinic is recommended. However, regular life-long follow-up is required at a local level and adult cardiologists must be aware of the cardiovascular issues that may arise in adult CHD patients and recognize problems which warrant referral to an adult congenital heart disease clinic. Many patients with important residua or sequelae from their CHD are asymptomatic, and the first symptom is often an arrhythmia (Table 14.2) [3].

This chapter is written to aid adult cardiologists caring for CHD patients in the community. This review of CHD will include a range of problems frequently seen in adult cardiology, such as a brief discussion of bicuspid aortic valve

Table 14.2 Management strategies in the follow-up of adult congenital heart disease patients.

Follow-up of stable CHD patients for non-cardiac problems
1. Endocarditis prophylaxis
2. Preoperative evaluation for non-cardiac surgery
3. Contraceptive counseling
4. Pregnancy counselling – usually requires referral to Adult CHD clinic
5. Guidelines for exercise and competitive sports

Follow-up of disease progression and detection of complications
1. RV enlargement and dysfunction
2. Increased pulmonary flow and subsequent pulmonary hypertension
3. Atrial and ventricular arrhythmias
4. LV dysfunction and heart failure
5. Sudden death
6. Erythrocytosis and hyperviscosity due to cyanotic CHD

Problems for follow-up after corrective surgery
1. Major residual valve lesions: severe pulmonary, aortic and mitral valve regurgitation, severe RV or LV outflow tract obstruction
2. Prosthetic valves, conduits – obstruction or regurgitation, infection
3. Postoperative forestation – hypertension, heart failure, coronary artery disease, bicuspid aortic valve disease progression, aortic aneurysm (ascending or at the site of coarctation repair), intracranial aneurysm
4. Repaired single ventricle
5. Systemic RV (d-TGA with atrial baffle, l-TGA) increased risk for systemic ventricular dysfunction and progressive heart failure
6. Coronary artery problems after an arterial switch for TGA

Socio-economic problems
1. Employment
2. Health insurance
3. Life insurance
4. Psychosocial issues

l-TGA, congenitally corrected transposition of the great arteries; CHD, congenital heart disease; d-TGA, complete transposition of the great arteries; LV, left ventricular; RV, right ventricular.

with aortic stenosis or regurgitation, to a more comprehensive review of those disorders infrequently seen in cardiology practice such as tetralogy of Fallot (TOF). Simple and complex hemodynamic problems will also be reviewed. An organizational chart is shown in Table 14.3.

Simple Obstructive Lesions

Bicuspid Aortic Valve and Associated Disorders

Bicuspid aortic valve (BAV) occurs in about 1–2% of the population. Some patients with BAV have an associated cardiovascular abnormality such as aortopathy and less frequently aortic coarctation. Early in life, there may be no hemodynamic abnormalities related to the BAV, but the BAV is a site of possible endocarditis with its inherent concerns. Endocarditis prophylaxis is recommended for all patients with BAV, regardless of the function of the valve.

Table 14.3 Classification of congenital heart disease for adult cardiologists.

1. *Simple obstructive lesions*
    (a) Aortic stenosis
        Bicuspid aortic valve with aortic stenosis, regurgitation and aortopathy
        Subvalvular aortic stenosis
        Supravalvular aortic stenosis
    (b) Pulmonary valve stenosis
    (c) Coarctation of the aorta
    (d) Coronary anomalies
2. *Left-to-right shunts*
    (a) Ventricular septal defect (VSD)
    (b) Atrial septal defect (ASD)
    (c) Patent ductus arterious (PDA)
    (d) Atrioventricular septal defect
3. *Complex corrected lesions*
    (a) Ebstein's anomaly
    (b) Tetralogy of Fallot (TOF)
    (c) Complex pulmonary valve atresia
    (d) Transposition of great arteries (d-TGA)
    (e) Single ventricle physiology

The medial layer of the aorta above the valve is often abnormal in patients with BAV, this predisposes patients to develop aortic root dilation and dissection. BAV is a common cause of dissection in young patients, especially in pregnant woman [4–6]. It is recognized that BAV demonstrates a high degree of heritability. Family echocardiographic screening is now recommended. Asymptomatic aortopathy may be identified in family members, in the absence of a BAV [7].

In middle adult life, about 65% of BAV's degenerate to cause aortic regurgitation or calcify and cause aortic stenosis. Due to the recognized progression of valve stenosis and regurgitation, regular cardiovascular evaluation is recommended to monitor for the development of symptoms, progressive valve disease, ventricular dysfunction, and aortic root enlargement.

Intervention must be individualized, the non-calcified stenotic bicuspid aortic valve may be amenable to balloon or surgical valvoplasty. Operative intervention is eventually required in the majority of BAV patients. The type of operative intervention depends on the primary lesion [8].

Subvalvular Aortic Stenosis

A special category of adult patients who need continued follow-up are those with discrete subvalvar aortic stenosis. These patients usually have a discrete fibrous ridge and/or fibromuscular tissue ridge located from 2–5 mm below the aortic valve. Frequently, the ridge is circumferential and attached both to the ventricular septum and the anterior leaflet of the mitral valve. Less commonly, a longer, tunnel-type of subvalvular obstruction is noted. These lesions usually progress during childhood and adolescence, and can cause a secondary thickening of the aortic valve resulting in aortic valve regurgitation.

Despite a number of different surgical techniques to remove the discrete stenosis with septal myotomy or myomectomy, recurrence – and the need for reoperation – occur frequently. In addition, aortic valve regurgitation can progress, despite adequate relief of the subaortic gradient [8].

Supravalvular Aortic Stenosis

Patients with discrete supravalvar aortic stenosis (AS) usually have good operative results with patch repair of the aortic root just above the valve. Residual valvular and supravalvar abnormalities, however, can occur and need long term follow-up. Supravalvar aortic stenosis can be familial and associated with the Williams syndrome. Genetic counseling is extremely important for this group of patients [8]. When late repair is accomplished, there is concern regarding progressive coronary artery disease, since the coronary arteries are in the high pressure region. Some syndromes involving congenital cardiac lesions are listed in Table 14.4.

Table 14.4 Syndromes associated with congenital heart disease.

1. Williams syndrome	Hypercalcemia, elfin facies, mental retardation, supravalvar PS, supraoartic AS, peripheral pulmonic stenosis
2. Lutembacher's syndrome	ASD, with rheumatic MS
3. Down's syndrome	Trisomy of chromosome 21, frequently with atrioventricular canal defect or ventricular septal defect
4. Noonan's syndrome	PS due to valve dysplasia, short stature, webbed neck, low nuchal hairline, low set ears, cubitus valgus, hypertrophic cardiomyopathy
5. Turner's syndrome	Short stature, webbed neck, low nuchal hairline, low set ears, cubitus valgus, coarctation of the aorta, aortic stenosis, propensity to aortic dissection
6. Holt-Oram syndrome	Heart–hand syndrome with autosomal dominant inheritance is characterized by upper limb and cardiac septal defects

AS, aortic stenosis; ASD, atrial septal defect; CHD, congenital heart disease, MS, mitral stenosis; PS, pulmonary stenosis

Pulmonary Stenosis

Right ventricular outflow tract obstruction is valvular in 90% of cases, and supravalvar or subvalvar in 10%. Supravalvar pulmonary stenosis (PS) results from the narrowing of the pulmonary trunk, its bifurcation, or its peripheral branches; it often coexists with other congenital cardiac abnormalities (valvular PS, atrial septal defect (ASD), ventricular septal defect (VSD), patent ductus arterious (PDA), or TOF, especially if there is pulmonary atresia). Subvalvar PS, caused by narrowing of the right ventricle (RV) infundibulum or sub infundibulum, usually occurs in association with a VSD. The severity of PS is shown in Table 14.5.

Table 14.5 Classification of pulmonary stenosis.

Severity of pulmonary stenosis	Peak gradient
1. Mild	<30 mmHg
2. Moderate	30–49 mmHg
3. Severe	>50 mmHg

The severity of symptoms and the prognosis are influenced by the severity of PS, RV systolic function, and the competence of the tricuspid valve. The condition may be initially identified in the asymptomatic adult after detection of a murmur. When the PS is severe, dyspnea on exertion, fatigability, or less commonly chest pain and syncope may occur. Eventually right heart failure develops. If the foramen ovale is patent, right-to-left (R-to-L) shunting may occur and cause cyanosis and clubbing [4,5].

Valvular PS may be associated with Noonan syndrome, which is an autosomal dominant disorder characterized by short stature, intellectual impairment, unique facial features, neck webbing, and congenital heart defects. Noonan syndrome should always be considered in a patient with valvular PS.

The jugular venous pressure demonstrates a prominent "A" wave. An RV lift is common. An ejection click is common and increased proximity of the click to the first heart sound suggests increasing severity of PS. A systolic murmur with delayed pulmonary component of the second heart sound is noted. With severe PS the pulmonary component of the second heart sound disappears. Right ventricular hypertrophy and right axis deviation are noted on the electrocardiogram.

The diagnosis of PS is confirmed by transthoracic echocardiography. Echo-Doppler evaluation determines the severity of PS, and the degree of right ventricular hypertrophy. Intervention is recommended when the peak gradient is over 50 mmHg in the setting of a normal cardiac output or when right ventricular hypertrophy is present.

Asymptomatic adults with mild PS do not need intervention other than endocarditis prophylaxis. The treatment of choice for PS is pulmonary balloon valvuloplasty. Re-intervention is more commonly required in patients treated with balloon rather than surgical intervention [9,10]. Recurrence is rare unless the patient has a dysplastic and immobile pulmonary valve, which may require surgical valvectomy. If there is severe pulmonary valve regurgitation, surgery is indicated.

In the past, surgical pulmonary valvotomy was routinely performed. Despite near-normal life expectancy, patients with operated PS have an increased risk of cardiovascular events related to long-standing pulmonary valve regurgitation and pulmonary valve replacement if often required [11].

Coarctation of the Aorta

Coarctation of the aorta (CoA) typically consists of a discrete diaphragm-like ridge extending into the aortic lumen just distal to the left subclavian artery at the site of the aortic ductal attachment (the ligamentum arteriosum) [4,5]. Isolated CoA is occasionally diagnosed in adults, presenting with a systolic murmur and upper extremity hypertension or leg fatigue. Hypertension in the upper extremities with reduced blood pressure in the lower extremities is classically noted resulting in radial to femoral artery delay in pulse appearance. Rarely, an aberrant right subclavian artery arises below the CoA so there is no difference between right upper and lower extremity pressures [8]. Bicuspid aortic valve occurs in over 50% of patients with CoA [4,5].

Disorders associated with CoA of the aorta include: (1) Turner syndrome (45, X karyotype) which is characterized by a short female, broad chest, with wide-spaced nipples, webbed neck, and cardiac defects (20%), most commonly CoA; (2) Shone syndrome which is characterized by multiple left-sided obstructive lesions including supravalvar mitral ring, subaortic stenosis, bicuspid aortic valve, and CoA; and (3) cerebral aneurysms [12].

CLINICAL PEARLS

Clinical clues for coarctation of the aorta A systolic ejection murmur is common in CoA. When the CoA is severe the murmur may be continuous.

A continuous murmur may be audible or palpable in the left axilla and back if well-developed collaterals from the internal thoracic, subclavian, and scapular arteries are present.

There may also be a murmur and click related to the bicuspid aortic valve.

Most adults with CoA are asymptomatic, but there may be symptoms of hypertension including headache, epistaxis, dizziness, palpitations and rarely lower extremity claudication due to reduced lower extremity blood flow.

The chest radiograph may demonstrate rib-notching secondary to large collateral vessels from the intercostal vessels of the posterior 3rd through 8th ribs. Notching is not seen in the anterior ribs, since the anterior intercostal arteries are not located in the costal grooves. The coarctation may be seen as an indentation of the aorta, one may see prestenotic and poststenotic dilatation of the aorta, producing the "figure 3-sign" [4,5]. The ECG demonstrates left ventricular hypertrophy. Echocardiography is often the initial diagnostic test which confirms the presence of CoA and associated features such as bicuspid aortic valve. When echocardiographic imaging is suboptimal, consider magnetic resonance or computerized tomographic imaging which clearly delineates the location and severity of CoA and the presence of collateral vessels.

CLINICAL PEARLS

Long term follow-up after surgery Patients with repaired CoA are at an increased risk of cardiovascular morbidity and mortality.

The late complications after CoA intervention, even after successful repair, include residual or recurrent hypertension (occurs in 50–75%), congestive heart failure, recurrent CoA, aortic dissection, infective endocarditis, cerebro-vascular accidents (CVA) due to rupture of an intracerebral aneurysm, and possible sequelae of a bicuspid aortic valve [4,5]. Age at the time of initial repair is the most important predictor of long-term survival.

Women considering pregnancy should have an extensive evaluation to detect any recurrence of CoA or aneurysm formation which is seen more frequently after prosthetic patch angioplasty. There is a risk of aortic dissection in pregnant women with CoA due to the recognized abnormality of the aorta [8,13].

Patients with CoA need endocarditis prophylaxis.

Coarctation intervention is usually recommended when the gradient is over 30 mmHg. Surgical treatment for CoA has been successfully performed for over six decades. Percutaneous intervention with balloon and stent dilation of native and recoarctation is increasingly performed. Balloon angioplasty and stenting is usually reserved for patients with recoarctation and has a success rate of approximately 80%, with success defined as a post procedural gradient <20 mmHg. Absence of significant collateral vessel may increase the risk of paraplegia with repeat operations. Residual obstruction can be due to a small transverse arch [8]. Percutaneous intervention was thought to be less invasive and caused less morbidity with equal long term results. However, a recent review compared the results of endovascular therapy (stenting and angioplasty) with surgical techniques. The immediate improvement in hypertension and the morbidity were similar across both groups. Surgical therapy was associated with a very low risk of restenosis and recurrence, whereas endovascular therapy had a much higher incidence for subsequent aneurysm formation (20%), recoarctation and need for repeat interventions [14].

Coronary Artery Anomalies

The single coronary artery is defined as an artery that arises from an arterial trunk and nourishes the entire myocardium. A left or right coronary artery originated from the posterior sinus or from the ascending aorta is rare [15]. Besides an ectopic origin, its anatomical course is usually normal. This anomaly is considered benign.

The most common coronary anomaly is the left circumflex coronary artery (LCX) arising from the proximal right coronary artery (RCA). When the LCX arises from the right coronary cusp or the proximal RCA, it invariably follows a retroactive course, with the LCX passing posteriorly around the aortic root. This variant is benign.

When a dominant RCA, the left main-, or the left anterior descending artery (LAD) originates from the contralateral sinus, it courses to its normal position through four pathways: interarterial, septal, retroaortic or anterior. The last three courses are benign. The interarterial course is most severe because it can cause ischemia, syncope and sudden death at young age [16]. Revascularization in young patients is indicated. However, the surgical indication for asymptomatic elderly patients is not clear because, at older ages, the arteries are less compressible, unless there is concomitant obstructive coronary artery disease [16]. In some adult patients with favorable echocardiographic windows, transthoracic echocardiography (TTE) can delineate the origin of the left main (LM), thus detecting coronary anomalies which may trigger sudden cardiac death [17]. Magnetic resonance coronary angiography or computerized tomographic angiography also can be used to define the course of abnormal coronary arteries, in patients with or without known CHD [18].

Coronary artery fistula is anomalous communication between a coronary artery and a cardiac chamber or vessel [19]. It can cause heart failure, pulmonary hypertension related to L-to-R shunt, arrhythmias or ischemia due to a coronary steal phenomenon. Treatment options include transcatheter closure by embolization with coils, Rashkind double-umbrella devices (USCI Angiographics, CR Bard, Bellerica, MA) or Amplatzer Duct Occluder (AGA Medical, Golden Valley, MN). Occasionally, a large fistula requires surgical intervention. The persistence of fistula leakage after coil embolization is problematic because of risk of endocarditis due to foreign body. A repeat attempt to close the fistula is suggested in select cases. Following occlusion of the fistula, there may be persistent coronary artery dilation, antiplatelet agents are used to prevent thrombus formation. Warfarin may be recommended for marked vessel dilatation. Cardiac surgical intervention is limited to fistulas with large branch vessels that could be compromised using embolization, or those lesions with multiple fistulous communications without a single narrow restrictive drainage site into a cardiac chamber or vessel [20].

Left-to-right Shunts

Ventricular Septal Defect

VSDs may be subdivided into membranous and muscular defects. Muscular VSDs (10–20%) are described according to their location on the ventricular septum. They have a higher rate of spontaneous closure than membranous VSD. The majority of VSDs, (70–80%) are located in the membranous portion of the interventricular septum. Less common VSD types include outlet VSD (~5%) located just below the aortic and pulmonary valves. The outlet VSD, also known as doubly committed, subaortic and subpulmonic or supracristal VSD, accounts for 30–35% of VSDs in Asian patients [3]. The atrioventricular septal defects (~5%) located near the junction of the mitral and tricuspid valves [4,5].

Large VSDs are usually detected in childhood due to a murmur or the presence of congestive heart failure. Without closure, large VSDs cause pulmonary hypertension with irreversible pulmonary vascular disease and eventual reversal of the shunt from right-to-left (Eisenmenger syndrome) [8]. Children and adults with isolated small VSDs rarely require closure, and follow-up suggests a low risk of complications [21]; however, endocarditis prophylaxis is recommended. The management of VSD depends on the size of the defect and the pulmonary vascular resistance. Surgery is recommended for patients with moderate or large VSD if the magnitude of pulmonary vascular obstructive disease is not prohibitive. Once the ratio of pulmonary to systemic vascular resistance exceeds 0.7, the risk associated with surgery is very high [4,5].

The small VSD causes a loud systolic murmur, which obliterates the second heart sound. A displaced apical left ventricular impulse and mitral diastolic flow rumble suggests a hemodynamically important VSD, causing volume overload. The features observed in the cardiac examination are listed in Table 14.6 [4,5]. Transthoracic echocardiography demonstrates the size, number, location and hemodynamic impact of the VSD.

Patients with VSD who have had repair during the first few years of life usually have normal hemodynamics, no residual shunt and no elevation of pulmonary artery pressure. During follow-up, if there is a residual murmur, cardiomegaly, or questionable increased pulmonary artery pressure, Doppler echocardiography is recommended. In the presence of an important residual VSD or pulmonary hypertension, cardiac catheterization is recommended [8]. Ideally this should be performed under the care of an Adult Congenital Cardiologist.

Table 14.6 Features of cardiovascular examination in patients with ventricular septal defect.

Size of the defect	Flow direction	Features
1. Small	(L-to-R)	High-frequency ejection murmur (this murmur terminates before the end of systole as the defect is occluded by contracting myocardium)
2. Moderate-to-large	(L-to-R)	Holosystolic murmur loudest at the left lower sternal border (usually accompanied by a palpable thrill); hyperactive left ventricle; bounding pulses with a normal pulse pressure
Short mid-diastolic apical murmur (caused by increased flow through mitral valve)
Decrescendo aortic diastolic murmur of AR (if the VSD undermines the valve annulus)
3. Moderate-to-large	(R-to-L)	This occurs as pulmonary hypertension develops
RV heave and pulsation over the pulmonary trunk
Holosystolic murmur and thrill diminishes and eventually disappears as flow through the defect decreases
New pulmonary regurgitation murmur (Graham Steel murmur) may appear
Finally, cyanosis and clubbing

AR, aortic valve regurgitation; L, left; PS, pulmonary stenosis; R, right; RV, right ventricle; VSD, ventricular septal defect.

Atrial Septal Defect

ASD is the most common form of CHD to escape detection in childhood due to the subtle physical findings and lack of symptoms present early in life [2]. ASD's are classified according to their location in the atrial septum. The most common ASD is the secundum defect which is located in the mid-portion of the atrial septum and is usually an isolated defect. Most patients with a large ASD have had intervention early in life. Others with a small ASD may have minimal hemodynamic disturbance, and thus were not identified or referred for intervention. The ostium primum ASD is located in the lower part of the atrial septum and is usually associated with abnormalities of the atrioventricular valves, particularly a cleft in the anterior mitral leaflet causing mitral regurgitation. A VSD or aneurysm of the membranous ventricular septum may also occur. The electrocardiogram in patients with primum ASD typically demonstrates left axis deviation. The sinus venosus type ASD is located in the upper part of the atrial septum and is usually associated with one or more anomalous pulmonary veins [4,5].

From the defect in the atrial septum, an L-to-R shunt develops and produces volume overload of the right atrium and right ventricle with increased pulmonary blood flow. If the right ventricle fails or its compliance diminishes in magnitude, R-to-L shunting may occur [4,5]. Adults with unrepaired ASDs may be asymptomatic and present with a murmur or present with fatigue, dyspnea, palpitations, atrial fibrillation or right heart failure. Pulmonary hypertension occurs in less than 10% of ASDs.

Occasionally an ASD is identified when right ventricular pressure increases or right ventricular compliance decreases and persistent hypoxia not responsive to supplemental oxygen is noted. Right to left shunting through an ASD should be suspected in this situation [22].

The jugular venous pressure may be normal or equal "A" and "V" waves may be noted. Cardiac examination demonstrates a right ventricular impulse. Fixed split second heart sound is the characteristic physical examination finding in patients with ASD. A pulmonary systolic ejection murmur due to increased flow across the pulmonary valve is common. If the shunt is large, a tricuspid diastolic rumble is heard at the right lower sternal border. Sinus arrhythmia is characteristically absent.

Chest radiograph will demonstrate right heart enlargement, prominent pulmonary arteries are and there is peripheral pulmonary pattern of "shunt vascularity" where the small pulmonary arteries are especially well visualized in the periphery of both lungs.

The transthoracic echocardiogram is the diagnostic test of choice for most patients, but some patients with poor echocardiographic windows require a transesophageal echocardiogram for diagnosis and definitive measurement of the ASD size and the tissue rims. The sinus venosus ASD with anomalous pulmonary venous drainage may be difficult to visualize by transthoracic echocardiography.

Treatment of ASD depends on the size, hemodynamic impact, location in the atrial septum, and available treatment modalities. An ASD should be closed if there is evidence of a systemic to pulmonary shunt (Qp:Qs) greater than or equal to 1.5:1, volume overload of right-sided cardiac chambers or symptoms related to the defect. ASD closure is performed in an effort to prevent right heart failure, arrhythmias and paradoxical embolism. Studies have demonstrated improvement in survival even with ASD closure in patients over 40 years of age [23]. However, the rate of late atrial fibrillation after surgical ASD closure increases according to age at the time of intervention, with up to 60% of patients having late atrial arrhythmias when ASD closure is performed later than age 40 years [24]. Anticoagulation early after surgical ASD closure may be recommended, depending on patient characteristics and surgical preferences.

The exact determination of the size, shape, and location of the ASD and the presence or absence of associated lesions, is essential for eligibility for percutaneous transcatheter closure. Secundum ASD is the only type of ASD currently amenable to transcatheter occlusion techniques [8]. Catheterization may be needed to determine the degree and direction of the shunt, as well as presence and severity of pulmonary hypertension. When catheterization is performed, it should be done in conjunction with ASD device closure if possible. A small ASD of <0.5 cm in diameter, with minimal L-to-R shunting (ratio of pulmonary to systemic flow <1.5) usually causes no hemodynamic disturbances and may not require closure unless there have been episodes of paradoxical embolization. A defect of >2 cm in diameter associated with a substantial shunt (Qp:Qs > 1.5) and a dilated right heart will need repair. The indications for ASD closure are listed in Table 14.7.

Table 14.7 Indication for atrial septal defect closure.

1. Symptoms of dyspnea, fatigue or right heart failure
2. Recurrent pulmonary infections
3. Paradoxical embolism
4. Atrial arrhythmia even in the presence of a small defect
5. Moderate pulmonary hypertension without pulmonary vascular disease
6. Asymptomatic patients with large ASD (Qp:Qs > 1.5:1.0), right heart volume overload and no pulmonary hypertension

ASD, atrial septal defect

Adult patients usually prefer percutaneous closure of the ASD if feasible. The summary data of over 1390 patients with devices implanted world-wide demonstrates an implantation rate of 96%, a complete closure rate of 91% and a total success rate of 99% at one month. These closure rates are high and compare favorably with surgical series. The exclusion criteria for percutaneous closure are listed in Table 14.8.

Most patients who have ASD surgery in early childhood have no significant cardiovascular problems as adults, and in general, do not require long term

Table 14.8 Exclusion criteria for percutaneous atrial septal defect closure.

1. Associated CHD requiring cardiac surgery
2. Partial anomalous pulmonary venous connection
3. Pulmonary vascular resistance greater than 7 Woods units
4. R-to-L shunting at atrial level with a systemic saturation of less than 94%
5. Recent myocardial infarction
6. Unstable angina
7. Decompensated heart failure or left ventricular decompensation with an ejection fraction of less than 30%
8. Active sepsis
9. Life expectancy of less than 2 years
10. Large ASD (>35 mm) or multiple ASDs

ASD, atrial septal defect; CHD, congenital heart disease, L, left; R, right

follow-up. In contrast, patients who have undergone repair as adults, those who have elevated pulmonary pressure and vascular resistance prior to surgery, and those who have had arrhythmia or ventricular dysfunction preoperatively do require long term follow-up [8,24]. Atrial arrhythmias can occur late, after surgery, especially if there is residual atrial enlargement. Endocarditis prophylaxis is not required for patients with secundum ASD but is required for most ostium primum ASD following repair because of the abnormalities of the atrioventricular valves. All patients with ostium primum ASD have abnormalities of the mitral valve, and most have residual mitral regurgitation post-operatively. A few have severe mitral regurgitation and may later require valve replacement.

Patent Ductus Arteriosus

The arterial duct connects the descending aorta to the left pulmonary artery near its junction with the main pulmonary artery in fetal life and normally closes after birth. Persistence of the ductus arteriosis after birth is associated with prematurity and maternal rubella.

CLINICAL PEARLS

Differentiation between small and large PDA A small PDA in the adult produces an arterial venous fistula. A continuous murmur which envelopes the second heart sound is heard beneath the left clavicle as the aortic pressure is consistently greater than the pulmonary artery pressure, allowing continuous flow from the aorta to the pulmonary artery.

Patients with a moderate-sized PDA may present with symptoms of heart failure with enlarged left-sided cardiac chambers. Bounding pulses and a wide pulse pressure are common findings. Prominent suprasternal and carotid pulsations are notable. A left ventricular heave or lift may be present.

When severe pulmonary hypertension is present, the clinical features include loss of the diastolic murmur and wide pulse pressure; the single second heart sound is increased in intensity, and there is a forceful right ventricular heave felt at the left lower sternal border.

The chest radiograph may demonstrate left ventricular enlargement and left atrium (LA) enlargement if there is volume overloading due to a large L-to-R shunt. The main pulmonary artery may be prominent and there will be increased pulmonary vascular markings [2]. With pulmonary vascular disease the main pulmonary artery segment is dilated but the peripheral vessels are scanty (pruning, or "tree in winter").

Transcatheter closure of a tiny PDA, not audible on auscultation remains controversial and should not be routinely performed. A small PDA is considered for prophylactic closure to eliminate the very small risk of endarteritis. Closure is recommended in patients with a past episode of endarteritis. The presence of volume overloading of the left atrium and left ventricle is a clear indication for intervention [1]. Percutaneous device closure of a moderate sized PDA with left heart enlargement is recommended to avoid progressive heart failure. PDA closure should be avoided in patients with irreversible pulmonary vascular disease [25].

Surgical or percutaneous closure of PDA is safe and effective [1]. The indications for PDA closure are listed in Table 14.9. Once severe pulmonary vascular obstructive disease develops, closure is contra-indicated [4,5]. PDA with associated pulmonary hypertension may be difficult to visualize by echocardiography. All patients with severe pulmonary hypertension should be evaluated for a cardiac cause as this may change treatment and prognosis.

Table 14.9 Indication for patent ductus arterious closure.

1. PDA and evidence of volume overload (LA and LV enlargement)
2. Congestive heart failure due to long-standing volume overload of LV
3. Aneurysm of the PDA (surgical closure)
4. Calcified PDA (percutaneous closure)
5. Moderate pulmonary hypertension without pulmonary vascular disease

LA, left atrium, LV, left ventricle, PDA, patent ductus arterious

Atrioventricular Septal Defect

Many patients with Down's syndrome have an atrioventricular septal defect also known as complete atrioventricular canal or endocardial cushion defect. They had surgery during infancy and survived into adulthood without major hemodynamic complications. The problems for follow-up are listed in Table 14.10. Endocarditis prophylaxis is indicated in all of these patients with evidence of residual shunt or valvular abnormalities [8].

Table 14.10 Follow-up of patients with corrected atrioventricular septal defects.

1. Late heart block
2. Progression of mitral or tricuspid regurgitation
3. Late left ventricular outflow tract obstruction
4. Progression of pulmonary vascular disease

Complex Lesion

Ebstein's Anomaly

Ebstein's anomaly consists of a downward displacement of the septal and the anterior leaflets of the tricuspid valve related to incomplete delamination from the right ventricle. The true right ventricular cavity is small, and the proximal part of the right ventricle above the tricuspid valve forms the atrialized right ventricle. There is usually tricuspid valve regurgitation and an ASD. If the anomaly is very severe early operation is needed if the patient is to survive. Milder forms of Ebstein's anomaly may be diagnosed as mitral valve prolapse or an ASD.

Classical features of this anomaly include marked dilatation of the right atrium and a tendency to atrial arrhythmias, related to atrial enlargement and an increased frequency (~20%) of one or more accessory conduction pathways. The anomaly is diagnosed definitively by echocardiography.

Treatment in older children and adults includes repair or replacement of the tricuspid valve in conjunction with the closure of the ASD [3,8]. If valve replacement is indicated, bioprosthetic valve is usually preferable to mechanical valve [26]. Other aspects of the management include prophylaxis against infective endocarditis and treatment of right and left heart failure.

The treatment of arrhythmia consists of medications or catheter ablation, if an accessory pathway is present. The success with ablation is lower than in patients without Ebstein's anomaly and the recurrence is higher [27]. Despite these procedures, right ventricular dysfunction, complete heart block, persistent or recurrent supraventricular arrhythmias, stenosis or regurgitation of the tricuspid valve, and prosthetic valve dysfunction, all can occur late after surgery and require close follow-up [3,8].

Congenitally Corrected Transposition of the Great Arteries

In congenitally corrected transposition (left transposition of the great arteries, l-TGA), the right atrium is connected to an anatomic left ventricle that ejects into a pulmonary artery, and the left atrium is connected to an anatomic right ventricle that ejects blood into the aorta. The discordant connection between ventricles and great arteries is the hallmark of a congenitally corrected transposition or l-TGA, but the added discordance of the atrioventricular connection ensures that venous blood goes to the lungs and arterial blood goes to the aorta, hence the term "corrected transposition". Most patients with this anomaly have an associated VSD and PS. These patients have often had operative intervention early in life. Abnormalities of the systemic tricuspid valve are also common causing regurgitation. An Ebstein-like anomaly of the systemic tricuspid valve may occur, contributing to the degree of regurgitation.

The diagnosis of l-TGA is usually made by echocardiography, but patients may present with an abnormal electrocardiogram or arrhythmias. Patients with l-TGA are prone to heart block, occurring at a rate of 1–2% each year or commonly complicating operative intervention.

CLINICAL PEARLS

Clinical clues in the physical examination of a patient with TGA The ECG is abnormal in these patients because of the ventricular inversion, the ventricular septum is activated abnormally from left to right, thus giving a Q wave in the anterior and inferior chest leads, which may lead to the misdiagnosis of myocardial infarction.

The systemic right ventricle often demonstrates reduced function, and patients may present with heart failure.

Because the aortic valve is placed high in the left chest, the aortic component of the second heart sound is heard best at the upper sternal border; this may be the only clinical sign in congenitally corrected transposition without associated cardiac anomalies [3,28,29]. The prominent aortic closure sound may be mistaken for a prominent pulmonary valve closure sound and pulmonary hypertension.

The morphologic left ventricle is located under the sternum and a parasternal impulse may be present – further increasing the clinical suspicion of pulmonary hypertension.

Adult patients often present with systemic atrio-ventricular valve regurgitation and require valve replacement. The systemic tricuspid valve should not be repaired. Surgery should therefore be carried out only by a congenital cardiac surgeon [3,28,29].

Tetralogy of Fallot

The anatomic features of TOF include a large subaortic VSD and obstruction to pulmonary outflow at infundibular or pulmonary valve level. Secondary features include right ventricular hypertrophy and overriding of the aorta over the VSD. Other associated abnormalities include right aortic arch in 25% of patients [4,5], ASD in 10% (so called pentalogy of Fallot) [30] and coronary arterial anomalies in 10% [31]. About 25% of these patients have a Di George syndrome (chromosome 22q11 deletion, associated with hypocalcemia and impaired T cell function). About 10% have an absent pulmonary valve with mild infundibular obstruction; these patients usually have hugely dilated main, right and left pulmonary arteries [28].

TOF is the most common form of cyanotic CHD. Identification of an unoperated adult is uncommon since successful surgical repair (closure of the VSD and relief of PS) has been performed since the 1950s.

CLINICAL PEARLS

Clinical clues in the examination of patients with TOF Patients with unrepaired TOF have cyanosis and digital clubbing, the severity of which is determined by the degree of obstruction of the right ventricular outflow tract.

A right ventricular lift is palpable. In some patients, a systolic thrill caused by turbulent flow across the right ventricular outflow tract is present.

The first heart sound is normal, but the second heart sound is single, since P2 is inaudible from PS. An aortic ejection click due to a dilated, overriding aorta may be heard. A systolic ejection murmur, audible along the left sternal border, is caused by the obstruction of right ventricular outflow. The intensity and duration of the murmur is inversely related to the severity of the obstruction of right ventricular outflow; a soft, short murmur suggests severe obstruction [4,5].

The ECG demonstrates right ventricular hypertrophy, right axis deviation, tall peaked P waves and after repair, right bundle branch block is universally noted. The chest radiograph demonstrates a normal or small heart size, and diminished lung markings. The heart is classically "boot-shaped", with an upturned right ventricular apex and a concave main pulmonary arterial segment. A right-sided aortic arch may be present. Arterial oxygen desaturation is evident as is compensatory erythrocytosis, the magnitude of which is proportional to the severity of desaturation [4,5]. The diagnosis of TOF is usually suspected clinically and confirmed by echocardiography. Cardiac catheterization may be required to evaluate the pulmonary artery anatomy and coronary anatomy.

In the past, infants with TOF underwent one of three palliative procedures to increase pulmonary blood flow, thereby reducing the severity of cyanosis and improve exercise tolerance (Table 14.11). Currently, surgical repair which includes VSD closure and relief of the right ventricular outflow obstruction, is performed in the very young [4,5]. Residual abnormalities, as seen by adult cardiologists, are listed in Table 14.12 [32].

Table 14.11 Palliative surgery for infants with tetralogy of Fallot.

1. Blalock–Taussig (BT)	End-to-side anastomosis of subclavian artery to PA
2. Modified BT	Subclavian artery to PA connection using a GoreTex graft
3. Pott's shunt	Side-to-side anastomosis of descending AO to LPA
4. Waterson's shunt	Side-to-side anastomosis of ascending AO to RPA

AO, aorta; BT, Blalock–Taussig; LPA, left pulmonary artery; PA, pulmonary artery; RPA, right pulmonary artery.

Table 14.12 Postoperative residua after tetralogy of Fallot repair.

1. Pulmonary regurgitation – related to RVOT patch
2. Pulmonary stenosis
3. Atrial arrhythmias
4. Ventricular arrhythmias with propensity for sudden death
5. Right ventricular dysfunction, systolic and diastolic
6. Tricuspid valve regurgitation related to long-standing PR and RV dilatation
7. Residual pulmonary artery stenosis usually related to prior BT shunt
8. Aortic root dilatation
9. Aortic valve regurgitation
10. Left ventricular dysfunction, related to inadequate myocardial preservation or coronary artery injury at operation

BT, Blalock–Taussig; PR, pulmonary valve regurgitation; RV, right ventricle; RVOT, right ventricular outflow tract.

Supraventricular and ventricular arrhythmias frequently develop in repaired TOF patients and may be life-threatening. They may originate from the area of the right ventriculotomy and outflow patch. Ablation therapy is an option if pharmacotherapy is not effective [2]. Recommendations for device placement should be individualized.

Pulmonary valve regurgitation is the most common postoperative complication that requires intervention in TOF patients. This occurs as consequence of surgical repair of the right ventricular outflow tract by placement of a transannular pulmonary patch used to relieve right ventricular outflow tract (RVOT) obstruction. PR is usually tolerated well for many years, but eventually causes enlargement of the right ventricle, leading to important right ventricular volume overload, dysfunction and tricuspid valve regurgitation [4,5,12]. All patients with repaired TOF should be seen regularly at an established adult congenital heart disease clinic. The timing of pulmonary valve replacement must be individualized, however, patients with symptoms related to PR, right ventricular enlargement, arrhythmias, and progressive tricuspid regurgitation (TR) should be considered for operative intervention. When pulmonary valve replacement if performed, a porcine valve is usually placed, these valves have a reasonable record for longevity [2]. Percutaneous pulmonary valves have been used in TOF patients with pulmonary valve regurgitation, the appropriate patient characteristics are being established [33]. An aneurysm may form at the site of the right ventricular outflow tract patch. Although such aneurysms are usually identified incidentally, rupture has been reported in rare patients [34].

Patients with palliated and repaired TOF and elevated RV systolic pressure should be evaluated for discrete pulmonary artery stenosis. These stenoses are usually related to the prior shunt procedures. When pulmonary artery stenosis is present, it can be treated with balloon dilation and/or stenting.

Patients with repaired or unrepaired TOF are at risk for endocarditis and should therefore receive prophylaxis with antibiotics before dental or elective surgical procedures.

Complex Pulmonary Atresia

Complex pulmonary atresia is similar to a severe form of TOF, but due to the absence of a connection between the right ventricle and pulmonary arteries, there are other sources of pulmonary blood flow. Major systemic to pulmonary collaterals provide pulmonary blood flow early in life. These connections can eventually cause the development of pulmonary vascular disease.

Many patients with complex pulmonary atresia and ventricular septal defect are repaired using a homograft (valved or non-valved) conduit to provide continuity between the right ventricle and pulmonary artery. Unfortunately, no perfect conduit or graft has been developed, and obstruction to these conduits is expected with time. Obstruction can be due to sternal compression, the development of intimal growth in the graft or conduit, homograft valvular stenosis, or narrowing at the site of insertion of the graft or conduit onto the ventricle or onto the pulmonary artery. Patients with severe conduit obstruction, will require replacement of the conduit or graft. This can be a difficult operative procedure because the conduit is often located directly below the sternum and sometimes imbedded in the sternum, such that access for cardiopulmonary bypass can be exceedingly difficult [2]. Percutaneous intervention is occasionally possible for patients with conduit obstruction.

Right ventricular dysfunction and arrhythmias are problems that can occur with progressive right ventricular pressure overload. Some patients, however, will have systemic or near systemic right ventricular pressure with minimal or no symptoms.

Patients with right ventricular to pulmonary artery conduits need at least yearly echocardiographic evaluation to assess whether or not conduit obstruction or regurgitation is progressive [2]. These patients require individualized care with regular visits to an established adult congenital heart disease clinic. Operative intervention should only be performed by an experienced congenital heart surgeon.

Patients with repaired or unrepaired complex pulmonary atresia are at risk for endocarditis and should therefore receive prophylaxis with antibiotics before dental or elective surgical procedures.

Complete Transposition of the Great Arteries

Complete d-TGA consists of the origin of the aorta arising from the morphological right ventricle and the pulmonary artery from the morphological left ventricle. Nearly 40% of d-TGA patients have an associated VSD. Without surgery, the prognosis of d-TGA is very poor; the patients can only survive if there is communication between the two circulations or by balloon atrial septostomy.

In patients with d-TGA and an intact ventricular septum, the arterial switch repair is now the treatment of choice. This consists of transfer of the pulmonary artery to communicate with the morphologic right ventricle and the aorta to communicate with the morphologic left ventricle. The two coronary arteries are also transferred to the new aortic root. The arterial switch operation was first performed in the 1970's, so we are only now seeing adult patients who have had this operation. Unique concerns include coronary ostial problems resulting in reduced or abnormal coronary blood flow. This appears to be uncommon but periodic non-invasive coronary assessment is suggested. The pulmonary artery or aortic anastamoses may also become obstructed [35].

Atrial switch surgery, once the preferred procedure, is now rarely performed. Adult patients who have had the atrial switch operation (Mustard or Senning) commonly have complications which include atrial arrhythmias due to the extensive atrial repair, systemic ventricular dysfunction and systemic tricuspid valve regurgitation. Right ventricular dysfunction is expected in patients after the atrial switch operation [4,5,12].

CLINICAL PEARLS
Follow-up after surgery and indication for further intervention
Standard heart failure treatment should be instituted when systemic ventricular dysfunction is present but all of these patients should be regularly seen at an established adult congenital heart disease clinic. If they do not respond to medication, they should be considered for transplantation or double switch [8].

Pulmonary venous obstruction can cause pulmonary hypertension, as the hemodynamic effects are similar to mitral stenosis. Reoperation or catheter based intervention may be effective [3,17,18]. Balloon and stenting is also used for systemic venous baffle obstruction [8].

The complications of the atrial and arterial switch surgeries are listed in Tables 14.13 and 14.14 [36]. The arterial switch surgery is now the procedure of choice for patients with d-TGA due to the late complications of atrial switch operation. In experienced hands it carries a low morbidity and mortality rate and excellent long-term outcome [4,5].

Table 14.13 Complications after the atrial switch surgery (Mustard or Senning).

1. Atrial arrhythmias
2. Heart block
3. Increased risk of sudden death
4. Right ventricular dysfunction with associated heart failure
5. Systemic tricuspid valve regurgitation
6. Leakage of atrial baffle – especially important for patients who require pacemaker placement
7. Obstruction of the pulmonary or systemic venous baffle

Table 14.14 Complications after the arterial switch surgery.

1. Neo-aortic valve regurgitation
2. Anastamotic supravalvar pulmonary or aortic stenosis
3. Tricuspid valve regurgitation
4. Coronary arterial obstruction

One of the problems in the follow-up of these patients is the occurrence of sudden cardiac death. Which are the predictors of sudden cardiac death (SCD) in these patients?

CRITICAL THINKING

Warning signs of sudden cardiac death. A retrospective, multicenter, case-controlled study including 47 patients after Mustard or Senning operation for d-TGA and experienced a SCD event (34 SCD, 13 near-miss SCD) was reported [37]. The presence of arrhythmia or heart failure symptoms at most recent follow-up and history of documented arrhythmia atrial flutter/atrial fibrillation (AFL/AF) were found to increase the risk of SCD in TGA patients. Neither medication nor pacing was found to be protective. Most SCD events (81%) occurred during exercise. Ventricular tachycardia/ventricular fibrillation (VT/VF) were the recorded rhythm during SCD in 21 of 47 patients. In patients presenting with symptoms of heart failure and those with documented AFL/AF, electrophysiologic study for inducible VT/VF should be seriously considered. When VT/VF is inducible using moderately aggressive pacing protocols, an implanted cardioverter defibrillator (ICD) should be considered.

In patients with TGA associated with VSD, operative intervention often consists of VSD closure with a patch so as to redirect left ventricular blood to the aorta (Rastelli operation). The pulmonary artery is sacrificed and a right ventricular to pulmonary artery conduit is placed. These patients are prone to left ventricular outflow tract obstruction due to the configuration of the VSD patch and right ventricular to pulmonary artery conduit obstruction. Different types of procedures for patients with TGA are shown in Table 14.15.

Table 14.15 Surgical or percutaneous procedure for patients with transposition of great arteries.

Type of procedure	Operative technique
1. Rashkind procedure	Percutaneous balloon atrial septostomy; done in the first week of life as palliative procedure while waiting for definitive surgery, if the native ASD is inadequate
2. Atrial switch surgery (Mustard or Senning)	Atrial baffles redirect venous blood through the mitral valve to the anatomical LV then to the pulmonary artery and the oxygenated blood through the tricuspid valve to the anatomical RV and then to the aorta
3. Arterial switch surgery	The aorta and pulmonary artery are transected above the valves, switched and reconnected. The coronary arteries are relocated to the neo-aorta

ASD, atrial septal defect; LV, left ventricle; RV, right ventricle

Single Ventricle Physiology

There are a number of complex congenital heart lesions that all lead to the patient having only one effective pumping ventricle. They include:

1 Double inlet left ventricle, or double inlet right ventricle (Single ventricle).
2 Hypoplastic left heart: aortic or mitral atresia, or critical aortic stenosis.
3 Hypoplastic right heart: tricuspid atresia.

The combination of a single ventricle with moderate pulmonary stenosis is one of the commoner causes of untreated cyanotic CHD in an adult. Because it is usually not possible to get the hypoplastic ventricle to grow enough to support a circulation, all these lesions are treated by the so-called single ventricle repair that often involves three stages.

Stage 1

1 In early infancy there may be a need to band the pulmonary artery to reduce excessive pulmonary blood flow that causes congestive heart failure and then pulmonary vascular disease (double inlet ventricles without PS, tricuspid atresia with transposition of the great arteries, mitral atresia).

2 If there is a markedly reduced pulmonary blood flow and cyanosis, some form of aorto-pulmonary shunt is needed (double inlet ventricles with PS, tricuspid or pulmonary atresia).

3 In aortic atresia or critical aortic stenosis the hypoplastic aorta is anastomosed to the main pulmonary artery to provide a conduit to the descending aorta, and the distal pulmonary arteries are cut off the main pulmonary artery and supplied from the aorta via a small conduit (Norwood procedure).

Stage 2

A bidirectional Glenn procedure is done by cutting off the superior vena cava (SVC) at its entry into the right atrium, and then connecting the proximal SVC to the junction of the right and left pulmonary arteries. In this way all upper body venous drainage perfuses the lungs, and arterial saturation increases without any added volume loading of the single ventricle.

With time, arterial oxygen saturation begins to decrease:

1 As the proportion of the lower body increase with growth, more desaturated venous blood returning through the inferior vena cava (IVC) bypasses the lungs.

2 Collateral venous connections between SVC and IVC steal blood away from the lungs. Sometimes these collaterals can be occluded at catheterization.

3 Arteriovenous fistulae in the lungs bypass alveoli and so reduce oxygenation in the lungs. Sometimes these fistulae can be occluded at catheterization.

Stage 3

The inferior vena caval blood is directed to the pulmonary arteries by a conduit inside or outside the right atrium (Fontan–Kreutzer procedure). This removes cyanosis, but at the cost of a higher than normal systemic venous pressure.

Most patients are improved by the Fontan–Kreutzer procedure, even though their exercise capacity is below normal. However, complications are common.

1 Atrial arrhythmias impair the function of the one pumping ventricle.

2 Atrial thrombi may embolize to the lung. Many patients are put onto warfarin or aspirin to reduce this risk.

3 Progressive mitral or tricuspid valve disease may develop and impair ventricular function. If atrial pressure rises, then so does systemic venous pressure, and this impairs blood flow.

4 Protein losing enteropathy is usually a late complication with a poor prognosis.

With all these complications, the likelihood of good health more than 15–20 years after the single ventricle repair is low. Many of these patients will require a heart transplant [3,17,18]. All patients with palliated single ventricle require regular (preferably annual) evaluation by an adult congenital cardiologist.

Eisenmenger Syndrome

Eisenmenger syndrome remains a common cause of cyanosis in the adult and involves irreversible pulmonary vascular disease due to long-standing cardiac shunt with eventual reversal of the shunt [4,5]. Presenting symptoms are listed in Table 14.16. Patients with Eisenmenger syndrome often have hemoptysis but this is rarely fatal. They can have pulmonary artery rupture, thromboembolism, and local thrombosis.

The findings of the physical examination are listed in Table 14.17. Eisenmenger patients often do well with conservative medical management for many years. When clinical deterioration is noted, pulmonary vasodilator therapy [38,39] and lung transplantation with intracardiac repair or heart-lung transplantation [40] can be considered. The management is listed in Table 14.18. Systemic vasodilators with more effect on the systemic than the pulmonary vasculature will increase R-to-L shunt, simultaneously decrease cerebral oxygen supply and may cause sudden death. Patients with Eisenmenger syndrome should be seen regularly by an adult congenital cardiologist to review recognized complications, and new treatment options.

Table 14.16 Symptoms of Eisenmerger syndrome.

Symptoms	Causes
1. Cyanosis	R-to-L shunting
2. Palpitations	Atrial fibrillation and flutter
3. Erythrocytosis	Oxygen desaturation
4. Hyperviscosity	Visual disturbance, fatigue, headache, dizziness, paresthesia
5. Hemoptysis	Pulmonary infarction, rupture of dilated pulmonary veins
6. Stroke	Paradoxical embolism, venous thrombosis of cerebral vessel, intracranial hemorrhage
7. Brain abscess	Septic paradoxical embolism
8. Syncope	Low cardiac output or arrhythmias
9. Risk of sudden death	

L, left; R, right

Table 14.17 Physical findings in Eisenmerger syndrome.

1. Digital clubbing
2. Cyanosis
3. Jugular venous distension if there is CHF
4. Prominent A wave, and V wave if TR present
5. Right parasternal heave
6. Loud P2
7. Murmur of VSD, ASD, PDA disappears
8. Decrescendo diastolic murmur of PI (Graham Steel murmur)
9. Holosystolic murmur of TR
10. Edema and ascites if right heart failure is present

ASD, atrial septal defect; CHF, congestive heart failure; L, left; PDA, patent ductus arterious; PI, pulmonic insufficiency; R, right; TR, tricuspid valve regurgitation; VSD, ventricular septal defect

Table 14.18 Management of patients with Eisenmenger syndrome.

1. Avoid intravascular volume depletion (increased R-to-L shunt)
2. Avoid heavy exertion (increased R-to-L shunt)
3. Avoid high altitude (decreased oxygen saturation)
4. Avoid peripheral vasodilators (increased R-to-L shunt)
5. Avoid pregnancy (high maternal and fetal morbidity and mortality)
6. Phlebotomy with isovolumic replacement for symptomatic hyperviscosity in the absence of dehydration
7. Watch for iron deficiency from repeat phlebotomy
8. In patient going for non-cardiac surgery:
    avoid intravascular volume depletion (increased R-to-L shunt)
    prevention of paradoxical embolism with intravenous line air filters
    prophylactic phlebotomy to improve hemostasis
    avoid anticoagulant and antiplatelet agents (exacerbate hemorrhagic diathesis)
9. Pulmonary vasodilators
10. Lung or combined heart–lung transplantation in patients with high risk markers:
    syncope
    refractory right heart failure
    advanced NYHA function class
    severe hypoxemia

L, left; NYHA, New York Heart Association; R, right.

Difficult Situations and Suggested Solutions

Real World Question How to Treat Left Ventricular Failure in CHD Patients?

There are limited data on the appropriate medical treatment options for adult congenital cardiac patients with symptomatic systemic ventricular dysfunction. Standard medical therapy, including angiotensin converting enzyme (ACE) inhibitor, angiotensin II receptor blockers (ARB), carvedilol, diuretic, and digoxin is routinely instituted. For patients with more advanced symptoms, additional medical therapy including spironolactone, and nesiritide can be used. Cardiac resynchronization therapy has been beneficial for adult patients with poor LV function and intraventricular conduction delay, if dyssynchrony is present, the patient would benefit bi-ventricular pacing.

EMERGING TREND

Cardiac resynchronization therapy in CHD A multi-center, retrospective evaluation of cardiac resynchronisation therapy (CRT) in 103 patients with CHD, poor LV function and intraventricular conduction delay was reported [41]. The median age at time of implantation was 12.8 years (3 months to 55.4 years). The median duration of follow-up was four months (22 days to 1 year). The diagnosis was CHD in 73 patients (71%), cardiomyopathy in 16 (16%), and congenital complete atrioventricular block in 14 (13%). The QRS duration before pacing was 166.1 ± 33.3 ms, which decreased after CRT by 37.7 ± 30.7 ms ($P < 0.01$). Pre-CRT systemic ventricular ejection fraction (EF) was $26.2 \pm 11.6\%$. The EF increased by 12.8 ± 12.7 EF with a mean EF after CRT of $39.9 \pm 14.8\%$ ($P < 0.05$). Of 18 patients who underwent CRT while listed for heart transplantation, three improved sufficiently to allow removal from the transplant waiting list, five underwent transplant, two died, and eight others are currently awaiting transplant.

Real World Question How to Treat Pulmonary Hypertension and Right Ventricular Failure in CHD Patients?

Pulmonary arterial hypertension (PAH) related to Eisenmenger syndrome carries a better prognosis that primary PAH. With appropriate medical care prolonged survival is possible. Alternative treatment options include pulmonary vasodilator therapy. There are limited data available on the impact of pulmonary vasodilators in patients with Eisenmenger syndrome, however, small series report optimistic results. These agents are recommended for class III or IV symptoms [40,42]. Lung transplantation with intracardiac repair or heart-lung transplantation are additional options for Eisenmenger patients with advanced symptoms unresponsive to standard therapy [43].

Treatment of non-systemic ventricular failure in CHD patients should focus on treating the underlying cause. When non-systemic ventricular outflow tract obstruction is causing non-systemic ventricular failure, intervention is indicated. When valvular regurgitation causes non-systemic ventricular failure, valve intervention is recommended. Treatment for severe non-systemic ventricular systolic and or diastolic dysfunction, which is not related to a mechanical problem can be difficult. Symptomatic benefit from medical therapy is limited. Medical therapy includes diuretics, and occasionally digitalis. Patients should be monitored for arrhythmias.

EMERGING TREND

Pulmonary arterial hypertension on Bosentan The long-term outcome of children with PAH treated with bosentan therapy, with or without concomitant prostanoid therapy was retrospectively reviewed [44]. 86 children with PAH (idiopathic, associated with CHD or connective tissue disease) started bosentan with or without concomitant intravenous epoprostenol or subcutaneous treprostinil therapy. Hemodynamics, World Health Organization (WHO) functional class, and safety data were collected. At the cut-off date, 68 patients (79%) were still treated with bosentan, 13 (15%) were discontinued, and 5 (6%) had died. Median exposure to bosentan was 14 months. In 90% of the patients ($n = 78$), WHO functional class improved (46%) or was unchanged (44%) with bosentan treatment. Mean pulmonary artery pressure and pulmonary vascular resistance decreased ($64 \pm 3\,mmHg$ to $57 \pm 3\,mmHg$, $P = 0.005$ and $20 \pm 2\,Um^2$ to $15 \pm 2\,Um^2$, $P = 0.01$, respectively; $n = 49$). Kaplan–Meier survival estimates at one and two years were 98% and 91%, respectively. The risk for worsening PAH was lower in patients in WHO functional class I/II at bosentan initiation than in patients in WHO class III/IV at bosentan initiation. These data suggest that bosentan, an oral endothelin ET_A/ET_B receptor antagonist, with or without concomitant prostanoid therapy, is safe and efficacious for the treatment of PAH in children.

Real World Question How to Treat Atrial Arrythmias in Adult CHD Patients?

Atrial arrhythmias are common in patients with CHD. Adults with atrial septal defects often come to medical attention after the onset of atrial fibrillation. Treatment of atrial arrhythmias should be individualized and therapy depends on the type of CHD present and the need for intervention. When operative intervention is recommended for CHD, a simultaneous Maze procedure may be beneficial. Medical therapy and cardioversion should be considered for others. The rate of late atrial fibrillation after surgical ASD closure increases according to age at the time of intervention, with up to 60% of patients having late atrial arrhythmias when ASD closure is done later than age 40 years [26]. These patients require anticoagulation for stroke prevention and either heart rate control or medical and electrical therapy for atrial fibrillation conversion.

Patients with operated CHD may also present with atrial fibrillation. It is imperative to perform a comprehensive anatomic evaluation in these patients to exclude a lesion that requires intervention. Patients with repaired TOF and severe pulmonary valve regurgitation may be asymptomatic for many years. The initial symptom related to right heart enlargement and secondary progressive tricuspid valve regurgitation may be atrial fibrillation. A comprehensive evaluation by a congenital cardiologist is recommended when patients present with atrial fibrillation prior to considering ablation or other intervention. There should be a high index of suspicion that the atrial fibrillation is due to residua or sequela of CHD [45].

Atrial tachycardia and atrial flutter are also common after operation for CHD and may be scar dependent. A comprehensive evaluation by a congenital cardiologist is recommended for residua or sequela. If the atrial arrhythmia is due to scar, catheter ablation is the recommended treatment.

Real World Question How to Treat Ventricular Arrhythmias in Adult CHD Patients?

Ventricular arrhythmias are not uncommon in patients with operated CHD or severe ventricular dysfunction. Treatment of ventricular arrhythmias should be individualized and therapy depends on the type of CHD present and the need for intervention. When operative intervention is recommended for CHD, preoperative electrophysiology study may help to guide therapy. ICDs should be used in adult CHD patients with severe systemic ventricular dysfunction associated with ventricular tachycardia and in other select patients. Adult CHD patients who are at risk for arrhythmias, or have clinical arrhythmias, should be referred to an adult CHD clinic for evaluation and management. The complex cardiac anatomy warrants specialized care and intervention [46].

Real World Question How to Manage Hematological Complications of Cyanosis?

The characteristic features of cyanosis include decreased oxygen saturation and increased hemoglobin and hematocrit. The resulting physical features include central cyanosis and digital clubbing. Erythrocytosis occurs due to tissue hypoxia; this is distinctly different from polycythemia (increase in cellular mass including white cells and platelets). The increase of hematocrit improves oxygen-carrying capacity for patients with cyanotic heart disease, but decreases systemic oxygen transport because the increased blood viscosity decreases cardiac output. Common problems encountered in patients with cyanotic CHD include scoliosis, painful arthropathy or arthritis, gallstones, pulmonary hemorrhage or thrombus and renal dysfunction. Rarely, hyperviscosity symptoms occur and are manifest by fatigue, paresthesias, headaches, and reduced concentration. Dehydration should be excluded before considering phlebotomy. When required, phlebotomy should be accompanied by fluid administration, especially in Eisenmenger patients to avoid hypotension and associated risks.

Erythrocytosis can be compensated or decompensated, defined in terms of erythrocyte indices and symptoms of hyperviscosity. Patients with compensated erythrocytosis establish an equilibrium-hematocrit level in an iron-replete state, and usually have no symptoms of hyperviscosity even at high hematocrit levels. On the other hand, some patients with uncompensated erythrocytosis manifest unstable rising hematocrit levels and experience severe hyperviscosity symptoms. This imbalance may be iatrogenic and related to excess phlebotomy and subsequent iron administration. In order to decrease the symptoms, cessation of phlebotomy is advised. When symptoms of hyperviscosity occur with a hematocrit (Hct) less than 65%, iron deficiency must be sought, as symptoms of the latter may closely resemble of those of

Table 14.19 Indications for phlebotomy.

1. Symptomatic hyperviscosity in an adequately hydrated patient (usually Hct $>$ 65%)
2. Asymptomatic patients with Hct $>$ 65% prior to surgery

Hct, hematocrit

hyperviscosity [42]. Iron deficiency, often caused by phlebotomy, increases the risk of stroke in cyanotic patients. Dehydration also aggravates the condition. For cyanotic patients with hemoglobin levels less than 18 g, or Hct levels less than 62, iron therapy is recommended for seven to 10 days. This should be discontinued when hemoglobin and hematocrit levels increase. The indications for phlebotomy are listed in Table 14.19. Unlike children, cyanotic adults do not appear to be at risk for cerebral arterial thrombosis [43].

Cyanotic patients should be counseled to avoid pregnancy which carries a very high risk of maternal and fetal mortality if cyanosis is related to pulmonary hypertension and a very high risk of fetal morbidity and mortality if cyanosis is not associated with pulmonary hypertension. With expert management and conservative care, prolonged survival is possible for patients with cyanotic heart disease.

Real World Question **How to Prescribe Exercise Protocols for Patients with CHD?**
Patients with CHD who seek exercise counseling should be carefully evaluated for structural and high risk cardiovascular disease. Special attention should be directed to pulmonary hypertension, severe obstructive lesions, arrhythmias, myocardial dysfunction, and symptoms including exercise induced syncope, chest pain or dizziness [42]. The guidelines for exercise and competitive sports are listed in Table 14.20. If there is uncertainty, or if professional athletes require counseling, a consultation with an adult congenital cardiologist is suggested.

Real World Question **How to Manage Non-cardiac Surgery in CHD Patients?**
Patients with acyanotic CHD require meticulous intraoperative and postoperative care for non-cardiac procedures. The problems that need to be closely followed during surgery include: hemodynamic status, ventilation, blood coagulation, renal function, and anesthesia care. In the high risk patient, referral to a tertiary center is appropriate even for a minor operative intervention. Patients will be followed by an adult congenital cardiologist and cared for by a cardiovascular anesthesiologist.

Perioperative management of patients with cyanotic CHD and those with pulmonary vascular disease is very complex and carries a high risk. Special precaution to prevent dehydration and hypovolemia is critical. Large fluctuations of systemic vascular resistance should be avoided. Systemic hypotension can lead to an increase of R-to-L shunting with a decrease of pulmonary

Table 14.20 Guidelines for exercise and competitive sports.

Conditions	Level of activity
1. Patients 6 months after repair of L-to-R shunt lesion (no pulmonary hypertension, arrhythmias, myocardial dysfunction)	All sports allowed
2. Patients with residual shunts (PAP <40 mmHg, no myocardial dysfunction or arrhythmias)	All sports allowed
3. Patients with elevated pulmonary vascular resistance	No competitive sports
4. Patients with aortic and pulmonary stenosis	Varied (according to degree of stenosis)
5. Patients with uncomplicated CoA	Competitive sports (allowed if gradient <20 mmHg and normal systolic BP with exercise)
6. Patients after repair of TOF (with marked PR, residual RV systolic hypertension > 50% of systemic, significant rhythm disturbance)	Low-intensity sports
7. Patients with TGA after atrial switch procedure, or Fontan operation	Varied (according to residual ventricular function and arrhythmias)

BP, blood pressure; CoA, coarctation of aorta; L, left; PAP, pulmonary artery pressure; R, right; d-TGA, complete transposition of the great arteries; TOF, tetralogy of Fallot

blood flow. Hypercapnia and hypoxia can stimulate an increase of pulmonary vascular resistance. Close monitoring of intravascular blood volume and cautious use of vasodilators, including regional anesthesia, are mandatory [42]. An enlarged pulmonary artery secondary to L-to-R shunt or pulmonary hypertension can result in chronic compression of a bronchus resulting in recurrent or chronic atelectasis, pneumonia or emphysema. The patients can have diaphragmatic palsy due to phrenic nerve injury from previous surgery. They can have scoliosis that is not severe enough to impair pulmonary function but restrictive airway obstruction is well recognized [42].

If the hematocrit is more than 65%, patients should have prophylactic phlebotomy in order to improve hemostasis and minimize post-operative bleeding [21]. The bleeding time is prolonged while the partial thromboplastin time is normal. In addition, a special method of partial thromboplastin time monitoring is required.

In the presence of intracardiac shunt, special devices should be used to prevent cerebral embolization or brain abscess. Filters should be placed in intravenous lines with scrupulous attention in maintaining all venous lines free of air or bubbles to reduce the risk of paradoxical embolization [45].

Real World Question How to Manage Endocarditis Prophylaxis for Adult Patients with CHD?

Infection most commonly affects sites of turbulent flow on the low-pressure side of gradients; they are listed in Table 14.21. The risk of endocarditis associated with isolated low-pressure lesions in the right heart is low [42].

Table 14.21 Indications for antibiotic prophylaxis.

1. Restrictive VSD
2. PDA
3. Cleft mitral valve
4. Aortic coarctation at the coarctation site or at the site of an associated bicuspid aortic valve
5. Prosthetic valves, shunts, conduits

PDA, patent ductus arterious; VSD, ventricular septal defect

Real World Question How to Approach Pregnancy in Patients with CHD?

Clinical decisions regarding pregnancy should be coordinated between the primary care physician, the adult congenital cardiologist, and an high-risk obstetrician associated with a major obstetrical center where support in perinatology and anesthesia is available [40]. The facets of management before, during and following pregnancy that need to be covered are listed in Table 14.22. The reported genetic transmission of maternal congenital heart disease to offspring varies from 4–16% [46].

The more pregnancy is contraindicated, the more fail-safe the method of contraception chosen should be. The guideline for selection of contraception methods is shown in Table 14.23.

Patients with elevated pulmonary vascular resistance are at markedly increased risk of cardiovascular complications and death during pregnancy and should not become pregnant. Those with marginal ventricular function, or class III or IV heart failure should be discouraged from getting pregnant due to the risk of progressive heart failure, and the inability to safely use the

Table 14.22 Facets of management before, during and after pregnancy.

1. Advice on contraception
2. Counseling on risks of pregnancy to the mother and fetus
3. Surveillance during pregnancy and delivery
4. Postpartum reassessment

Table 14.23 Guidelines for selection of contraception methods.

Method	Failure rate (%)	Problems
1. Barrier	10–20	
2. Intrauterine device	4	Infection
3. Hormonal suppression	<3	Thromboembolism (avoid in patients with R-to-L shunts)
4. Male or female sterilization	<1	Procedural and psychological

L, left; R, right

usual heart failure medications during pregnancy. Patients with cyanotic lesions are at increased risk for fetal loss, prematurity and small for gestational age infants [47].

Operated patients with CHD may be able to have a safe and successful pregnancy but careful pre-pregnancy counseling is mandatory. This counseling should be performed by a specialized adult congenital heart clinic in conjunction with a high-risk obstetrics clinic and genetics evaluation when appropriate. Although the risk of CHD in the offspring of patients with CHD is low (4–5%), there are select groups in which the frequency of inheritance is increased such as conotruncal abnormalities with 22q11 (up to 50%), Noonan's syndrome (50%), familial ASDs (up to 50%) and even bicuspid aortic valves.

Postoperative patients who have good ventricular function and normal pulmonary artery pressure, no history of significant cardiovascular complications including arrhythmias may be reasonable candidates for pregnancy.

The most difficult question a young woman with CHD can ask is whether or not she can hope to have her own children. The final *recommendation* will be based on many aspects of risk assessment to herself and the fetus. The final *decision* always comes from the patient and her partner [42].

References

1 Care for the adults with congenital heart disease. Presented at the 32nd Bethesda Conference, Bethesda, Maryland, October 2–3, 2000. J Am Coll Cardiol 2000; 37:1161–1198.

2 Waight D, Cao Q, Hijazi Z. Percutaneous interventions in patients with congenital heart disease. Armonk, NY: Futura, 2000.

3 Somerville J (2000) Cardiac problems of adults with congenital heart disease. In: James H Moller and Julian IE Hoffman (eds), *Pediatric Cardiovascular Medicine*, pp. 687–705. Churchill Livingstone, New York.

4 Brickner M, Hillis L, Lange R. Congenital heart disease in adults. First of two parts. N Engl J Med 2000;342:256–263.

5 Brickner M, Hillis L, Lange R. Congenital heart Disease in adults. Second of two parts. N Engl J Med 2000;342:334–342.

6 Januzzi J, Isselbacher E, Fattori R *et al*. Characterizing the young patient with aortic dissection: results from the International Registry of Aortic Dissection (IRAD). J Am Coll Cardiol 2004;43:665–669.

7 Cripe L, Andelfinger G, Martin L *et al*. Bicuspid aortic valve is heritable. J Am Coll Cardiol 2004;44:138–143.

8 Graham T. Long term care of patients with congenital cardiac abnormalities. Advances in Cardiovascular Medicine 1998;5:2.

9 Peterson C, Schilthuis J, Dodge-Khatami A *et al*. Comparative long-term results of surgery versus balloon valvuloplasty for pulmonary valve stenosis in infants and children. Ann Thorac Surg 2003;76:1078–1082.

10 Chen C, Cheng T, Huant T *et al*. Percutaneous balloon valvuloplasty for pulmonic stenosis in adolescents and adults. N Engl J Med 1996;335:21–25.

11 Earing M, Connolly HM, Dearani J *et al*. Long-term follow-up of patients after surgical treatment for isolated pulmonary valve stenosis. Mayo Clin Proc 2005;80:871–876.

12 Connolly H, Huston J 3rd, Brown R Jr. *et al.* Intracranial aneurysms in patients with coarctation of the aorta: a prospective magnetic resonance angiographic study of 100 patients. Mayo Clin Proc 2003;78:1491–1499.

13 Beauchesne L, Connolly H, Ammash N *et al.* Coarctation of the aorta: outcome of pregnancy. J Am Coll Cardiol 2001;38:1728–1733.

14 Carr JA. The results of catheter-based therapy compared with surgical repair of adult aortic coarctation. J Am Coll Cardiol 2006;47:1101–1107.

15 Choi J, Kornblum R. Pete Maravich's incredible heart. J Forensic Sci 1990;35:981–986.

16 Yamanaka O, Hobbs R. Coronary artery anomalies in 126,595 patients undergoing coronary arteriography. Cathet Cardiovasc Diagn 1990;21:28–40.

17 Nowak B, Voigtlander T, Kolsch B *et al.* Echocardiogarphic visualization of anomalous left main coronary arteries originating from the right sinus of Valsalva. Int J Cardiol 1994;46:67–73.

18 Taylor A, Thorne S, Rubens M *et al.* Coronary artery imaging in grown up congenital heart disease: complementary role of magnetic resonance and XR coronary angiography. Circulation 2000;101:1670–1678.

19 Hoffman J. Congenital anomalies of the coronary vessels and the aortic root. In: Emmanouilides G, Riesenschneider TA, Allen H, Gutgesell H, eds. Heart disease in infants, children and adolescents including the fetus and young adult. Baltimore: Williams and Wilkins, 1995:78–782.

20 Okubo M, Nykamen D, Bensen L. Outcomes of transcatheter embolization in the treatment of coronary artery fistulas. Cathet Cardiovasc Intervent 2001;52:510–517.

21 Gabriel H, Heger M, Innerhofer P *et al.* Long-term outcome of patients with ventricular septal defect considered not to require surgical closure during childhood. J Am Coll Cardiol 2002;39:1066–1071.

22 Mannon B, Bemis C, Carver J. Right ventricular infarction complicated by right to left shunt. J Am Coll Cardiol 1983;1:554–557.

23 Attie F, Rosas M, Granados N *et al.* Surgical treatment for secundum atrial septal defect in patients > 40 years old. A randomized clinical trial. J Am Coll Cardiol 2001;38:2035–42.

24 Murphy J, Gersh B, McGoon M *et al.* Long–term outcome after surgical repair of isolated atrial septal defect. Follow-up at 27 to 32 years. N Engl J Med 1990;323:1645–50.

25 Therrien J, Connelly M, Webb G. Patent Ductus Arteriosus. Curr Treat Options Cardiovasc Med 1999;1:341–346.

26 Kiziltan H, Theodoro D, Warnes C *et al.* Late results of bioprosthetic tricuspid valve replacement in Ebstein's anomaly. Ann Thorac Surg 1998;66:1539–45.

27 Cappato R, Schlutter M, Weiss C *et al.* Radiofrequency current catheter ablation of accessory atrioventricular pathways in Ebstein's anomaly. Circulation 1996;94:376–83.

28 Hoffman J. Congenital Heart Disease. In: Rosendorff C, ed. Essential Cardiology: Principles and Practice. Philadelphia: W. B. Saunders Company, 2001:391–409.

29 Perloff J, Child J. Congenital heart disease in adults. Philadelphia: W. B. Saunders Company, 1998.

30 Rao B, Anderson R, Edwards J. Anatomic variations in the tetralogy of Fallot. Am Heart J 1971;81:361–71.

31 Rowe R, Vlad P, Keith J. Experiences with 180 cases of tetralogy of Fallot in infants and children. CMAJ 1955;73:23–30.

32 Oechslin E, Harrison D, Harris L *et al.* Reoperation in adults with repair of tetralogy of Fallot: indications and outcomes. J Thorac Cardiovas Surg 1999;118:245–51.

33 Khambadkone S, Coats L, Taylor A *et al.* Percutaneous pulmonary valve implantation in humans: results in 59 consecutive patients. Circulation 2005;112:1189–97.

34 Feldt R, Avasthey P, Yoshimasu F *et al*. Incidence of congenital heart disease in children born to residents in Olmsted County, Minnesota, 1950–1969. Mayo Clin Proc 1971;46:794–9.

35 Prifti E, Crucean A, Bonacchi M *et al*. Early and long term outcome of the arterial switch operation for transposition of the great arteries: predictors and functional evaluation. Eur J Cardiothorac Surg 2002;22:864–73.

36 Wilson N, Clarkson P, Barratt–Boyes B *et al*. Long term outcome after the Mustard repair for simple transposition of the great arteries: 28 year follow–up. J Am Coll Cardiol 1998;32:758–65.

37 Kammeraad JAK, Deurzen HMV, Sreeram N *et al*. Predictors of sudden cardiac death after mustard or senning repair for transposition of great arteries. J Am Coll Cardiol 2004;44:1095–1029.

38 Christensen D, McConnell M, Book W *et al*. Initial experience with bosentan therapy in patients with the Eisenmenger syndrome. Am J Cardiol 2004;94:261–3.

39 Rosenzweig E, Kerstein D, Barst R. Long-term prostacyclin for pulmonary hypertension with associated congenital heart defects. Circulation 1999;99:1858–65.

40 de Perrot M, Chaparro C, McRae K *et al*. Twenty-year experience of lung transplantation at a single center: Influence of recipient diagnosis on long-term survival. J Thorac Cardiovasc Surg 2004;127:1493–501.

41 Dubin AN, Janousek J, Rhee E *et al*. Resynchronization therapy in pediatric and congenital heart disease patients. An International MultiCenter Study. J Am Coll Cardiol, 2005; 46:2277–2283.

42 Marelli A, Moodie D. Adult congenital heart disease. In: Topol E, Califf R, Isner J, Editors; Textbook of Cardiovascular Medicine. Lippincott-Raven, 1998.

43 Perloff J, Marelli A, Miner P. Risk of stroke in adults with cyanotic congenital heart disease. Circulation 1993;87:1954–1959.

44 Berman Rosenzweig E, Dunbar I, Widlitz A. Effects of long-term bosentan in children with pulmonary arterial hypertension. J Am Coll Cardiol 2005;46:697–704

45 Ammash N, Connolly H, Abel M *et al*. Noncardiac surgery in Eisenmenger syndrome. J Am Coll Cardiol 1999;33:222–227.

46 Whittemore R, Hobbins J, Engle M. Pregnancy and its outcome in women with and without surgical treatment of congenital heart disease. Am J Cardiol 1982;50:641.

47 Siu S, Sermer M, Colman J *et al*. Prospective multicenter study of pregnancy outcomes in women with heart disease. Circulation 2001;104:515–521.

Index

Note: Page numbers in italics refer to a figure; page numbers ending in a *t* refers to a table.